M. Hori · Y. Maruyama · R.S. Reneman (Eds.)

Cardiac Adaptation and Failure

With 208 Figures

Springer

Masatsugu Hori, M.D., Ph.D.
Chief, Division of Cardiology, The First Department of Medicine,
Osaka University School of Medicine
2-2 Yamadaoka, Suita, Osaka, 565 Japan

Yukio Maruyama, M.D., Ph.D.
Professor and Chairman, The First Department of Internal Medicine,
Fukushima Medical College
1 Hikarigaoka, Fukushima, 960-12 Japan

Robert S. Reneman, M.D., Ph.D.
Professor of Physiology/Scientific Director CARIM, Department of Physiology,
University of Limburg
P.O. Box 616, 6200 MD Maastricht, The Netherlands

ISBN 4-431-70133-8 Springer-Verlag Tokyo Berlin Heidelberg New York
ISBN 3-540-70133-8 Springer-Verlag Berlin Heidelberg New York Tokyo
ISBN 0-387-70133-8 Springer-Verlag New York Berlin Heidelberg Tokyo

Printed on acid free paper

Typesetting: Best-set Typesetter Ltd., Hong Kong
Printing and binding: Permanent Typesetting & Printing Co., Ltd., Hong Kong

Preface

Ischemia and heart failure are the two major cardiac diseases that cause the majority of cardiac deaths. Myocardial infarction caused by coronary atherosclerosis still results in high mortality in the prime of life. Recent progress in reperfusion techniques such as coronary thrombolysis (PTCR), coronary angioplasty with balloon and laser (PTCA), and directional coronary atherectomy (DCA) has greatly contributed to reducing the risk of infarction in patients with coronary artery disease. However, reperfusion injury and restenosis of the coronary artery are now causing a new round of headaches among cardiologists and their patients. As a new strategy for the treatment of chronic heart failure, numerous inotropic agents have recently been developed. However, despite the tremendous effort invested in the development of these new drugs, most have failed to prolong the life span of patients with chronic heart failure. These dilemmas are drawing our attention to the biological response of the heart to various types of stresses.

Indeed, extensive previous research, both basic and clinical, has already succeeded in disclosing the underlying pathophysiology of myocardial ischemia and failure. The techniques to measure pressure and cardiac chamber dimensions have progressed, as seen in cardiac catheterization, echocardiography and Doppler techniques, and radionuclide imaging. Most of these efforts, however, have been directed at understanding cardiovascular hemodynamic impairment. In contrast, recent advances in cellular physiology and molecular biology have revealed further important aspects of the pathophysiology of the heart, e.g., subcellular signal transduction, intracellular metabolic changes, and adaptive responses of the myocardium to various kinds of stresses such as ischemic and mechanical overload. It is becoming increasingly clear that the adpative response of the myocardial cells must be taken into account in the development of new forms of treatment for heart disease. This book discusses a variety of interesting aspects of this new approach, including the molecular regulation of myocardial proteins in mechanical overload, the alteration of adrenoceptors in the stressed heart, metabolic adaptation in cardiac hypertrophy, and intracellular calcium handling.

In the ischemic heart, metabolic adaptation results in ischemic tolerance. Ischemic preconditioning establishes ischemic tolerance against ischemic injury in animals, although the clinical validity of this observation has not been established. Disclosure of the underlying mechanism and the key mediators of ischemic tolerance will undoubtedly promote effective treatment for the ischemic heart in the near future. In the pressure-overloaded heart, cardiac proteins and structures also show a remarkable adaptation to mechanical stress, yielding cardiac hypertrophy. However, these adaptive mechanisms are partially or totally decompensated in failing hearts, and mechanical and metabolic functions further deteriorate in a vicious cycle. Treatment should be directed at augmenting the compensatory mechanisms and inhibiting maladaptation of the heart to maintain its intrinsic homeostasis.

In recent years, cardiologists have attained a profound understanding of the pathogenesis of maladaptation of the heart to various conditions. Few other medical fields have experienced as spectacular an explosion in knowledge in as brief a period as has the field of cardiology in the past few years. Since tremendous progress has been made in specialized fields, it is a daunting task to digest and absorb the flood of new information. The editors believe that this book will provide a helpful guide for clinical researchers and practitioners to the recent advances in the these new fields.

This book was planned in conjunction with the Tenth International Conference of the Cardiovascular System Dynamics Society held in Kobe, Japan, on September 23–25, 1992, followed by a satellite symposium in Fukushima (chaired by Prof. Y. Maruyama). Prof. R.S. Reneman, an editor of this book, was a Starr lecturer at the conference. Although the contents of the book were planned independently of the conference program, many of the active participants contributed to this book. We heartily thank Dr. Klassen, President of the Society, who made it possible for us to host such a fruitful meeting and to publish this book. Finally, I would like to thank Dr. M. Kitakaze, Osaka University, and the editorial staff of Springer-Verlag Tokyo for their continuous support in the publication of this book.

MASATSUGU HORI
July, 1994

Contents

Treatment of Chronic Heart Failure

List of Contributors

Part 1

Cardiac Adaptation to Coronary Insufficiency

Coronary Perfusion Pressure and Myocardial Metabolism

1.1 Cardiac Contractility and Oxygen Consumption Under Altered Coronary Perfusion

Yoichi Goto[1]

Summary. Left ventricular contractility and the energetic cost of contraction were assessed in various conditions of altered coronary perfusion in isolated, cross-circulated dog and rabbit hearts utilizing frameworks of E_{max} (left ventricular contractility index) and pressure–volume area (PVA, a measure of total left ventricular mechanical energy expenditure). PVA has been shown to correlate linearly with myocardial oxygen consumption per beat (V_{O_2}) in a load-independent manner, and the reciprocal of the slope of the V_{O_2}–PVA relation is considered to indicate "contractile efficiency" (the energy transduction efficiency from oxygen to total mechanical energy), while the V_{O_2} intercept (PVA-independent V_{O_2}) reflects V_{O_2} for nonmechanical activities such as excitation–contraction coupling and basal metabolism. Contractile efficiency was not affected by depressed contractility with mildly decreased coronary perfusion pressure or stunned myocardium, or by enhanced contractility during increased coronary blood flow with adenosine. However, contractile efficiency seemingly increased during severely decreased coronary perfusion pressure, because the V_{O_2}–PVA relation tilted down, probably due to load-dependent depression of E_{max}. On the other hand, the "oxygen cost of contractility," the ratio of an increase in PVA-independent V_{O_2} to an increase in E_{max}, was higher in stunned myocardium than in normal hearts, suggesting that the energy cost of calcium handling is elevated in stunned myocardium. The oxygen cost of contractility was similar with propranolol treatment, decreased coronary perfusion pressure, or increased coronary blood flow. Furthermore, the "wall tension–regional area" area (TAA), a measure of total mechanical energy of a ventricular region obtained by analogy with PVA, was found to have a highly linear correlation with regional V_{O_2} in a load-independent manner. Thus, using the frameworks of E_{max}, PVA, and TAA, we can interconnect ventricular

[1] Division of Cardiology, Department of Medicine, National Cardiovascular Center, 5-7-1 Fujishiro-dai, Suita, Osaka, 565 Japan

mechanics and energetics and better understand the pathophysiology and pathogenesis of various conditions of altered coronary perfusion.

Key words: Coronary perfusion pressure—Myocardial oxygen consumption—Pressure–volume area (PVA)—Tension–area area (TAA)—Gregg's phenomenon—Stunned myocardium—Contractility

Introduction

It is well known that decreased coronary perfusion pressure (CPP) and blood flow (CBF) depresses left ventricular (LV) contractile function and oxygen consumption (V_{O_2}) [1–3]. Furthermore, reperfusion after coronary occlusion results in stunned myocardium, which is characterized by a prolonged, but reversible, contractile dysfunction without residual myocardial ischemia or necrosis [4,5]. In contrast, increased CPP and CBF enhances LV contractile function and V_{O_2}, which is known as Gregg's phenomenon [1,2,6,7]. Therefore, there is a consensus that altered coronary perfusion exerts striking and physiologically important influences on both LV contractile function and V_{O_2}. However, because the relation between changes in LV contractile function and V_{O_2} has not been systematically analyzed, it is still unclear whether the energy cost of LV contraction is also affected under various conditions of altered coronary perfusion.

In recent decades, E_{max}, the slope of the LV end-systolic pressure–volume relation (ESPVR), has been used as a load-independent measure of LV contractility [8,9]. Also, the LV pressure–volume area (PVA), a specific area in the pressure–volume diagram circumscribed by the end-systolic and end-diastolic pressure–volume relations and the systolic segment of the pressure–volume trajectory (Fig. 1a), has been shown to correlate linearly with LV V_{O_2}, representing the total mechanical energy generated by the LV [10] (Fig. 1b). Using the frameworks of E_{max} and the V_{O_2}–PVA relation, one can assess the relation between LV contractile function and its energy cost during various inotropic interventions.

In this article, we present our data on E_{max} and the V_{O_2}–PVA relation in the excised, cross-circulated dog and rabbit hearts under various conditions of altered coronary perfusion and discuss the physiological implications of the results. To this end, we employed three pathological conditions of altered coronary perfusion: decreased CPP and CBF, stunned myocardium after reperfusion, and increased CBF with adenosine (Gregg's phenomenon).

The second purpose of this article relates to assessment of regional myocardial mechanoenergetics. Conventionally, regional myocardial contractile function has been quantified by the amount of segmental shortening [11], wall thickening [12], or the regional work index [13]. All these variables decrease during myocardial ischemia [11–13], and Ross [14] recently suggested that there is a tight coupling between oxygen supply and regional myocardial con-

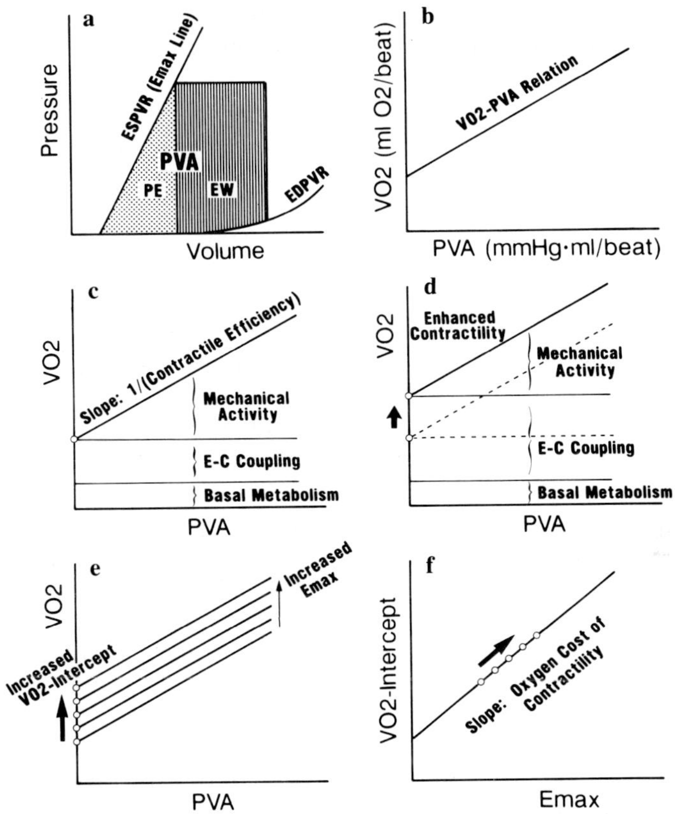

Fig. 1a–f. Schematic illustrations of left ventricular pressure–volume (P–V) area (*PVA*) and the related mechanoenergetic indexes. PVA is the area surrounded by the end-systolic (*ESPVR*) and end-diastolic P–V relations (*EDPVR*) and the systolic P–V trajectory. It consists of both potential energy (*PE*) and external work (*EW*) in an ejecting contraction (**a**). The V_{O_2}–PVA relation is linear (**b**), and the reciprocal of the slope indicates contractile efficiency, while the V_{O_2}-intercept (or PVA-independent V_{O_2}) reflects V_{O_2} for excitation–contraction (*E–C*) coupling and basal metabolism (**c**). When ventricular contractility (E_{max}) is enhanced by catecholamines or calcium, the V_{O_2}–PVA relation shifts upward in a parallel manner with an increased V_{O_2} for E–C coupling (**d**). As E_{max} is progressively enhanced in multiple steps, the V_{O_2}–intercept also increases progressively (**e**), constructing a linear relation between V_{O_2} intercept and E_{max} (**f**). The slope is called the oxygen cost of contractility. V_{O_2}, cardiac oxygen consumption per beat. (From [33] with permission)

traction ("myocardial perfusion–contraction matching"). However, the relation between regional V_{O_2} and the regional mechanical variables under various loading conditions is not fully understood. Therefore, we describe our new method to assess regional myocardial contraction and energetics of the LV using the relation between "wall tension–regional area" area (TAA) and regional V_{O_2} by analogy with the V_{O_2}–PVA relation.

Methods

Background

Previous studies have shown that PVA linearly correlates with V_{O_2} per beat in a load-independent manner [10,15] (Fig. 1b). The reciprocal of the slope of the linear V_{O_2}–PVA relation is called "contractile efficiency" [10,16], and has been considered to indicate the chemomechanical energy transduction efficiency of contractile machinery from oxygen to total mechanical energy generated by a LV contraction (Fig. 1c). On the other hand, the V_{O_2}-intercept of the V_{O_2}–PVA relation (PVA-independent V_{O_2}) consists of V_{O_2} for nonmechanical activities such as excitation–contraction (E–C) coupling and basal metabolism [15].

Enhanced ventricular contractility (E_{max}) with calcium or epinephrine increases V_{O_2} for E–C coupling without affecting contractile efficiency, resulting in a parallel upward shift of the V_{O_2}–PVA relation [15] (Fig. 1d). However, enhanced contractility with calcium or epinephrine does not affect V_{O_2} for basal metabolism [15]. When LV contractility is enhanced in several steps as in Fig. 1e, the increases in PVA-independent V_{O_2} linearly correlate with the increases in E_{max} (Fig. 1f). The slope of the linear relation between PVA-independent V_{O_2} and E_{max} is called "oxygen cost of contractility" [17], which indicates the oxygen requirement in E–C coupling for a unit increase in E_{max}.

In addition to these frameworks in the whole ventricle, "wall tension–regional area" area (TAA), a regional version of PVA, has been defined in the wall tension–regional area (T–A) diagram as a measure of regional total mechanical energy generated by myocardial contraction of a ventricular region [18] (Fig. 2). The basis for TAA is a notion that the T–A diagram for a ventricular region is energetically equivalent to the pressure–volume diagram for the whole ventricle, because we have demonstrated that LV regional work can be reliably quantified by the area within a T–A loop with the correct dimensions of energy (joules) [19,20]. Both PVA and TAA have the dimensions of energy (joules).

Heart Preparation

Experiments were performed in isolated, blood-perfused dog or rabbit hearts supported by cross-circulation with an intact animal. The surgical procedures for the cross-circulated heart preparation of the dog or rabbit have been described previously [9,15]. After cross-circulation was started, a thin balloon was inserted into the LV of the isolated heart and connected to our custom-made volume servo pump (dog study) or to a microsyringe (rabbit study) to

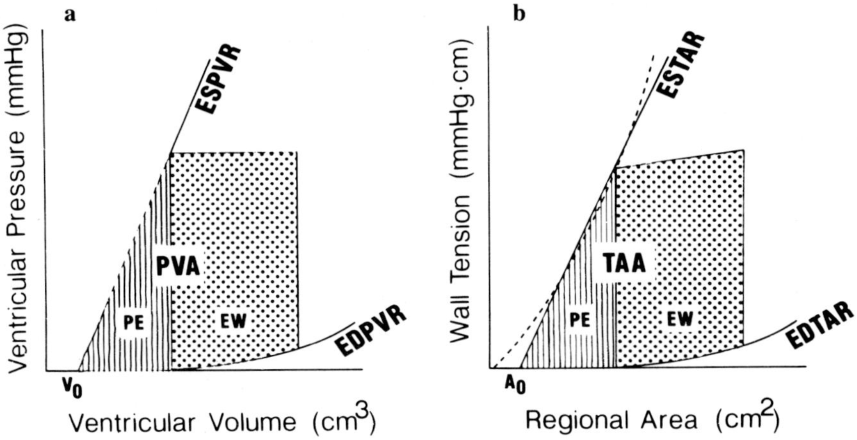

Fig. 2. Schematic illustration of pressure–volume area (*PVA*) (**a**) and "wall tension–regional area" area (*TAA*) (**b**). By analogy with PVA, TAA is defined as the area surrounded by the end-systolic (*ESTAR*) and end-diastolic T–A relation (*EDTAR*) and systolic T–A trajectory. It consists of two portions of external work (*EW*) and potential energy (*PE*). Although theoretical analysis predicts that the ESTAR is nonlinear with downward convexity, actual measurements have shown that the ESTAR is virtually linear (see Fig. 9)

control and measure the LV volume. CBF and coronary arteriovenous oxygen content difference were measured to calculate V_{O_2} per beat.

In a separate series of isolated dog heart experiments for regional mechanoenergetics, two pairs of ultrasonic crystals were placed in the LV subendocardium to measure orthogonal segment lengths in the anterior wall region to determine regional area during the cardiac cycle [18]. CBF into the left anterior descending artery and arteriovenous oxygen content difference between the left anterior descending artery and the anterior interventricular vein were measured to calculate the regional V_{O_2} of the anterior wall region.

Experimental Protocol

In the dog study, LV pressure, volume, CBF, and arteriovenous oxygen content difference were measured during either isovolumic or ejecting contractions under various LV end-diastolic volumes to calculate LV E_{max}, PVA, and V_{O_2}. In the rabbit study, similar measurements were made during only isovolumic contractions. The pathological conditions we examined were: (1) decreased CPP and CBF produced by constricting the coronary arterial perfusion tube (dog), in comparison with the effect of propranolol which elicits a direct negative inotropic effect without an alteration of coronary perfusion [21]; (2) stunned myocardium produced by 15-min global ischemia followed by 120-min reperfusion (dog) [22]; (3) increased CBF (Gregg's phenomenon) induced by intracoronary adenosine infusion (20–200 μg/min) at a constant CPP (rabbit) [23].

In the regional energetics study, measurements were made for regional area and regional V_{O_2} as well as LV pressure and volume under altered preload and afterload conditions using a volume servo pump at a constant contractility.

Data Analysis

In each pathological condition, contractile efficiency was determined from the reciprocal of the slope of the V_{O_2}–PVA relation. The oxygen cost of contractility was calculated from the ratio of the change in PVA-independent V_{O_2} to the change in E_{max}, except for the stunned myocardium protocol, in which the cost was determined from the slope of the relation between PVA-independent V_{O_2} and E_{max} during $CaCl_2$ infusion before and after producing stunned myocardium.

In the regional mechanoenergetics protocol, the relation between regional V_{O_2} and TAA was assessed in each loading condition in each heart. Calculation of wall tension, regional area, and TAA has been described previously [18–20]. By analogy with the ventricular contractile efficiency, "regional contractile efficiency" was calculated from the reciprocal of the slope of the regional V_{O_2}–TAA relation.

Results and Discussion

Decreased CPP and CBF

Figure 3 shows the pressure–volume loops (upper panels) and the V_{O_2}–PVA relations (lower panels) during the control period and mildly decreased and severely decreased CPP in a representative dog heart [21]. With mildly decreased CPP, E_{max} moderately decreased and the V_{O_2}–PVA relation shifted slightly downward in a parallel manner. With severely decreased CPP, E_{max} markedly decreased and the V_{O_2}–PVA relation shifted further downward with a decrease in the slope. The averaged data obtained in 11 hearts are shown in Table 1. Mean CPP was 82 ± 8 mmHg during the control period, 51 ± 6 mmHg during mildly decreased CPP, and 32 ± 6 mmHg during severely decreased CPP.

The decreased slope of the V_{O_2}–PVA relation and the consequent high contractile efficiency value during severely decreased CPP were in contrast to the unchanged slope and contractile efficiency during mildly decreased CPP and with propranolol (Table 1). Although the decreased slope of the V_{O_2}–PVA relation literally indicates an increased contractile efficiency, it may be explained in another way, as follows. During severely decreased CPP, E_{max} progressively decreased with increases in PVA (Fig. 4), indicating that LV contractility was more severely depressed at higher LV volumes (or greater

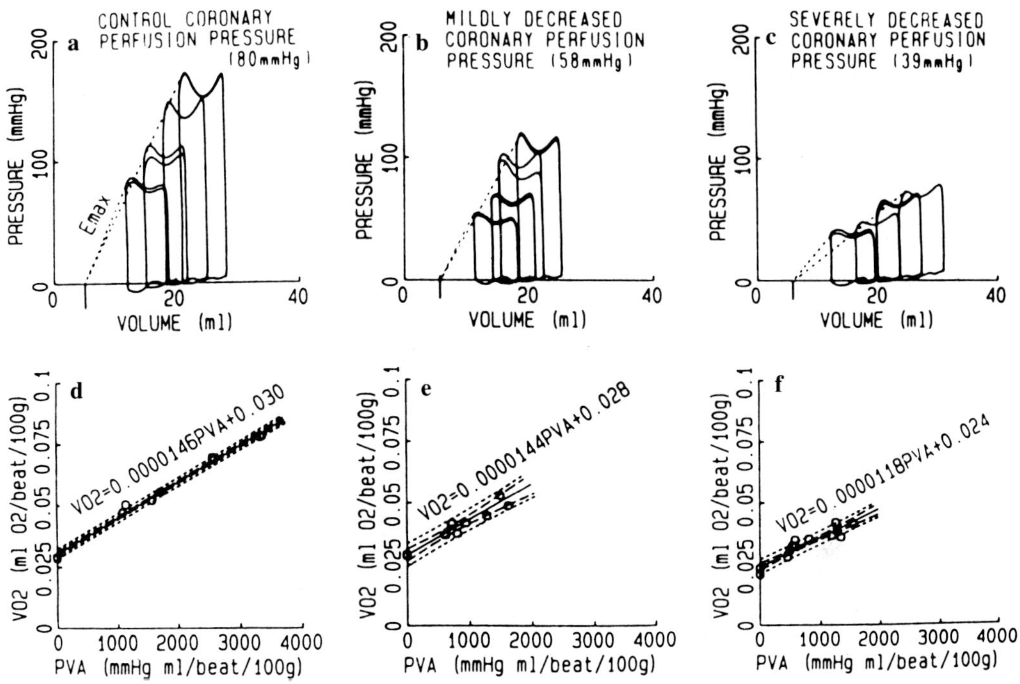

Fig. 3. Left ventricular pressure–volume loops (**a–c**) and the V_{O_2}–PVA relations (**d–f**) during control (**a** and **d**), mildly decreased coronary perfusion pressure (**b** and **e**) and severely decreased perfusion pressure (**c** and **f**) in a representative dog heart. (From [21] with permission)

PVA) under severely decreased CPP, probably due to progressive subendocardial hypoperfusion at higher LV volumes. The progressive decreases in LV contractility at a greater PVA range would be accompanied by proportional reductions of the E–C coupling energy, and hence, by proportional decreases in PVA-independent V_{O_2}, leading to tilting down of the resultant V_{O_2}–PVA relation at a greater PVA range (Fig. 5). Therefore, the decreased slope of the V_{O_2}–PVA relation during severely decreased CPP may not necessarily indicate a true increase in contractile efficiency at the level of contractile machinery, but may simply be a consequence of the load-dependent decreases in both LV contractility and PVA-independent V_{O_2}.

However, because we have recently observed a decreased slope value of the V_{O_2}–PVA relation in other pathological conditions at a normal CPP (such as soon after postischemic reperfusion [22] and respiratory acidosis [24], there could be some unknown mechanisms for a true increase in contractile efficiency via changes in crossbridge kinetics or anaerobic metabolism. Further studies will be needed to address this issue.

Table 1. Vo_2–PVA relation under altered coronary perfusion.

Condition	E_{max} ($mmHg \cdot ml^{-1} \cdot 100\,g$)	Slope ($10^{-5} \cdot ml\,O_2 \cdot mmHg^{-1} \cdot ml^{-1}$)	PVA-independent Vo_2 ($O_2 \cdot beat^{-1} \cdot 100\,g^{-1}$)	Contractile efficiency (%)	Oxygen cost of contractility ($ml\,O_2 \cdot ml \cdot mmHg^{-1} \cdot 100\,g^{-2}$)
Decreased coronary perfusion pressure					
Control	8.3 ± 3.0	1.66 ± 0.24	0.028 ± 0.005	40.8 ± 6.1	
Mild	6.8 ± 2.1*	1.59 ± 0.24	0.025 ± 0.004	42.5 ± 6.2	0.0026 ± 0.0027
Severe	3.7 ± 1.8*	1.26 ± 0.28*	0.021 ± 0.003*	55.1 ± 11.3*	0.0018 ± 0.0009
Propranolol					
Control	11.6 ± 3.2	1.76 ± 0.57	0.027 ± 0.013	41.7 ± 13.2	
Propranolol	5.6 ± 0.9*	1.64 ± 0.53	0.019 ± 0.007*	44.3 ± 12.9	0.0013 ± 0.0009
Stunned myocardium					
Control	7.8 ± 2.6	1.84 ± 0.38	0.024 ± 0.006	37.9 ± 8.6	0.0011 ± 0.0003
Stunned	4.9 ± 1.5*	1.64 ± 0.34	0.022 ± 0.004	43.2 ± 7.3	0.0023 ± 0.0005*
Increased coronary blood flow					
Control	7.9 ± 4.5	2.18 ± 0.61	0.030 ± 0.004	32.1 ± 6.5	
Adenosine	9.2 ± 5.0*	2.19 ± 0.60	0.036 ± 0.005*	32.1 ± 7.6	0.0049 ± 0.0042

Vo_2, cardiac oxygen consumption per beat; E_{max}, left ventricular contractility index.
* $P < 0.05$ compared with the respective control value.

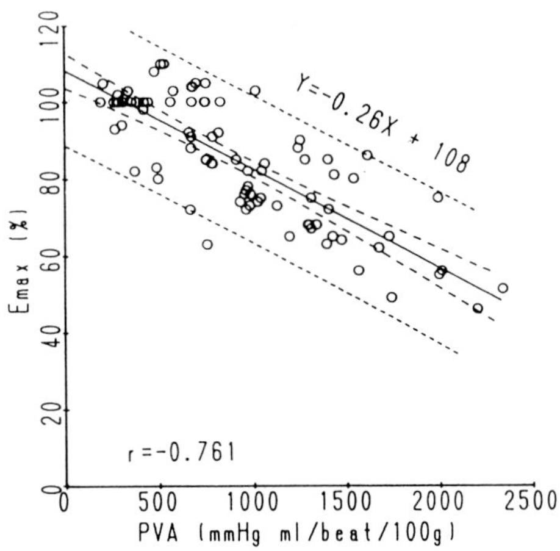

Fig. 4. Correlation between percent E_{max} and PVA during severely decreased coronary perfusion pressure in 11 hearts. With increases in PVA, E_{max} linearly decreased. The *inner pair of dashed lines* indicate the 95% confidence limit of the regression line and the *outer pair of dashed lines* indicate the 95% confidence limit for sampled data (From [21] with permission)

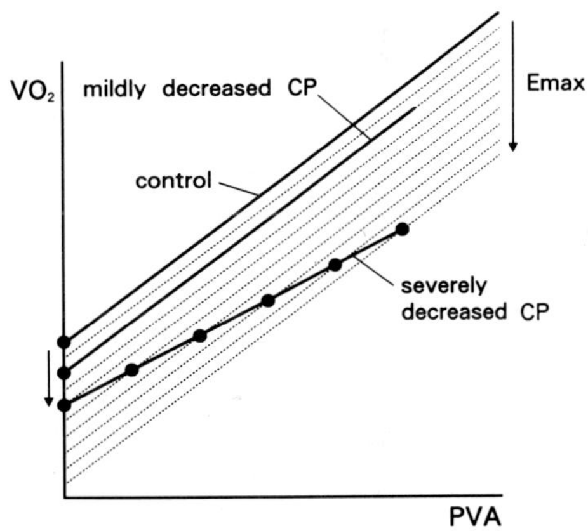

Fig. 5. Schematic illustration of the V_{O_2}–PVA relations during control and mildly and severely decreased coronary perfusion pressure (*CP*). With decreases in CP, the V_{O_2}–PVA relations shift downward in a parallel manner in proportion to decreases in E_{max} (mildly decreased CP). However, because E_{max} progressively decreases with increases in PVA during severely decreased CP, the resultant V_{O_2}–PVA relation has a low slope value during this period

The decrease in PVA-independent V_{O_2} was in proportion to the decrease in E_{max} during mildly decreased and severely decreased CPP and with propranolol (Table 1). As a result, the oxygen cost of contractility during severely decreased CPP did not significantly differ from that during propranolol treatment. This suggests that decreased CPP (and CBF) depresses LV contractility by reducing E–C coupling in a similar manner to propranolol. These results are in accordance with a recent report of Kihara et al. [25] that a reduction of LV contractility during hypoxia is accompanied by a proportional decrease in peak intracellular Ca^{2+} transients detected by aequorin.

Stunned Myocardium

Figure 6 indicates the pressure–volume loops (upper panels) and the V_{O_2}–PVA relations (lower panels) during the control period and with 20 min, 60 min, and

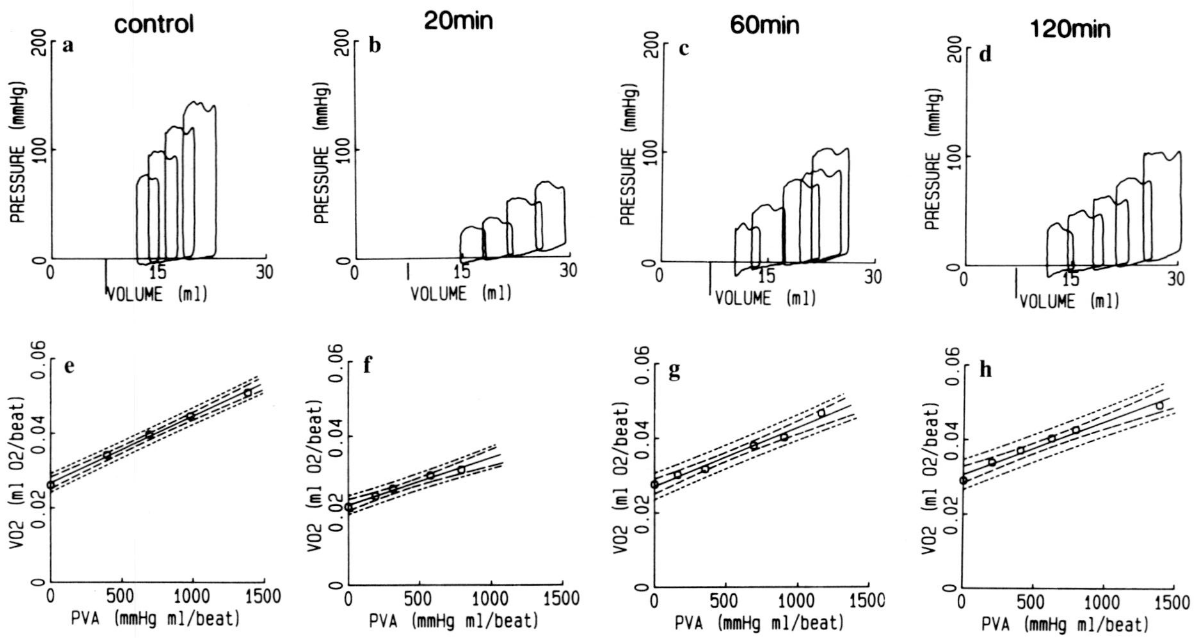

Fig. 6. Left ventricular pressure–volume loops (**a–d**) and the V_{O_2}–PVA relations (**e–h**) during the control period (**a** and **e**) and 20 min (**b** and **f**), 60 min (**c** and **g**), and 120 min reperfusion (**d** and **h**) after 15 min global ischemia in a representative heart. (From [22] with permission)

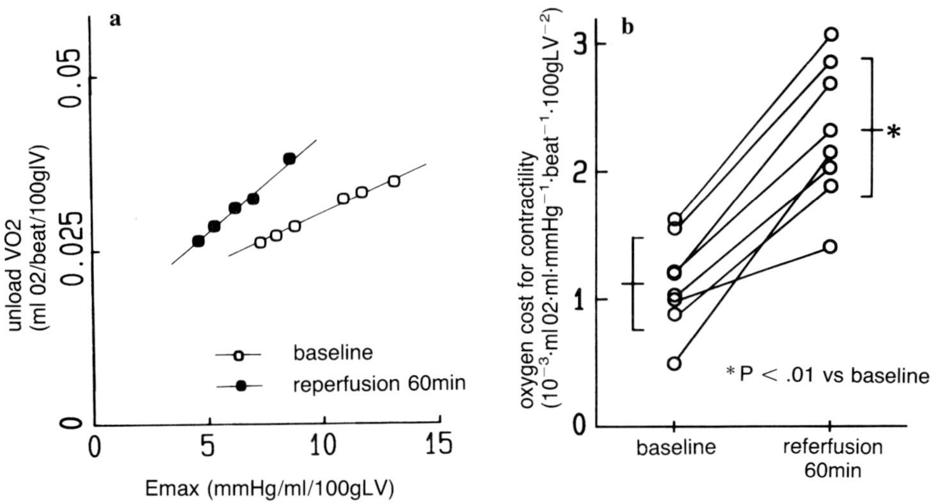

Fig. 7. **a** The relation between PVA-independent V_{O_2} (unloaded V_{O_2}) and E_{max} before and after postischemic reperfusion in a representative heart. The steeper slope of the linear relation after reperfusion indicates an elevated oxygen cost of contractility in stunned myocardium. **b** Changes in oxygen cost of contractility before and after reperfusion in all eight hearts

120 min reperfusion after 15 min global ischemia in a representative dog heart [22]. At 20 min after ischemia and reperfusion, E_{max} markedly decreased and the V_{O_2}–PVA relation shifted downward strikingly. In contrast, at 120 min of reperfusion, the V_{O_2}–PVA relation was almost superimposable on the control relation, while E_{max} remained considerably depressed. Based on the average of 8 hearts, E_{max} was significantly lower in stunned myocardium than in the control, whereas PVA-indenpdent V_{O_2} was not significantly different between the two conditions (Table 1). This indicates that stunned myocardium requires disproportionately high oxygen consumption despite the decreased contractility.

Furthermore, the oxygen cost of contractility assessed from the relation between PVA-independent V_{O_2} and E_{max} was twofold higher in stunned myocardium than in control (Fig. 7), indicating that the energy cost of E–C coupling is markedly elevated in stunned myocardium. This disproportionately high V_{O_2} for E–C coupling can be explained by either a decreased molar coupling ratio of Ca^{2+} to ATP in the Ca^{2+} uptake process of sarcoplasmic reticulum (SR) [26] or a decreased Ca^{2+} responsiveness of contractile protein [5], or both, in stunned myocardium.

Contractile efficiency in stunned myocardium was lower than that in the preischemic control myocardium, but did not significantly differ from that in the sham group heart in which the elapsed time from the control measurement was matched [22]. Therefore, it is unlikely that contractile efficiency is importantly affected by postischemic stunning per se.

Gregg's Phenomenon

Figure 8 shows the end-systolic pressure–volume relations (panel a) and V_{O_2}–PVA relations (panel b) obtained during control and adenosine infusion in a cross-circulated rabbit heart. During increased CBF with adenosine at a constant CPP, E_{max} increased and the V_{O_2}–PVA relation shifted upward in a parallel manner. Based on the average of nine hearts, while CBF increased by 99% ± 76% with adenosine, E_{max} and PVA-independent V_{O_2} increased by 18% ± 15% and 22% ± 18%, respectively [23] (Table 1). In contrast, contractile efficiency was unchanged during increased CBF. These increases in E_{max} and PVA-independent V_{O_2} were not eliminated by pretreatment with propranolol (data not shown).

The oxygen cost of contractility during the enhancement of E_{max} with increased CBF appeared 2–3 times greater than that with other interventions in the dog heart (Table 1). However, this oxygen cost value was not significantly different from that reported previously for epinephrine (0.0035 ± 0.0014 ml $O_2 \cdot ml \cdot mmHg^{-1} \cdot 100\,g^{-2}$) or calcium (0.0054 ± 0.0053 ml $O_2 \cdot ml \cdot mmHg^{-1} \cdot 100\,g^{-2}$) in the dog heart [15] or isoproterenol in the rabbit heart [27] (0.0064 ± 0.0021 $O_2 \cdot ml \cdot mmHg^{-1} \cdot 100\,g^{-2}$).

There are several possible mechanisms for increased E_{max} and PVA-independent V_{O_2} with increased CBF. However, adenosine at this dose does not have a direct positive inotropic effect on the rabbit ventricular muscle.

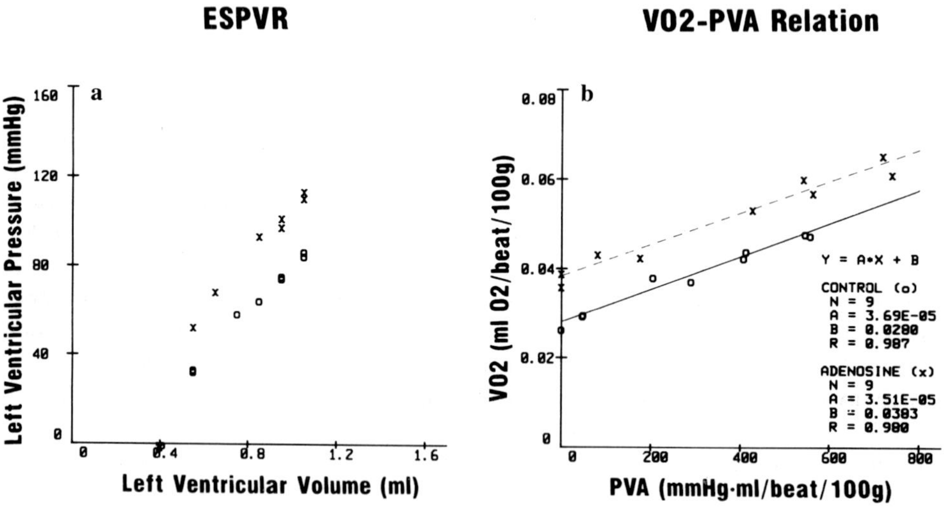

Fig. 8. Examples of the end-systolic pressure-volume relation (*ESPVR*) (**a**) and the V_{O_2}–PVA relation (**b**) obtained before (*circles*) and during (*crosses*) adenosine perfusion in one heart. Increased coronary blood flow with adenosine resulted in both an increase in the slope of the ESPVR (E_{max}) and a parallel upward shift of the V_{O_2}–PVA relation, indicating an enhancement of ventricular contractility and increase in PVA-independent V_{O_2} with a constant contractile efficiency

Also, the fact that β-blockade did not eliminate the increases in E_{max} and V_{O_2} indicates that circulating catecholamines from the support animals were not responsible for this phenomenon. In this context, previous studies reported that increased CPP and CBF increases ventricular wall thickness [28], epicardial circumference [29], and sarcomere length [30]. Because adenosine preferentially dilates coronary microvessels (i.e., intramyocardial capacitance vessels between arterioles <170 μm in diameter and venules <150 μm in diameter) [31], intramyocardial blood volume would increase with adenosine. The increased intramyocardial blood volume should result in a stretch of myocardial fiber in the mid and outer layers of the ventricular wall at a constant LV chamber volume. Thus, the increased myocardial fiber length would at least in part contribute to the increases in both generated force and V_{O_2} via the Frank-Starling mechanism.

In contrast, Kitakaze and Marban [32] recently reported an increase in the intracellular calcium transient during systole when CPP and CBF were elevated in isolated, crystalloid-perfused ferret hearts. A positive inotropic effect caused by increased intracellular calcium could reasonably explain both the parallel upward shift of the V_{O_2}–PVA relation and the close agreement of the oxygen cost of contractility between increased CBF and calcium. However, whether intracellular calcium similarly increases with increased CBF in a more physiological preparation (e.g., a blood-perfused heart with intact coronary autoregulation) and more importantly, the primary mechanism of the increase in intracellular calcium, are still to be determined. Clearly, further studies are needed to elucidate the subcellular mechanism of Gregg's phenomenon.

Regional Myocardial Contractility and Energetics

The correlations between regional V_{O_2} and myocardial shortening (regional area shrinkage), regional work, or TAA were compared under the following loading conditions: (1) increased preload, (2) decrease afterload, (3) increased preload and afterload (increased end-diastolic volume at a constant stroke volume), and (4) altered mode of contraction (ejecting versus isovolumic contractions) [18]. During increased preload, all three variables correlated positively with regional V_{O_2} ($r = 0.78$ to 1.00). During decreased afterload, the correlation was negative for area shrinkage ($r = -0.65$ to -0.91) and variable for regional work ($r = -0.55$ to 0.98) but positive and highly linear for TAA ($r = 0.80$ to 0.99). During increased preload and afterload (Fig. 9), the correlation was again negative for area shrinkage ($r = -0.77$ to -0.97) but positive for regional work ($r = 0.83$ to 0.93) and TAA ($r = 0.95$ to 0.99). During the altered mode of contraction, the correlation was insignificant for area shrinkage ($r = 0.24$ to 0.57) and moderate for regional work ($r = 0.50$ to 0.79), whereas again highly linear for TAA ($r = 0.95$ to 0.98). Thus, only TAA correlated closely with regional V_{O_2} under any loading conditions.

Furthermore, the slope ($2.22 \pm 0.78\ 10^{-5} \cdot ml\,O_2 \cdot mmHg^{-1} \cdot ml^{-1}$) and regional V_{O_2} intercept ($0.037 \pm 0.009\,ml\,O_2 \cdot beat^{-1} \cdot 100\,g^{-1}$) of the regional

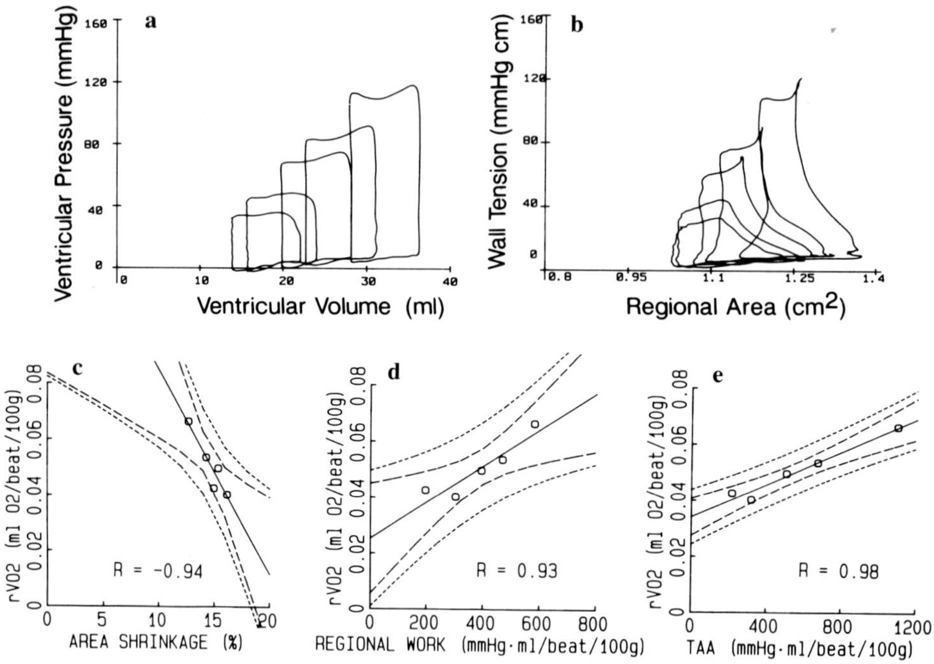

Fig. 9. Examples of left ventricular pressure–volume loops (**a**) and wall tension–regional area loops (**b**) measured during the increased preload and afterload protocol. **c–e** Correlations between regional V_{O_2} and percent area shrinkage (**c**), regional work (**d**), and TAA (**e**). (From [18] with permission)

V_{O_2}–TAA regression line were remarkably consistent among the different hearts and loading conditions. The "regional contractile efficiency" calculated from the slope of the regional V_{O_2}–TAA relation averaged 33% ± 10.1% in all eleven hearts, which is close to the reported value for the contractile efficiency of the whole heart obtained from the slope of the V_{O_2}–PVA relation [9,10,16]. This indicates that TAA has the same energetic meaning as PVA and correctly represents total mechanical energy generated by myocardial contraction of a region regardless of ventricular loading conditions.

In summary, left ventricular mechanoenergetics is variously affected during altered coronary perfusion. Decreased CPP depresses E_{max} and PVA-independent V_{O_2} proportionally, probably by reducing E–C coupling. The seemingly increased contractile efficiency during severely decreased CPP may be caused by tilting down of the resultant V_{O_2}–PVA relation due to progressive decreases in contractility. Postischemic stunned myocardium results in an oxygen cost of contractility double that of the normal heart, probably because of the Ca^{2+}/ATP uncoupling in SR and/or a decreased Ca^{2+} responsiveness of contractile protein. Doubled CBF enhanced both E_{max} and PVA-independent V_{O_2} without changing contractile efficiency, although the subcellular mechanism of this phenomenon remains to be determined. Thus, using the frameworks of E_{max} and the V_{O_2}–PVA relation, as well as the regional V_{O_2}–TAA relation, we can interconnect mechanics and energetics in both the LV and a ventricular region to approach the pathophysiology and pathogenesis of various conditions of altered coronary perfusion.

Acknowledgment. Supported in part by Research Grants for Cardiovascular Diseases (4A-1 and 4C-4) from the Ministry of Health and Welfare of Japan.

References

1. Opie LH (1965) Coronary flow rate and perfusion pressure as determinants of mechanical function in oxidative metabolism of isolated perfused rat heart. J Physiol (Lond) 180:529–541
2. Arnold G, Morgenstern C, Lochner W (1976) The autoregulation of the heart work by the coronary perfusion pressure. Pfluegers Arch 321:34–55
3. Downey JM (1976) Myocardial contractile force as a function of coronary blood flow. Am J Physiol 230:1–6
4. Braunwald E, Kloner RA (1982) The stunned myocardium: Prolonged, postischemic ventricular dysfunction. Circulation 66:1146–1149
5. Kusuoka H, Porterfield JK, Weisman HF, Weisfeldt ML, Marban E (1987) Pathophysiology and pathogenesis of stunned myocardium: depressed Ca^{2+} activation of contraction as a consequence of reperfusion-induced cellular calcium overload in ferret hearts. J Clin Invest 79:950–961
6. Gregg DE (1958) Regulation of the collateral and coronary circulation of the heart. In: McMichael J (ed) Circulation Proceedings of the Harvey Tercentenary Congress. Blackwell Oxford, UK, pp 163–186
7. Feigl EO (1983) Coronary physiology. Physiol Rev 63:13–18
8. Suga H, Sagawa K (1974) Instantaneous pressure–volume relationships and their ratio in the excised supported canine left ventricle. Circ Res 35:117–126
9. Goto Y, Slinker BK, LeWinter MM (1988) Similar normalized E_{max} and O_2 consumption–pressure–volume area relation in rabbit and dog. Am J Physiol 255:H366–H374
10. Suga H (1990) Ventricular energetics. Physiol Rev 70:247–277
11. Theroux P, Franklin D, Ross J Jr, Kemper WS (1974) Regional myocardial function during acute coronary artery occlusion and its modification by pharmacologic agents in the dog. Circ Res 35:896–908
12. Gallagher KP, Matsuzaki M, Osakada G, Kemper WS, Ross J Jr (1983) Effect of exercise on the relationship between myocardial blood flow and systolic wall thickening in dogs with acute coronary stenosis. Circ Res 52:716–729
13. Forrester JS, Wyatt HL, Da Luz PL, Tyberg JV, Diamond GA, Swan HJC (1976) Functional significance of regional ischemic contraction abnormalities. Circulation 54:64–70
14. Ross J Jr (1991) Myocardial perfusion–contraction matching. Implications for coronary heart disease and hibernation. Circulation 70:247–277

15. Suga H, Hisano R, Goto Y, Yamada O, Igarashi Y (1983) Effect of positive inotropic agents on the relation between oxygen consumption and systolic pressure volume area in canine left ventricle. Circ Res 53:306–318
16. Goto Y, Slinker BK, LeWinter MM (1990) Decreased contractile efficiency and increased non-mechanical energy cost in hyperthyroid rabbit heart: Relation between O_2 consumption and systolic pressure–volume area or force–time integral. Circ Res 66:999–1011
17. Ohgoshi Y, Goto Y, Futaki S, Yaku H, Kawaguchi O, Suga H (1990) New method to determine oxygen cost for contractility. Jpn J Physiol 40:127–138
18. Goto Y, Futaki S, Kawaguchi O, Hata K, Takasago T, Saeki A, Nishioka T, Taylor TW, Suga H (1993) Coupling between regional myocardial oxygen consumption and contraction under altered preload and afterload. J Am Coll Cardiol 21: 1522–1531
19. Goto Y, Suga H, Yamada O, Igarashi Y, Saito M, Hiramori K (1986) Left ventricular regional work from wall tension–area loop in canine heart. Am J Physiol 250:H151–H158
20. Goto Y, Igarashi Y, Yasumura Y, Nozawa T, Futaki S, Hiramori K, Suga H (1988) Integrated regional work equals total left ventricular work in regionally ischemic canine heart. Am J Physiol 254:H894–H904
21. Suga H, Goto Y, Yasumura Y, Nozawa T, Futaki S, Tanaka N, Uenishi M (1988) O_2 consumption of dog heart under decreased coronary perfusion and propranolol. Am J Physiol 254:H292–H303
22. Ohgoshi Y, Goto Y, Futaki S, Yaku H, Kawaguchi O, Suga H (1991) Increased oxygen cost of contractility in stunned myocardium of dog. Circ Res 69:975–988
23. Goto Y, Slinker BK, LeWinter MM (1991) Effect of coronary hyperemia on E_{max} and oxygen consumption in blood-perfused rabbit hearts. Energetic consequences of Gregg's phenomenon. Circ Res 68:482–492
24. Hata K, Goto Y, Kawaguchi O, Takasago T, Saeki A, Nishioka T, Suga H (1994) Hypercapneic acidosis increases oxygen cost of contractility in the dog left ventricle. Am J Physiol 266:H730–H740
25. Kihara Y, Grossman W, Morgan JP (1989) Direct measurement of changes in intracellular calcium transients during hypoxia, ischemia, and reperfusion of the intact mammalian heart. Circ Res 65:1029–1044
26. Krause SM, Hess ML (1984) Characterization of cardiac sarcoplasmic reticulum dysfunction during short-term, normothermic, global ischemia. Circ Res 55:176–184
27. Goto Y, Slinker BK, LeWinter MM (1992) Effects of amrinone and isoproterenol on mechanoenergetics of blood-perfused rabbit heart. Am J Physiol 262:H719–H727
28. Gaasch WH, Bernard SA (1977) The effect of acute changes in coronary blood flow on left ventricular end-diastolic thickness: an echocardiographic study. Circulation 56:593–598
29. Vogel WM, Apstein CS, Briggs LL, Gaasch WH, Ahn J (1982) Acute alterations in left ventricular diastolic chamber stiffness. Circ Res 51:465–478
30. Poche R, Arnold G, Gahlen D (1971) Über den Einfluss des Perfusionsdruckes im Coronarsystem des stillgestellten, aerob perfundierten, isolierten Meerschweinchenherzens auf Stoffwechsel und Feinstruktur des Herzmuskels. Virchows Arch Abt B Zellpathol 8:252–262
31. Chilian WM, Layne SM, Klausner EC, Eastham CL, Marcus ML (1989) Redistribution of coronary microvascular resistance produced by dipyridamole. Am J Physiol 256:H383–H390

32. Kitakaze M, Marban E (1989) Cellular mechanism of the modulation of contractile function by coronary perfusion pressure in ferret hearts. J Physiol (Lond) 414: 455–472
33. Goto Y, Futaki S, Kawaguchi O, Hata K, Takasago T, Saeki A, Nishioka T, Suga H (1992) Left ventricular contractility and energetic cost in disease models. Jpn Circ J 56:716–721

1.2 Effect of Coronary Perfusion on Myocardial Contractility in the Heart

Masafumi Kitakaze[1], Tetsuo Minamino[1], Toshikazu Morioka[1], Koichi Node[1], Michitoshi Inoue[2], Masatsugu Hori[1], Takenobu Kamada[1], and Eduardo Marban[3]

Summary. Coronary perfusion pressure and blood flow are closely linked to myocardial metabolic states and contractility. When coronary perfusion pressure is decreased below the level of the coronary flow autoregulation, myocardial contractility is markedly decreased: myocardial ischemia causes accumulation of H^+ and inorganic phosphates, both of which decrease the myofilament sensitivity to Ca^{2+} and maximal response of myofilaments to Ca^{2+}. Furthermore, adenosine and endothelial-dependent relaxant factor (EDRF; NO), produced during ischemia, stimulate G_i proteins and guanylate cyclase, respectively, both of which have been reported to decrease myocardial contractility. In turn, norepinephrine is released according to the severity of myocardial ischemia, which tends to compensate the depression of myocardial contractility. On the other hand, even if myocardial ischemia is not apparent due to coronary flow autoregulation during mild reduction of coronary perfusion pressure, myocardial contractility is decreased, recognized as Gregg's phenomenon. There are several hypotheses to explain this phenomenon: (1) decreases in sarcomere length of the myofilaments; (2) reversal of latent myocardial ischemia; (3) release of cardiodepressive agents; and (4) decreases in Ca^{2+} transient and Ca^{2+} sensitivity. We measured Ca^{2+} transients in the ferret Langendorff preparation at various perfusion pressures. The amplitude of Ca^{2+} transients was decreased when coronary perfusion pressure was reduced within the range of coronary flow autoregulation. Considering these results together, we support the tight linkage between coronary perfusion and myocardial contractility in normal and ischemic hearts. The concerted interac-

[1] First Department of Medicine, Osaka University School of Medicine, 2-2 Yamadaoka, Suita, Osaka, 565 Japan
[2] Department of Information Science, Osaka University Hospital, Osaka, Japan
[3] Cardiology, Department of Medicine, Johns Hopkins University, Baltimore, MD, USA

tion between myocardial perfusion and intracellular Ca^{2+} contraction may be essential for maintaining homeostasis of myocardial cellular function.

Key words: Coronary perfusion pressure—Myocardial contractile force—Ca^{2+}—Gregg's phenomenon—Autoregulation—Ischemia

The Mechanisms of Coronary Flow Regulation

It is critically important to prevent myocardium from decreases in contractility when coronary perfusion pressure is reduced. Reductions of coronary perfusion pressure may result from systemic hypotension, or narrowing of the coronary artery diameter caused by atherosclerosis, thrombus, or vasospasm in clinical settings. It is essential for the heart to regulate coronary blood flow to meet myocardial oxygen consumption because a debt of myocardial oxygen supply easily induces myocardial ischemia and cardiac pump dysfunction. Myocardial tissue is less resistant to ischemia and hypoxia than the other organs except brain and kidney. In this sense, myocardial perfusion through coronary resistance vessels indirectly but strongly regulates myocardial contractility in the heart.

Metabolic Regulation of Coronary Blood Flow

Since myocardial oxygen demand in the heart is high relative to the other organs and tissues, myocardium becomes easily ischemic even if coronary blood flow is only moderately decreased. When myocardial oxygen consumption is augmented by exercise or sympathetic nerve stimulation, several vasoactive mechanisms to preserve myocardial perfusion work promptly. First of all, when tissue pO_2 is decreased, coronary blood flow is increased to maintain constant tissue pO_2, suggesting that tissue pO_2 may be the sensor to regulate coronary vasomotor tones [1–3]. Increases in pCO_2 are also reported to decrease the resistance of coronary vessels. Indeed, both decreases in O_2 [1] and increases in CO_2 [2] may account for 23% of coronary flow autoregulation [3]. However, the mechanism by which O_2 and CO_2 regulate the tones of coronary arteries is still unknown.

On the other hand, adenosine is another vasoactive substance for mediating coronary flow autoregulation [4–7]. There is no doubt that adenosine is released from the heart when oxygen supply is not adequate for oxygen needs, i.e., ischemia, hypoxia, and enhanced oxygen consumption [8–12]. Conversely, adenosine release is decreased when oxygen is excessively supplied by overperfusion [12]. These observations suggest that adenosine plays a crucial role in the local regulation of blood flow in normal and ischemic hearts. However, there are several lines of evidence against the role of adenosine in coronary flow autoregulation [13–16]. Adenosine deaminase is reported to have no effect on the coronary resistance in the unstressed heart [13]. Furthermore, adenosine deaminase does not affect the vascular resistance during graded reduction in perfusion pressure [14], indicating that adenosine does not play an essential role in coronary flow autoregulation. There are other findings which suggest that the interstitial adenosine concentration might be too low for coronary vasodilation [15,16]. Therefore, although release of adenosine increased during reduction of coronary perfusion pressure within the range of coronary flow autoregulation [12], adenosine does not seem to be involved in coronary flow autoregulation.

We reexamined whether coronary flow autoregulation is altered by 8-phenyltheophylline, an adenosine receptor antagonist. 8-Phenyltheophylline had little effect (10% attenuation of the coronary flow autoregulation) on coronary flow autoregulation, consistent with the previous results, although coronary venous adenosine concentration was increased according to the reduction of coronary perfusion pressure in the range of coronary flow autoregulation. However, regional myocardial contractility assessed by fractional shortening of the regional myocardium in the range of coronary autoregulation was markedly depressed by 8-phenyltheophylline administration (Fig. 1). The regional flow distribution, i.e., the flow ratio between endocardial and epicardial tissue (End/Epi flow ratio), was modified by 8-phenyltheophylline within the range of coronary flow autoregulation: 8-phenyltheophylline administration significantly decreased the End/Epi flow ratio within this range. This result indicates that endogenous adenosine plays an important role in maintaining endocardial flow at the expense of epicardial flow in the range of coronary flow autoregulation.

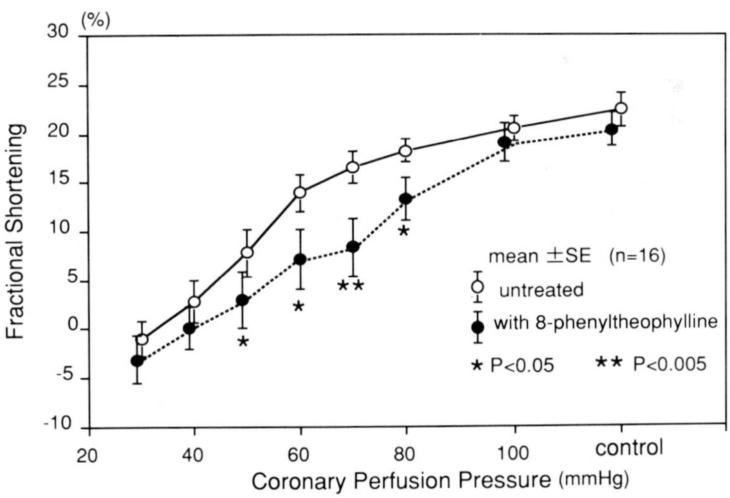

Fig. 1. Changes in fractional shortening during reduction of coronary perfusion pressure with and without intracoronary administration of 8-phenyltheophylline in the open chest dogs. Although 8-phenyltheophylline minimally changed the coronary blood flow during graded reduction of coronary perfusion pressure, it caused a downward shift in the coronary perfusion pressure and fractional shortening relationship

Endothelial-dependent relaxant factor (EDRF) is also released due to the flow dependent mechanism and thus, adenosine may accelerate the release of EDRF due to the vasodilatory action of adenosine. Recently, Ueeda et al. [17] reported that NO synthase inhibitors potently attenuate coronary flow autoregulation, suggesting that EDRF regulates the capacity of coronary flow autoregulation. Since they employed the rat Langendorff preparation, this hypothesis needs to be tested in the experimental model of the blood-perfused hearts because the rate of the removal of EDRF in the crystalloid solution and blood may be different. There are several lines of evidence that the basal resting coronary blood flow is reduced by inhibitors of NO synthase and conflicting evidence that resting coronary flow is unaffected by inhibitors of NO synthase. Taken together, the hypothesis of EDRF for regulating the coronary autoregulation is attractive; however, further investigation is required.

Recently, it has been reported that K^+ channels are involved in the regulation of coronary blood flow. Recent evidence indicates that ATP-sensitive K^+ channels play a crucial role in coronary vasodilation during hypoxia in isolated guinea pig hearts; the authors observed that an ATP-sensitive K^+-channel blocker inhibits the vasodilation during hypoxic condition [8]. Their findings suggest that the trigger of coronary vasodilation may be a decrease in intracellular ATP concentration, which augments the outward current through ATP-sensitive K^+ channels and causes hyperpolarization. Furthermore, glibenclamide attenuates the extent of the hyperemic flow due to beta-adrenoceptor stimulation [19] and ischemia [20] in the canine hearts. Komaru et al. [21] reported that vasodilation of small coronary arteries (diameter less than 100 μm) during reduction of coronary perfusion pressure within the range of coronary flow autoregulation is blunted by glibenclamide, suggesting that coronary flow autoregulation involves K^+ channels in the hearts. Under conditions of autoregulation of coronary flow, the stimulus to open K^+ channels during reduction of coronary perfusion pressure is not known. K^+ channels are known to open due not only to depletion of myocardial ATP content, but also acidosis and increases in intracellular Ca^{2+} concentration [22,23]. However, these factors do not seem to be altered during reduction of coronary perfusion pressure in the range of coronary flow autoregulation. Interestingly, adenosine and K^+ channels are tightly linked: ATP-sensitive K^+ channels modulate adenosine-induced coronary vasodilation. Aversano et al. [20] reported that the adenosine-induced coronary vasodilation is substantially attenuated by blockade of ATP-sensitive K^+ channels. This result suggests that adenosine A_2 receptors may also be affected by ATP-sensitive K^+ channels. In our preliminary study, adenosine-induced coronary vasodilation was strongly enhanced when we additionally administered nicorandil and cromakalim, K^+ channel openers. This potentiation of adenosine-induced coronary vasodilation may also be beneficial for the ischemic myocardium; however, how this linkage is related to coronary flow autoregulation is unknown.

As the mechanical factors which may regulate autoregulation, tissue pressure [24] and a myogenic mechanism [25] have been proposed. The tissue pressure hypothesis indicates that a rise in arterial pressure transiently increases fluid exudation at the capillaries and the perivascular fluid pressure increases vascular resistance by mechanical compression. The myogenic theory postulates the intrinsic mechanism of vascular muscle tone; when vascular muscle is stretched, the muscle constricts and when intravascular pressure is lowered, the vascular muscle may relax, probably due to the alteration of Ca^{2+} influx through the stretch-induced transmembrane potential changes. These two mechanisms, however, are not yet proved and additional contribution of metabolic factors may be more important.

Neural Regulation of Coronary Blood Flow

Alpha- and beta-adrenoceptors are reported to exist in coronary arteries, and their activation mediates coronary vasoconstriction and relaxation. Alpha-adrenoceptor stimulation contracts the isolated coronary arteries [26–28]. Zuberbuhler and Bohr [26] showed that exposure to norepinephrine under beta-adrenoceptor blockade contracts isolated canine coronary artery, and exposure to norepinephrine under alpha-adrenoceptor blockade relaxes it. Their results suggest that alpha-adrenoceptor stimulation mediates coronary vasoconstriction and beta-adrenoceptor stimulation mediates vasorelaxation. However, modulation of activity of beta-adrenoceptor does not seem to be realistic for mediating coronary flow autoregulation, and the role of alpha-adrenoceptor-mediated coronary vasoconstriction is also unclear for coronary flow autoregulation. Interestingly, alpha-adrenoceptor stimulation mediates redistribution of intramyocardial flow during mild reduction of coronary perfusion pressure, since it is reported that alpha-adrenoceptor stimulation favors an increase in endocardial flow at the expense of epicardial flow reduction during coronary hypoperfusion [29,30]. This effect is prominent during exercise and mild coronary hypoperfusion. Phenoxybenzamine slightly increased total coronary blood flow, but decreased endocardial flow, which may worsen overall myocardial perfusion. Recently, it was reported from our laboratory that the alpha$_1$-adrenoceptor antagonist prazosin markedly attenuates the release of adenosine from the ischemic myocardium (Fig. 2) either under hypoperfusion [31] or coronary embolization [32]; administration of a low dose of prazosin which does not affect basal coronary blood flow reduces the coronary blood flow in response to these stimuli and further deteriorates the ischemic changes, i.e., an increase in lactate production and a decrease in regional segment shortening. Although a contribution of alpha-adrenergic activity in the release of adenine nucleotide has been reported in endothelial cells [33], it is more likely that alpha$_1$-adrenergic activity plays a dominant role in the release of adenosine in ischemic myocardial cells [34,35].

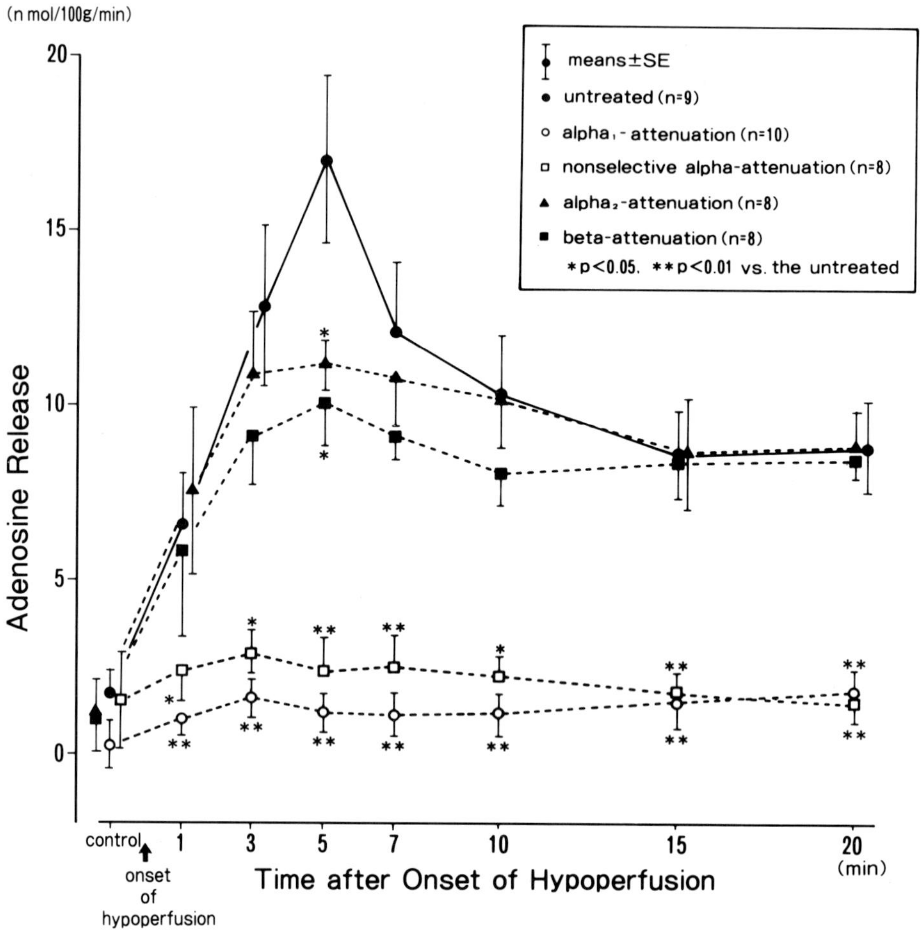

Fig. 2. Adenosine release during coronary hypoperfusion under alpha$_1$-(prazosin) (open circles), alpha$_2$-(yohimbine + propranolol) (solid triangles), nonselective alpha-(phentolamine + propranolol) (open squares), and beta-adrenoceptor (propranolol) (solid squares) attenuations. Note that both prazosin and phentolamine markedly reduced release of adenosine [30]

How Coronary Perfusion Regulates Myocardial Contraction

When coronary perfusion pressure is decreased, myocardial contractility is decreased due to several factors. When myocardial ischemia occurs, early contractile failure is reported to be attributable to the accumulation of phosphate (P_i) and H^+ in cardiomyocytes [36]. P_i is reported to decrease both the maximal force of contraction and the Ca^{2+} sensitivity of the myofilaments,

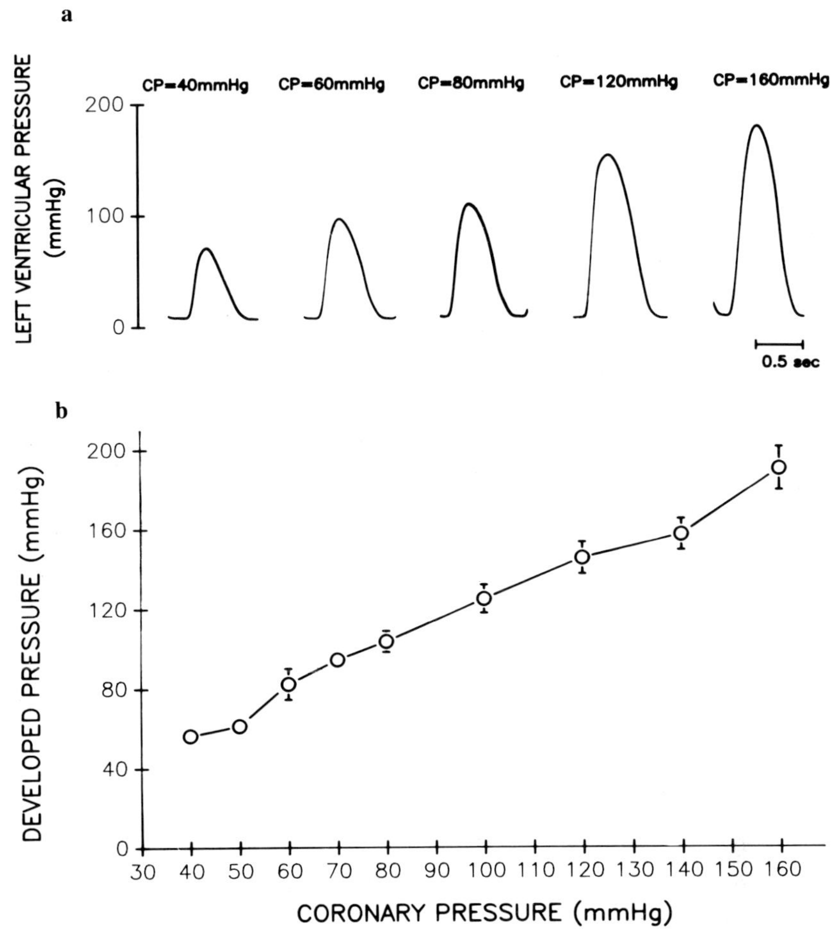

Fig. 3. Dependence of contractile pressure on coronary perfusion pressure (*CP*) in the Langendorff perfused heart excised from the ferret. **a** Representative records of left ventricular pressure during twitch contractions at the value of coronary perfusion pressure indicated above each record. At each coronary perfusion pressure tested, developed pressure was allowed to reach steady state before contractile or metabolic parameters were measured. **b** Pooled data from eight hearts (mean ± SEM) [38]

while H^+ decreases only Ca^{2+} sensitivity [36]. During the early phase of hypoxia, contractile dysfunction correlates well with increases in P_i and H^+. However, despite no changes in P_i and H^+ within the range of coronary flow autoregulation, myocardial contraction is decreased due to decreases in coronary perfusion pressure; this is known as Gregg's phenomenon. In 1963, Gregg reported that decreases in coronary perfusion pressure decrease myocardial oxygen consumption [37], and many researchers confirmed this

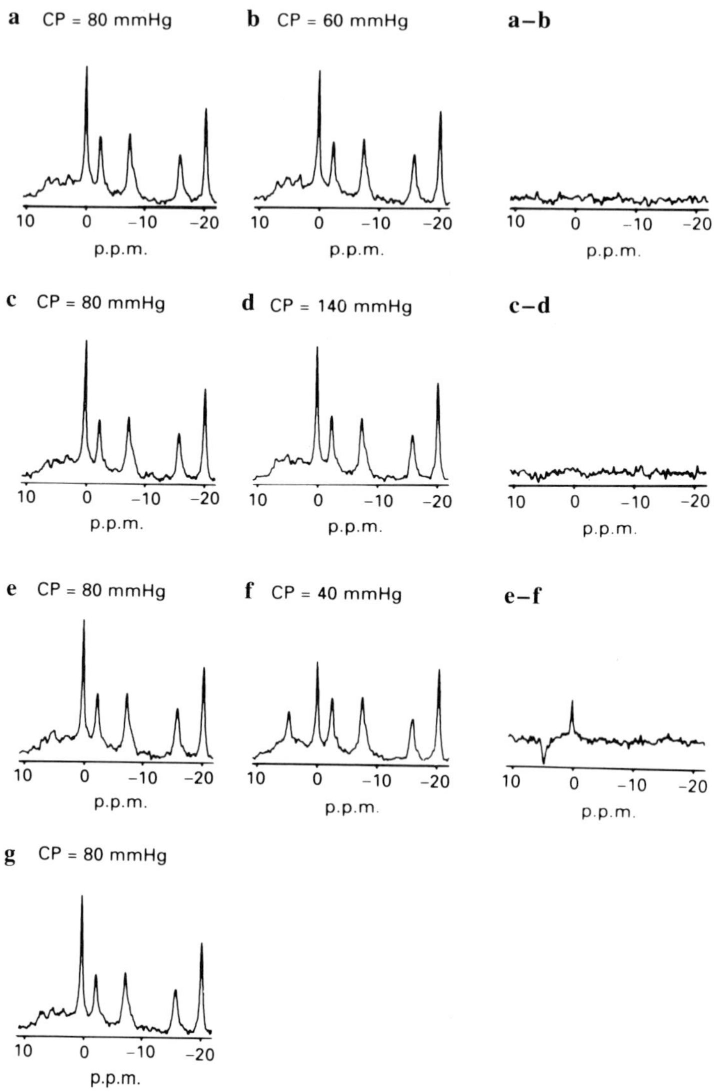

Fig. 4. Phosphorus nuclear magnetic resonance (NMR) spectra at various coronary perfusion pressures (*CP*) in a representative experiment. **a–g** (left and center columns) each spectrum is the average of 152 scans acquired at 2-s intervals at each of the coronary perfusion pressures indicated. From *left to right* within each panel, the identity of the peaks is as follows: inorganic phosphate (P_i; small except in **f**), phosphocreatinine (PCr, assigned to 0 ppm), the three peaks of ATP, and the magnesium trimetaphosphate standard at −20 ppm. The spectra were acquired in the same chronological as alphabetical order. *Right column*: spectra showing the difference between **a** and **b** (**a–b**, *top row*), **c** and **d** (**c–d**, *second row*) and **e** and **f** (**e–f**, *third row*). Only **e–f** exhibits an appreciable signal, which corresponds to an increase in P_i (shown *downward* here) and a decrease in PCr. These changes were fully reversible (compare **e** and **g**) [38]

Fig. 5. The absence or presence of metabolic evidence of ischemia at different coronary perfusion pressure. Pooled data from 5 hearts for lactate efflux (**a**), P_i and intramyocardial pH (pH_i) (**b**) and developed pressure (**c**). In **a**, only values for lactate efflux at 30 and 40 mmHg are significantly greater than the value at 80 mmHg. [P_i] is significantly elevated at and below a coronary perfusion pressure of 60 mmHg [38]

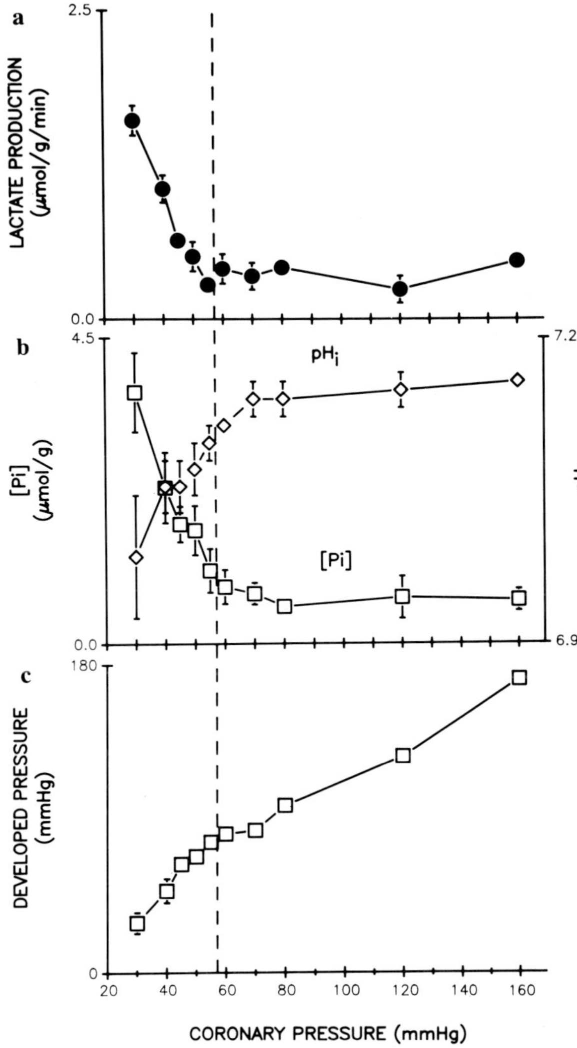

observation and further observed that myocardial contraction is likewise dependent on the coronary perfusion pressure [38,39].

Figure 3 shows the dependence of contractile pressure on coronary arterial pressure in the ferret Langendorff preparation. This phenomenon may contribute to the protection of myocardium from the occurrence of ischemia, and may constitute the cardioprotective mechanism because of energy-sparing effects due to decreased myocardial oxygen consumption and contractility. There are several possible mechanisms for this interesting observation [40]: (1) slight changes in P_i and H^+, (2) the presence of subtle myocardial ischemia, (3) increases in myocardial filament length (Frank-Starling mechanisms), (4)

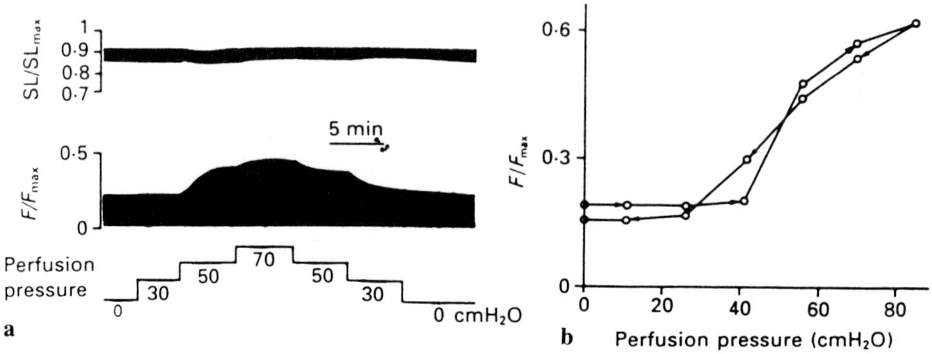

Fig. 6. Influence of perfusion pressure on peak force of contraction of rat papillary muscles. **a** Original recording of force (*F*) and segment length (*SL*) during stepwise changes in perfusion pressure. **b** Peak force–pressure relationship as obtained with a protocol comparable to that shown in **a**. The *arrows* indicate the sequence of increase in and subsequent decreasing pressure steps. When segment length was not changed as is indicated in SL/SL_{max}, the generated force (F/F_{max}) was altered by changing perfusion pressure [39]. *max*, maximal (segment length or force)

decreases in Ca^{2+}-sensitivity of myofilaments due to other causes, and (5) decreases in Ca^{2+} transient [38–40]. Any or all of these phenomena may well explain the decreased myocardial contractility. First of all, neither P_i nor H^+ measured by the ^{31}P NMR method changes during the mild reduction of coronary perfusion pressure in the range of coronary autoregulation, as shown in Figs. 4 and 5. Below the range of coronary flow autoregulation, both P_i and H^+ were increased; in this range, decreases in developed pressure became steeper compared with the range of coronary autoregulation. This observation suggests that although both P_i and H^+ can decrease myocardial contractility, decreases in contraction due to Gregg's phenomenon are not attributable to these metabolic changes.

Decreases in coronary perfusion pressure may cause subtle subendocardial ischemia. However, when lactate release from the hearts was measured during reduction of coronary perfusion pressure in the range of coronary autoregulation, lactate release could not be detected. This observation argues against latent subendocardial ischemia during the reduction of coronary perfusion pressure when Gregg's phenomenon is clearly observed, because lactate release is a sensitive index for the detection of anaerobic glycolysis.

The third possibility is the Frank-Starling mechanism: when myofilament is stretched, myocardial contractility is increased. However, this possibility is not likely. Figure 6 shows the results of experiments in papillary muscles by Schouten et al. [39]. When perfusion pressure is altered, myocardial contractility is further increased even if the myocardium contracts and relaxes at the level of maximum length (L_{max}). The fourth and fifth possibilities—modulation of Ca^{2+} sensitivity of the myofilaments and/or Ca^{2+} transients—

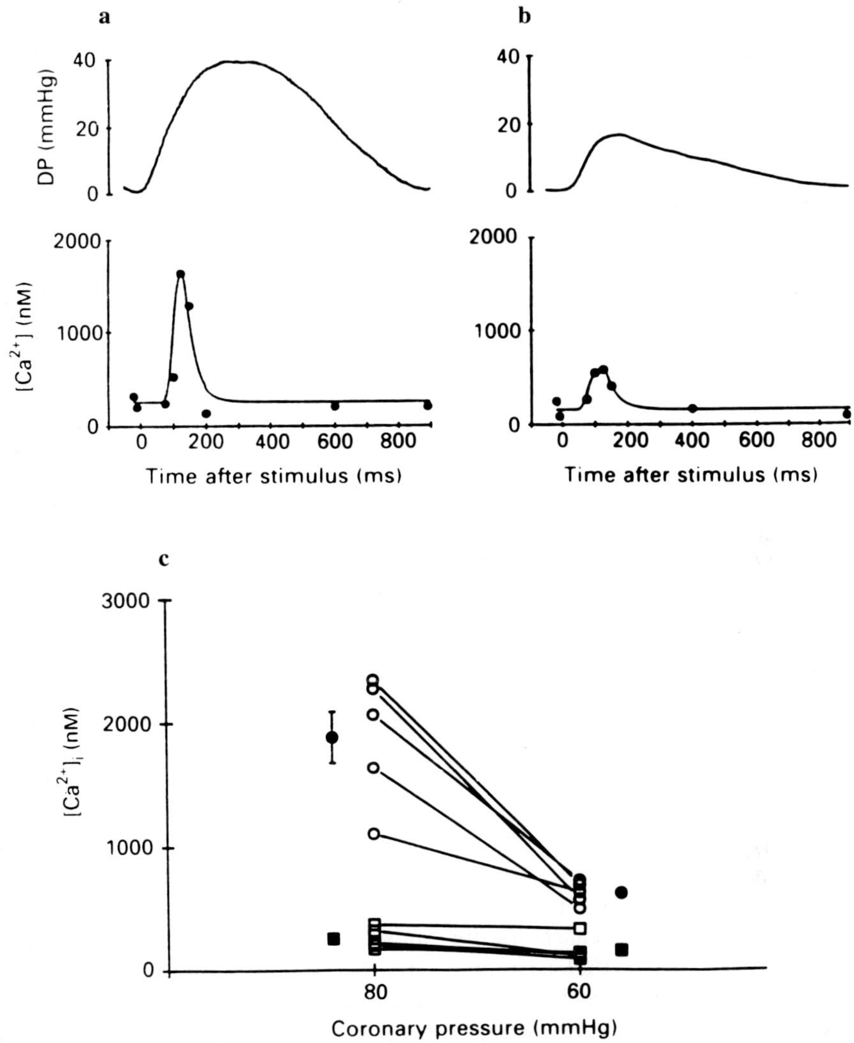

Fig. 7a–c. Changes in Ca^{2+} transients when coronary perfusion pressure is decreased. **a,b** Representative changes in one heart. Ventricular developed pressure (*DP, upper panel*) and Ca^{2+} transient (*lower panel*) during perfusion at 80 mmHg (**a**) or 60 mmHg (**b**) coronary perfusion pressure. The hearts were loaded with the 5,5′-difluoro derivative of 1,2-bis(o-aminophenoxy)ethylene-N,N,N′,N′,-tetraacetic acid (5F-BAPTA) and $[Ca^{2+}]_o$ was increased to 8 m*M* prior to the gated acquisition of the ^{19}F spectra used to calculate each value of $[Ca^{2+}]_i$ in **a**. The coronary perfusion pressure was then decreased to 60 mmHg and a new set of gated spectra was obtained after contractile pressure had reached steady state. ^{31}Phosphorus spectra from the same heart revealed to significant differences at the two coronary perfusion pressures. The differences in $[Ca^{2+}]_i$ were statistically significant by paired *t*-test. *Open circles* and *squares* are the data during systolic and diastolic phases (mean ± SEM) [38]

appear likely to explain Gregg's phenomenon. Figure 7 shows the modulation of the Ca^{2+} transient during either reduction or augmentation of coronary perfusion pressure, observed in the ferret hearts. When coronary perfusion pressure is decreased, the amplitude of Ca^{2+} transients is markedly decreased. This finding is consistent with the observation that ^{45}Ca uptake into perfused rat hearts is increased when coronary perfusion pressure is raised from 60 to 120 mmHg [41]. On the other hand, when coronary perfusion pressure is increased, the amplitude of Ca^{2+} transients is also increased. This observation explains the cellular mechanism for Gregg's phenomenon. Furthermore, as Schouten et al. [39] suggested, we cannot negate the possibility that the myofilament sensitivity to Ca^{2+} is modulated by the changes in perfusion pressure, although the maximal Ca^{2+}-activated force obtained during transient myocardial tetanus is not altered by coronary perfusion pressure [38].

The interesting issue is the subcellular mechanism for the modulation of Ca^{2+} transients at various levels of coronary perfusion pressure. Two general types of mechanism must be considered as potentially underlying the effects of an increase in perfusion pressure or flow; first, the accumulation of a positively inotropic mediator or second messenger; second, the wash-out of negatively inotropic compounds. In the first category, a prominent candidate is cyclic AMP. Activation of adenylate cyclase occurs within 10 min of acute pressure overload in guinea pig hearts [42]. The attendant increase in cyclic AMP concentration and cyclic AMP dependent protein kinase activity would be expected to increase Ca^{2+} transients and contractile force. If this were true, one might also expect the rate of relaxation of twitch contractions, and the spontaneous heart rate, to be accelerated; we observed neither tendency, but our experiments were not designed to detect subtle changes in either of these parameters [38]. As far as negatively inotropic compounds are concerned, adenosine may be capable of explaining at least some of the observed changes in calcium transients [43,44]. Adenosine increases steeply when coronary perfusion pressure is decreased in the range of coronary autoregulation [12] as well as during myocardial ischemia; this increase in adenosine concentration would tend to decrease Ca^{2+} current and contractile force. The negative inotropic action of adenosine is exerted only when beta adrenoceptors are stimulated; therefore, the adenosine theory cannot fully explain Gregg's phenomenon.

In the clinical situation, when coronary stenosis persists for a long time, myocardial contraction remains depressed; this is termed myocardial hibernation [45]. When percutaneous transluminal coronary angioplasy is performed for fixed coronary stenosis in patients with effort angina, myocardial contraction improves markedly [46]. This improvement may be at least partly attributable to Gregg's phenomenon: increased coronary perfusion pressure increases myocardial contractility.

Although further investigation is necessary to learn the role of Gregg's phenomenon in the pathophysiological situation, we need to take account of the linkage between myocardial contractile force and coronary circulation.

References

1. Chang AE, Detar R (1980) Oxygen and vascular smooth muscle contraction revisited. Am J Physiol 238:H716–H718
2. Case RB, Felix A, Wachter M, Kyriakidis G, Castellana F (1978) Relative effect of CO_2 on canine coronary vascular resistance. Circ Res 42:410–418
3. Broten TP, Feigl EO (1992) Role of myocardial oxygen and carbon dioxide in coronary autoregulation. Am J Physiol 262:H1231–H1237
4. Hori M, Kitakaze M (1991) Adenosine, the heart, and coronary circulation. Hypertension 18:565–574
5. Sparks H, Bardenheuer H (1986) Regulation of adenosine formation in the heart. Circ Res 58:193–201
6. Berne RM, Rubio R (1979) Coronary circulation. In: Berne RM, Sperelakis N, Geiger SR (eds) Handbook of physiology, Sec 2. The cardiovascular system. American Physiology Society, Washington DC, pp 873–952
7. Berne RM (1980) The role of adenosine in the regulation of coronary blood flow. Circ Res 47:807–813
8. Berne RM, Rubio R, Curnish RR (1974) Release of adenosine from ischemic brain: effect on cerebral vascular resistance and incorporation into cerebral adenine nucleotides. Circ Res 35:262–271
9. Berne RM, Winn HR, Knabb RM, Ely SW, Rubio R (1983) Blood flow regulation by adenosine in heart, brain and skeletal muscle. In: Berne RM, Rall TW, Rubio R (eds) Regulatory function of adenosine. Nijhoff, The Hague, pp 293–317
10. Fox AC, Reed GE, Glassman E, Kaltman AJ, Silk BB (1974) Release of adenosine from human hearts during angina induced by rapid atrial pacing. J Clin Invest 53:1447–1457
11. Watkinson WP, Foley DH, Rubio R, Berne RM (1979) Myocardial adenosine formation with increased cardiac performance in the dog. Am J Physiol 296: H13–H21
12. Schrader J, Haddy FJ, Gerlach E (1977) Release of adenosine, inosine and hypoxanthine from the isolated guinea pig heart during hypoxia, flow-autoregulation and reactive hyperemia. Pfluegers Arch 369:1–6
13. Kroll K, Feigl EO (1985) Adenosine is unimportant in controlling coronary blood flow in unstressed dog hearts. Am J Physiol 249:H1186–H1187
14. Dole WP, Yamada N, Bishop VS, Olsson RA (1985) Role of adenosine in coronary blood flow regulation after reductions in perfusion pressure. Circ Res 56:517–524
15. Gidday JM, Ely SW, Esther JW, Berne RM (1984) Progressive attenuation of coronary reactive hyperemia with increasing interstitial theophylline permeation. Fed Proc 43:1084
16. Hanley FL, Grattan MT, Stevens MB, Hoffman JIE (1986) Role of adenosine in coronary autoregulation. Am J Physiol 251:H558–H566
17. Ueeda M, Silvia S, Olsson RA (1992) Nitric oxide modulates coronary autoregulation in the guinea pig. Circ Res 70:1296–1303
18. Daut J, Maier-Rudolph W, von Beckerath N, Mehrke G, Gunther K, Goedel-Meinen L (1990) Hypoxic dilation of coronary arteries is mediated by ATP-sensitive potassium channels. Science 247:1341–1344
19. Narishige T, Egashira K, Akatsuka Y, Imamura Y, Takahashi T, Kasuya H, Takeshita A (1994) Glibenclamide prevents coronary vasodilation induced by β_1-adrenoceptor stimulation in dogs. Am J Physiol 266:H84–H92

20. Aversano T, Ouyang P, Silverman H (1991) Blockade of the ATP-sensitive potassium channel modulate reactive hyperemia in the canine coronary circulation. Circ Res 69:618–622
21. Komaru T, Lamping KG, Easthan CL, Dellsperger KC (1991) Role of ATP-sensitive potassium channels in coronary microvascular autoregulatory responses. Circ Res 69:1146–1151
22. Lederer WJ, Nichols CG (1989) Nucletoide modulation of the activity of rat heart ATP-sensitive K^+ channels in isolated membrane patches. J Physiol 419:193–211
23. Fan Z, Maleilski JC (1993) Intracellular H^+ and Ca^{2+} modulation of trypsin-modified ATP-sensitive K^+ channels in rabbit ventricular myocytes. Circ Res 72:715–722
24. Kuo L, Davis MJ, Chilian WM (1988) Myogenic activity in isolated subepicardial and subendocardial coronary arteries. Am J Physiol 255:H1558–H1562
25. Johnson PC, Intaglietta M (1976) Contributions of pressure and flow sensitivity to auto-regulation in mesenteric arterioles. Am J Physiol 231:1686–1698
26. Zuberbuhler RC, Bohr DF (1965) Responses of coronary smooth muscle to catecholamine. Circ Res 16:431–440
27. Murry PA, Vatner SF (1979) Alpha-adrenoceptor attenuation of the coronary vascular response to severe exercise in the conscious dog. Circ Res 45:654–660
28. Vatner SF (1983) Alpha-adrenergic regulation of the coronary circulation in the conscious dog. Am J Cardiol 52:15A–21A
29. Nathan HJ, Feigl EO (1986) Adrenergic vasoconstriction lessens transmural steal during coronary hypoperfusion. Am J Physiol 250:H645–H653
30. Buffington CW, Feigl EO (1983) Effect of coronary artery pressure on transmural distribution of adrenergic coronary vasoconstriction in the dog. Circ Res 53:613–621
31. Kitakaze M, Hori M, Tamai J, Iwakura K, Koretsune Y, Kagiya T, Iwai K, Kitabatake A, Inoue M, Kamada T (1987) $Alpha_1$-adrenoceptor activity release of adenosine from the ischemic myocardium in dogs. Circ Res 60:631–639
32. Hori M, Tamai J, Kitakaze M, Iwakura K, Gotoh K, Iwai K, Koretsune Y, Kagiya T, Kitabatake A, Kamada T (1989) Adenosine-induced hyperemia attenuates myocardial ischemia in coronary microembolization in dogs. Am J Physiol 257: H244–H251
33. Buxton ILO, Walther J, Westfall DP (1990) Purinergic mechanisms in cardiac blood vessels: Stimulation of endothelial cell alpha receptors in vitro by the neurotransmitter norepinephrine leads to the rapid release of ATP and its subsequent breakdown to adenosine (abstract). Heart Vessels 4(Suppl):27
34. Kitakaze M, Hori M, Iwakura K, Sato H, Gotoh K, Tada M (1989) Protein kinase C regulates production of adenosine in hypoxic myocytes of rats (abstract). Circulation 80:II-498
35. Kitakaze M, Hori M, Kamada T (1993) Role of adenosine and its interaction with alpha adrenoceptor activity in ischemic and reperfusion injury of the heart myocardium. Cardiovasc Res 27:18–27
36. Kusuoka H, Weisfeldt ML, Jacobus E, Zweier J, Marban E (1986) Mechanism of early contractile failure during hypoxia in intact ferret heart: Evidence for modulation of maximal Ca^{2+}-activated force by inorganic phosphate. Circ Res 59:270–282
37. Gregg DE (1963) Effects of coronary perfusion pressure or coronary flow on oxygen usage of the myocardium. Circ Res 13:497–500

38. Kitakaze M, Marban E (1989) Cellular mechanism of the modulation of contractile function by coronary perfusion pressure in ferret hearts. J Physiol 414:455–472
39. Schouten VJ, Allaart CP, Westerhof N (1992) Effect of perfusion pressure on force contraction in thin papillary muscles and trabeculae from rat heart. J Physiol 451:585–604
40. Feigl EO (1983) Coronary physiology. Physiol Rev 63:1–205
41. Haneda T, Morgan HE, Watson PA (1988) Effect of calcium uptake increased by elevated aortic pressure on total and ribosomal protein synthesis in rat heart. J Mol Cell Cardiol 20:[Suppl III]-S35
42. Schreiber SS, Klein IL, Oratz M, Rothschild MA (1971) Adenylate cyclase activity and cyclic AMP in acute cardiac overload: a method for measuring cyclic AMP production based on ATP specific activity. J Mol Cell Cardiol 2:55–65
43. Isenberg G, Cerbai E, Klockner U (1987) Ionic channels and adenosine in isolated heart cells. In: Gerlach E, Becker BF (eds) Topics and perspective in adenosine research. Berlin, Springer-Verlag, pp 323–335
44. Cerbai E, Klockner U, Isenberg G (1988) Ca-antagonistic effects of adenosine in guinea pig atrial cells. Am J Physiol 255:H872–H878
45. Rahimtoola SH, Griffith GC (1989) The hibernating myocardium. Am Heart J 117:211–221
46. Akins CW, Pohost GM, DeSanctis RW, Block PC (1980) Selection of angina-free patients with severe left ventricular dysfuction for myocardial revascularization. Am J Cardiol 46:695–700

1.3 Coronary Flow Regulation Following Ischemia

Howard J. Zimring and Robert L. Engler[1]

Summary. Coronary flow regulation following myocardial ischemia has become increasingly relevant given the increased use of coronary revascularization treatment for myocardial infarction and ischemia. Animal and human observations to date show that many of the usual humoral factors affecting coronary flow interact with the inflammatory response to the preceding ischemic injury and possibly reperfusion injury to determine reperfusion coronary flow. Hypotheses to explain these observations include neutrophil (PMN) adhesion to capillaries and venules, as well as oxygen free-radical injury leading to endothelial dysfunction. Future experimentation in this area will address the issue of whether decreased post-ischemic coronary flow is a cause or an effect of evolving ischemic myocardial injury.

Key words: Reperfusion—No reflow—Inflammatory response—Microcirculation—Ischemia

Coronary Flow Regulation Following Ischemia

Coronary flow regulation under normal conditions has been extensively reviewed [1,2]. Given increased clinical use of thrombolysis, percutaneous transluminal coronary angioplasty (PTCA), and coronary artery bypass graft (CABG) surgery in the treatment of acute myocardial ischemia, understanding coronary flow regulation in post-ischemic conditions has become increasingly relevant. Many of the complex regulatory systems determining coronary blood flow are listed in Table 1. Coronary flow is normally most dependent on oxygen consumption, autoregulation, and compressive myocardial factors, and

[1] V.A. Medical Center and U.C.S.D. Medical Center, 3350 La Jolla Village Drive, San Diego, CA 92161, USA

Table 1. Coronary flow regulation factors.

Categories of coronary flow regulation	Effectors
Metabolic regulation	MVO_2, adenosine, K^+, pH, pCO_2, K_{ATP}
Auoregulation	Coronary perfusion pressure
Extrinsic compression	Systolic contractility and twisting, tissue edema, collateral flow
Autonomic nervous system	Sympathetic, parasympathetic
Humoral (circulating and endothelial)	Catecholamine, thromboxane, NO, EDCF, prostacyclin, endothelin, vasopressin, angiotensin II, serotonin, histamine
Vascular obstruction	Macrovascular and microvascular

MVO_2, myocardial oxygen consumption; *K_{ATP}*, adenosine triphosphate release from endothelium; *NO*, nitric oxide; *EDCF*, endothelial derived contraction factor

less dependent on neural and humoral factors [1]. However, following conditions of acute myocardial ischemia, additional factors influencing coronary flow regulation are introduced. These include the effects of the inflammatory response to the preceding myocardial ischemic injury as well as alteration of some of the factors regulating microvascular coronary flow listed in Table 1. This review will focus on the relationship of these altered microvascular factors to the post-ischemic inflammatory response. We will first present the salient observations to date regarding coronary flow following ischemia in animals and man, and then discuss current hypotheses which integrate these observations.

Animal Evidence

In vivo animal preparations using various periods of ischemia and reperfusion have reported a significant decrease in coronary flow following acute ischemia. In 1979 Kloner demonstrated that after 90 min of ischemia in a dog preparation a significant portion of endocardium was unable to be reperfused as evidenced by a fluorescent Thiaflavin S stain technique [3]. Macroscopically, the areas of decreased reperfusion were associated with severe necrosis. Kloner termed this observation "no reflow." Subsequently in 1983 Engler et al. reported that, in a similar model of 2 h of ischemia/reperfusion, the areas of no reflow defined by carbon black injection were associated with significant microvascular neutrophil (PMN) accumulation in a ratio of 1 PMN/1 capillary [4]. These changes tended to localize to areas of myocyte and microvasculature damage. This same laboratory in 1986 observed that when reperfusion was performed with PMN-depleted blood (via leukopac filters), the post-ischemic endocardial coronary flow measured by microsphere injection was increased from baseline rather than decreased [5]. In addition, reperfusion with PMN-depleted blood prevented the changes of tissue edema and PMN accumulation. As in Kloner's observations, the areas of no reflow were in the more severely damaged myocardium. These observations have since been reproduced by several independent investigators using alternative methods to compromise PMN function [6–10]. A key component of PMN function involves its interaction with the endothelium. For example, when the PMN adhesion receptors ICAM-1 and CD-18 are blocked by specific antibody techniques in both dog and cat preparations, coronary flow following ischemia increases [10,11]. Likewise, no reflow in the cat is less apparent when the glycoprotein L-selectin, which participates in PMN rolling adhesion, is blocked by specific antibodies [12]. Thus the PMN-endothelial interaction has been shown to be an important contributor to decreased coronary flow following ischemia by different investigators, species, and techniques.

Ambrosio et al. extended these findings by demonstrating that in an ischemia reperfusion preparation, decreased coronary flow after reperfusion continued to decrease over a 4-h reperfusion period and was thus a dynamic process [13,14]. Furthermore, there were histologic differences between myocardium in the areas of late decreased flow as compared with myocardium in the areas of early decreased flow. Late no-reflow tissue was characterized by contraction band necrosis and PMN accumulation while early no-reflow tissue was associated with coagulation necrosis. Lastly, the degree of late no reflow appeared dependent on the amount of prior ischemic injury as evidenced by its proportionate relationship to the degree of collateral blood supply during the period of ischemia. They concluded that ischemic reperfused myocardium undergoes progressive vascular obstruction due to either reperfusion injury or delayed ischemic injury.

The post-ischemic role of myocardial oxygen consumption and autoregulation on coronary flow regulation is largely unknown. In a model of stunned myocardium utilizing a 20-min ischemic reperfused dog preparation, no change in autoregulatory gain was found [15]. However, there are numerous reports of other microvascular coronary flow regulation systems being affected by and interacting with the inflammatory response to ischemic reperfused myocardium. For example, Mehta et al. observed that coronary vascular reserve is impaired in proportion to the duration of ischemia in a dog ischemia/reperfusion preparation [16]. This is evidenced by a decreased reactive hyperemic response to acetylcholine stimulation which results in nitric oxide (NO) dependent vasodilation in the dog. As in the post-ischemic coronary flow response, the impaired post-ischemic reactive hyperemic response to acetylcholine is dynamic, worsening over time [17]. Furthermore, electron microscopy shows that PMNs become "sandwiched" between the endothelium and the elastic lamina of *large* ischemic-reperfused epicardial arteries [17]. These findings suggests a possible link between the inflammatory response and potential damage to the endothelium and, therefore, the NO and adenosine coronary flow regulation systems.

Many of the studies cited above, however, fail to differentiate between the macrovascular and microvascular NO response. Observations have been made both for and against the possibility that nitric oxide mediates the impaired reactive hyperemic response in the microcirculation. Groups have shown that both NO-dependent (acetylcholine) and -independent (nitroglycerin) vasodilation are impaired following ischemia in intact animal preparations [16,17]. Thus, although disruption of the NO coronary flow system through endothelial damage may contribute to microvascular no reflow, it cannot, on its own, account for the entire phenomenon. Part of nitric oxide's contribution is suggested by evidence in the cat showing that platelet activating factor (PAF) antagonists can increase the post-ischemic endothelium-dependent reactive hyperemic response. This implies that PAF, which is increased following ischemia, may participate in a chain of events leading to a decreased NO response by endothelial cells [18]. Also, post-ischemic impaired NO release precedes PMN adhesion in this same cat ischemia/reperfusion model [19]. This observation may be significant when examined in the context of the known inhibitory effects of NO on PMN chemotaxis, adherence, and stimulation.

Adenosine, a known endogenous regulator of coronary flow, has also been observed to modify post-ischemic flow. Increases in post-ischemic coronary flow have been reported in dog preparations when exogenous adenosine is infused for the first hour of reperfusion following 90 min of ischemia [20]. This increased coronary flow correlates with decreased PMN accumulation on histologic analysis. Furthermore, a reported shift in the exogenous adenosine-induced hyperemia dose response curve to higher adenosine concentrations following 20 min of ischemia in a reperfused dog preparation suggests an altered sensitivity to adenosine in ischemic reperfused areas [15]. Curiously, despite the decreased sensitivity, an increased maximal coronary flow response to the exogenous adenosine signal occurs in the same ischemic reperfused areas. Lastly, it has been shown that pretreatment with 5-amino-imidazole 4-carboxamide (AICA)-riboside (a potentiator of endogenous adenosine levels), increases coronary flow and decreases PMN accumulation in ischemic reperfused regions [21]. The explanation for these observations is not yet known; however, involvement of adenosine-related coronary flow regulation in ischemic reperfused myocardium is clear.

The complement cascade is activated during and following ischemia and may therefore affect post-ischemic coronary flow [22]. Findings in an isolated rat heart preparation suggest that complement is necessary for PMN *activation* in a 20-min ischemia/reperfusion preparation [23]. On the other hand, PMN *adherence* in this same preparation appears to be independent of the presence of complement, suggesting an indirect effect of complement on post-ischemic coronary flow [23]. In fact, we have observed that intracoronary C5a decreases coronary flow and increases coronary effluent thromboxane and histamine levels in pigs [24]. This response can be attenuated by lodoxamide, an inhibitor of mast cell degranulation, but not by histamine blockers or PMN depletion [25]. This suggests that in this model of intraarterial complement activation, the thromboxane/leukotriene release and subsequent decreased coronary flow response was due to an indirect complement-mediated cardiac *mast* cell release. However, this observation is of uncertain relevance to in vivo ischemia where the gradient of C5a is toward the interstitium [26].

In summary, in vivo preparations show a dynamic decrease in coronary flow and coronary reserve following coronary reperfusion which appears dependent on increased PMN adherence to the endothelium, the degree of preceding ischemic injury, and possible modulation by altered microvascular regulators of coronary flow.

Human Evidence

Over the past 10 years evidence has accumulated which indicates that the no-reflow phenomenon occurs in man. Since the description of decreased coronary flow following ischemia in animals, case reports of post-revascularization decreased coronary flow despite large vessel angiographic patency have been presented [27]. The first human experimental evidence for no reflow in the microcirculation was presented in 1985 by Schofer et al. who utilized intracoronary thallium and technetium before and after thrombolysis in 11 patients with acute myocardial infarction [28]. They observed that over one-half of patients had persistent perfusion defects following angiographic reperfusion via thrombolytic treatment. Interestingly, this decrease in post-ischemic perfusion was apparent for at least 2 to 4 weeks following thrombolysis despite continued coronary artery patency. A similar study in 1992 utilizing myocardial contrast echo before and after PTCA or thrombolysis in acute myocardial infarction patients observed that over 20% of patients who had successful angiographic revascularization did not have significant myocardial reflow [29]. In addition, the presence of no reflow at initial revascularization was shown to predict decreased ventricular function persisting at least four weeks after revascularization.

Histologic and biochemical evidence for the presence of no reflow in man have also been reported. Histologic observations regarding reperfusion in man have been made in a necropsy study by the thrombolysis in myocardial infarction (TIMI) group in 1990. This study examined clinical and histologic findings in 52 patients treated with thrombolysis who died 5 h to 260 days post-treatment [30]. Patients with nonocclusive thrombus (indicating reperfusion) had a higher incidence of hemorrhagic infarction. This hemorrhage, however, was not associated with poor clinical outcome (rupture or shock) and was confined to necrotic areas. PMN concentration and histologic configuration were not assessed. Biochemical observations of increased reduction/oxidation products in the clinical reperfusion setting of PTCA, thrombolysis, and CABG surgery have recently been reviewed by Kloner [31]. Whether this oxidative burst is related to no-reflow perhaps through endothelial damage is unknown.

Taken as a whole, the thallium, echo, histologic, and biochemical evidence supports the presence of no reflow in man.

Mechanisms

One possible mechanism for no reflow has been termed the "PMN plugging" hypotheses [4]. This was based primarily on histologic evidence showing PMN accumulation in severely ischemic areas in a ratio of 1 PMN/1 capillary. The obstruction of capillaries by PMNs was thought to be related to endothelial blebs in the ischemic areas and compression from tissue edema. This, in combination with the increased stiffness of activated PMNs, was thought to alter the rheologic properties of blood flow and account for the observed capillary no reflow. Since then, it has been demonstrated that PMN accumulation in capillaries and post-capillary venules is also highly dependent on the adhesiveness of the PMN to the underlying endothelium. Thus, the interaction between the PMN and endothelium appears to be the central mechanism responsible for PMN accumulation in ischemic reperfused tissue and possibly for no reflow. In theory, PMNs could be triggered to a more adhesive or activated condition when exposed to injured endothelium or blood-borne substances present in the post-ischemic setting such as PAF or complement. Conversely, certain substances which are often decreased in the post-ischemic setting such as adenosine and nitric oxide are known to inhibit PMN activation and adhesion. Thus the balance between PMN activation and inhibition may be modified by many of the usual effectors of coronary flow regulation.

Another possible mechanism for no reflow which potentially involves the PMN is the "oxidative burst" hypothesis. Immediately after reperfusion a large increase in oxygen free-radical formation occurs as evidenced by electron spin resonance trapping techniques [32,33]. The source of oxygen free radicals is controversial. Possibilities include the activated PMN NADPH oxidase system, mitochondrial cytochrome leak, and endothelial xanthine oxidase. The existence of xanthine oxidase in human myocardial coronary endothelium has been questioned [34]. Activated PMNs have also been shown to interact with platelets and erythrocytes to form the vasoconstrictors serotonin and leukotriene respectively. However, studies designed to protect against oxygen free-radical related effects using superoxide dismutase and catalase have had conflicting results regarding improved coronary flow and myocardial salvage [35–37]. Furthermore, recent evidence has shown that PMN adherence can occur independent of PMN activation [23]. Thus, the oxidative burst's relationship to no reflow is uncertain.

Erythrocyte (RBC) and platelet plugging have been postulated in the past to be related to no reflow. Several different lines of evidence argue against these theories. First, histologic evidence has repeatedly shown RBC rouleaux formation in sequence following a single PMN. Second, the TIMI group pathological analysis failed to correlate reperfusion hemorrhage with poor clinical outcome. Third, and most importantly, reperfusion with PMN-depleted blood ameliorates no reflow [28]. Similarly, platelet plugging has been though unlikely due to histologic evidence and experiments by Mullane et al. which demonstrated no reduction in infarct size despite reperfusion with platelet-deficient blood [38].

In conclusion, evidence supports the existence of decreased coronary flow and abnormal coronary flow reserve following reperfusion of ischemic myocardium. The mechanism of this decreased coronary flow and flow reserve remains unresolved; however, PMN adhesion to and damage of previously ischemic endothelium appears to be a central part of the process. No-reflow can be modulated by many of the usual effectors of microvascular coronary flow; however, these effectors may be altered by the prior ischemic or reperfusion injury. The degree to which the endothelium and myocardium are injured by the PMN adhesion and subsequent decreased coronary flow and flow reserve is undertermined. It has not been possible to definitely distinguish *irreversibly* injured endothelium and myocardium which would perish regardless of reperfusion from *reversibly* injured endothelium and myocardium which might be susceptible to further reperfusion injury. Future research will undoubtedly focus on this important question due to the possibility for augmented myocardial salvage following clinical reperfusion during thrombolysis, PTCA, and CABG surgery.

References

1. Feigl EO (1983) Coronary physiology. Physiol Rev 3:2–205
2. Marcus ML, Schelbert MR, Wolf GG, Shorton DJ (1991) Cardiac imaging: a companion to Braunwold's Heart Disease. Saunders, pp 6–23
3. Kloner RA, Ganote CE, Jennings RB (1974) The "no reflow" phenomenon after temporary coronary occlusion in the dog. J Clin Invest 54:1496–1508
4. Engler RL, Schmid-Schonbein GW, Pavelec PS (1983) Leukocyte capillary plugging in myocardial ischemia and reperfusion in the dog. Am J Pathol 111:98–111
5. Engler RL, Dahlgren M, Petersen M, Dobbs A, Schmid-Schoenbein GW (1986) Accumulation of polymorphonuclear leukocytes during 3 hour experimental myocardial ischemia. Am J Physiol 251:H93–H100
6. Romson JL, Hook BG, Kunkel SL, Abrams GD, Schork MA, Lucchesi BR (1983) Reduction of the extent of ischemic myocardial injury by neutrophil depletion in the dog. Circulation 67(5):1016–1023
7. Chatelain P, Latour JG, Tran D, Lorgeril M, Dupras G, Bourassa M (1987) Neutrophil accumulation in experimental myocardial infarcts: relation with extent to injury and effect of reperfusion. Circulation 75:1083–1090
8. Litt MR, Jeremy RW, Weisman HF, Winkelstein JA, Becker LC (1989) Neutrophil depletion limited to reperfusion reduces myocardial infarct size after 90 minutes of ischemia: evidence for neutrophil-mediated reperfusion injury. Circulation 80: 1816–1827
9. Kolodgie FD, Virmani R, Farb A (1991) Limitation of no reflow injury by blood-free reperfusion with oxygenated perfluorochemical (Fluosol-DA 20%). J Am Coll Cardiol 18:215–223
10. Tanaka M, Brooks SE, Richard VJ, FitzHarris GP, Stoler RC, Jennings RB, Arfors K-E, Reimer KA (1993) Effect of anti-CD18 antibody on myocardial neutrophil accumulation and infarct size after ischemia and reperfusion in dogs. Circulation 87:526–535
11. Ma X-L, Tsao PS, Lefer AM (1991) Antibody to CD-18 exerts endothelial and cardiac protective effects in myocardial ischemia and reperfusion. J Clin Invest 88(4):1237–1243

12. Weyrich AS, Ma X-L, Lefer AM (1992) Protective effects of a P-selectin specific monoclonal antibody in myocardial ischemia and reperfusion (abstract). Circulation 86:I
13. Westlin W, Mullane KM (1989) Alleviation of myocardial stunning by leukocyte and platelet depletion. Circulation 80:1828–1836
14. Guyton RA, McClenathan JH, MichaelisLL (1977) Evolution of regional ischemia-distal to a proximal coronary stenosis: self propagation of ischemia. Am J Cardiol 40:381–392
15. Ito B, Libraty DH, Engler RL (1991) Effect of transient coronary occlusion on coronary blood flow autoregulation, vasodilator reserve and response to adenosine in the dog. J Am Coll Cardiol 18(3):858–867
16. Nichols WW, Mehta JL, Donnelly WH, Lawson D, Thompson L, terRiet M (1988) Reduction in coronary vasodilator reserve following coronary occlusion and reperfusion in anesthetized dog: Role of endothelium-derived relaxing factor, myocardial neutrophil infiltration and prostaglandins. J Mol Cell Cardiol 20:943–954
17. Kloner RA, Giacomelli F, Alker KJ, Hale SL, Matthews R, Bellows S (1991) Influx of neutrophils into the walls of large epicardial coronary arteries in response to ischemia/reperfusion. Circulation 84(4):1758–1772
18. Ma XL, Weyrich AS, Krantz SL, Lefer AM (1992) Mechanisms of the cardioprotective actions of WEB-2170, bepafant, a platelet activating factor antagonist, in myocardial ischemia and reperfusion. J Pharmacol Exp Ther 260(3):1229–1236
19. Ma X-L, Weyrich AS, Lefer DJ, Lefer AM (1993) Diminished basal nitric oxide release after myocardial ischemia and reperfusion promotes neutrophil adherence to coronary endothelium. Circulation Res 72(2):403–412
20. Olafsson B, Forman MB, Puett DW, Pou A, Cates CU, Friesinger GC, Virmani R (1987) Reduction of reperfusion injury in the canine preparation by intracoronary adenosine: importance of the endothelium and the no-reflow phenomenon. Circulation 76:1135–1145
21. Engler RL (1987) Consequences of activation and adenosine mediated inhibition of granulocytes during myocardial ischemia. Fed Proc 46:2407–2412
22. Rossen RD, Michael LH, Kagiyama A, Savage HE, Hanson G, Reisberg MA, Moake JN, Kim SH, Self D, Weakley S, Giannini E, Entman ML (1988) Mechanism of complement activation after coronary artery occlusion: evidence that myocardial ischemia in dogs causes release of constituents of myocardial subcellular origin that complex with human C1q. Circ Res 62:572–584
23. Shandelya SML, Kuppusamy P, Weisfeldt ML, Zweier JL (1993) Evaluation of the role of polymorphonuclear leukocytes on contractile function in myocardial reperfusion injury. Evidence for plasma-mediated leukocyte activation. Circulation 87:536–546
24. del Balzo U, Engler RL, Ito BR (1993) Complement C5a mediated myocardial ischemia and neutrophil sequestration: two independent phenomena. Am J Physiol 33(3):H336–H344
25. Ito BR, Engler RL, del Balzo U (1993) Role of cardiac mast cells in complete C5a-induced myocardial ischemia. Am J Physiol 264(33):H1346–H1354
26. Weisman HF, Bartow T, Leppo MK, Marsh HC Jr, Carson GR, Concino MF, Boyle MP, Roux KH, Weisfeldt ML, Fearon DT (1990) Soluble human complement receptor type 1: in vivo inhibitor of complement suppressing post-ischemic myocardial inflammation and necrosis. Science 249:146–151

27. Feld H, Lichstein E, Schachter J, Shani J (1992) Early and late angiographic findings of the "no reflow" phenomenon following direct angioplasty as primary treatment for acute myocardial infarction. Am Heart J 123(3):782–784
28. Schofer J, Montz R, Mathey DG (1985) Scintigraphic evidence of the "no reflow" phenomenon in human beings after coronary thrombolysis. J Am Coll Cardiol 5:593–598
29. Ito H, Tomooka T, Sakai N, Yu H, Higashino Y, Fujii K, Masuyama T, Kitabatake A, Minamino T (1992) Lack of myocardial perfusion immediately after successful thrombolysis. Circulation 85:1699–1705
30. Gertz SD, Kalan JM, Kragel AH, Roberts WC, Braunwald E (1990) Cardiac morphologic findings in patients with acute myocardial infarction treated with recombinant tissue plasminogen activator. Am J Cardiol 65:953–961
31. Kloner RA (1993) Does reperfusion injury exist in human? J Am Coll Cardiol 21:537–545
32. Garlick PB, Davies MJ, Hearse DJ, Slater TF (1987) Direct detection of free radicals in the reperfused rat heart using electron spin resonance spectroscopy. Circ Res 61:757–760
33. Bolli R, Patel BS, Jeroudi M, Lai EK, McCay PB (1988) Demonstration of free radical generation in "stunned" myocardium of intact dogs with the use of the spin trap alpha-phenyl *N-tert*-butyl mitrone. J Clin Invest 82:476–485
34. Eddy LJ, Stewart JR, Jones HP, Engerson TD, McCord JM, Downey JM (1987) Free radical-producing enzyme, xanthine oxidase, is undetectable in human hearts. Am J Physiol 253:H709–H711
35. Mehta JL, Lawson DL, Nichols WW (1989) Attenuated coronary relaxation after reperfusion: effects of superoxide dismutase and TxA2 inhibitor U63557A. Am J Physiol 257:H1240–H1246
36. Tanaka M, Fitzharris GP, Stoler RC, Jennings RB, Reimer KA (1989) PEG-SOD plus catalase do not limit infarct size after 90 minutes of ischemia and four days of reperfusion in dogs. Circulation 80:II-296
37. Opie LH (1989) Reperfusion injury and its pharmacologic modification. Circulation 80(4):1049–1062
38. Bendar M, Smith B, Pinto A, Mullane KM (1985) Nafazatrom-induced salvage of ischemic myocardium in anesthetized dogs is mediated through inhibition of neutrophil function. Circ Res 57:131–141

1.4 Coronary Collateral Growth in Canine Model with Gradual Coronary Stenosis and with Repetitive Coronary Occlusions

Hitonobu Tomoike[1]

Summary. The time course of coronary collateral growth in gradual coronary stenosis due to an ameroid constrictor, and in repetitive coronary occlusions, was examined functionally in a canine model. Dogs were instrumented under sterile surgery with pairs of 5 MHz piezo-electric crystals at the left anterior descending artery (LAD) and left circumflex artery (LCX) perfusion area, and a miniature pressure transducer into the left ventricular cavity along with a flow probe and a cuff occluder on the LCX. In an ameroid model, an X-ray transparent ameroid constrictor was placed on the LCX. Repetitive coronary occlusions were controlled by an AM/AM telemetry system while left ventricular pressure and regional wall motion were continuously recorded via an FM/FM telemetry system. Regional wall motion before and during brief coronary occlusion was serially measured in an awake dog until the collateral growth reached the level of functional maturation. Amelioration of regional hypokinesis during transient coronary occlusion was augmented after a certain period of nonrecovery not only in the ameroid model, but also in the repetitive occlusion model. The duration of the lag phase in the model of gradual coronary stenosis was determined by the time needed for the progression of coronary stenosis to more than 80%. The lag phase was also noted in the repetitive occlusion model; however, the biological reason for the lag remains unclarified. A unifying mechanism for the growth of epicardial coronary collateral vessels in both the ameroid and the repetitive occlusion models will be examined over the time course of collateral vessel growth.

Key words: Chronic coronary stenosis—Myocardial ischemia—Collateral function—Regional wall motion—Reactive hyperemia

---

[1] First Department of Internal Medicine, Yamagata University Medical School, 2-2-2 Iida-Nishi, Yamagata, 990-23 Japan

Introduction

Recently, several acute adaptive phenomena in response to ischemia have been identified, affecting the coronary circulation and myocardial performance; examples include ischemic preconditioning, myocardial stunning, and myocardial hibernation. The coronary collateral vessels have long been known as one of the adaptive mechanisms in patients with more than 80% to 90% chronic coronary stenosis. It was experimentally and clinically confirmed that the myocardium, perturbed due to coronary stenosis, was functionally preserved by the presence of collateral vessels [1–4]. Despite vast amounts of clinical evidence concerning the pathophysiology of coronary collateral vessels, factors which modify the collateral development remained unclarified. Experimental studies confirmed the usefulness of artificial coronary stenosis for enhancing collateral development [5]. A model of gradual coronary stenosis using an ameroid constrictor needed 20–30 days to reach a nearly-occluded state [6]. The resistance to coronary blood flow assessed with the tracer microsphere technique fell from 3.52 to 0.22 $\mathrm{mmHg \cdot ml^{-1} \cdot min^{-1} \cdot 100\,g^{-1}}$ during collateral enlargement within a period of eight weeks after implantation of an ameroid constrictor [7]. In a model of repetitive coronary occlusions, we noted a large animal-to-animal variation in the number of 2-min occlusions needed to obtain the functionally mature level of collaterals [8]. However, the chronological characteristics of collateral development have not been rigorously analyzed. Thus, the goal of the present study was to clarify the time course of collateral development with gradual coronary stenosis and with repetitive ischemia. As serial observations for several weeks are needed to document the time course of collateral growth, studies are required in conscious animals, along with well-controlled hemodynamic recordings.

Functional Assessment of Collateral Development

Coronary arteriography and a tracer microsphere technique have been applied for assessing in vivo the anatomical presence of collateral channels and the collateral blood flow, respectively. The assessment of regional myocardial blood flow has been considered a gold standard in experimental studies for documenting the dynamic characteristics of collateral circulation. However, these methods need invasive procedures and the number of repeated measurements possible is limited. Functional aspects of coronary collateral blood flow can be represented by the level of reactive hyperemia during reperfusion or by the reduction of systolic wall motion during coronary occlusion [3,8]. Once the animal is instrumented with a coronary flow probe or a pair of 5 MHz piezo-electric crystals for transit time measurements between crystals in the myocardium, together with a coronary cuff occluder, repeated and noninvasive assessments of the functional state of the coronary collateral vessels are feasible. We confirmed an intimate linear relation between the reduction of reactive hyperemia and regional systolic wall motion during the time course of collateral growth in an ameroid model [3] as well as in a repetitive brief occlusion model [8].

Recently, it was demonstrated that a coronary artery occlusion per se affects vascular reactivity related to the endothelial function in both the conduit and resistance vessels [9]. Endothelium-dependent coronary dilatation was markedly inhibited after 10–30 min but not 2 min of ischemia. In addition, a 2-min coronary occlusion, which we preferentially applied in our studies of collateral development, did not modify the level of reactive hyperemia nor cause deterioration of the process of recovery of systolic wall motion after reperfusion. Accordingly, we monitored the level of collateral vessel development functionally by the level of systolic wall motion during a 2-min coronary occlusion. The drawbacks of the present technique were: (1) it was impossible to obtain information after the collateral growth levels off, because any further improvement of normal wall motion cannot be expected; (2) the level of collateral blood flow cannot be extrapolated solely from the level of systolic wall motion.

Animal Model of Collateral Vessel Development

The anatomy and distribution of the major vessels supplying the myocardium are different among species [10]. The pig and the dog are preferentially employed as animal models to investigate the pathophysiology of collateral development. There are dozens of reasons for the selection of an appropriate animal model. In the present series of studies, we chose a canine model to facilitate long-term observations in a physiological state. In the dog, the left side dominates in coronary arteries, a topography which is a little different from that of human and porcine coronary arteries. Collateral pathways in the dog reside mostly at the epicardium and are largely intracoronary connections between vessels derived from the anterior descending and circumflex arteries, which are also different from human and porcine coronaries [11]. Schaper summed up such differences in type of collateral development thus: "Dogs can be used to study the epicardial large vessel response, and pigs can be used to study the endomural numerous small vessel response" [12].

The other aspect of collateral development is that there is a choice of experimental procedures for studying collateral development. To enhance the epicardial large vessel response, an ameroid model and a repetitive brief occlusion model [13] are available. Endomural small vessel response is also reproducible in a canine model by an intracoronary injection of microspheres (25 μm). Chilian and his co-workers reported that microvessels had responded with growth to micro-embolization (25 μm), especially in the subepicardium, whereas necroses were noted frequently in the subendocardium [14]. We chose a model of the epicardial large vessel response. The advantages of the repetitive brief coronary occlusion model are (1) the amount of ischemic stimulus is quantifiable and based simply on the number of occlusions; (2) its stimulus is controllable, e.g., changes in duration, repetition, and rate or mode of coronary occlusion; and (3) there are clinical implications as a model of recurrent episodes in coronary spasm.

Instrumented conscious dog models were carefully prepared along with the construction of an automated command and recording system including FM/FM and AM/AM telemetry devices [15]. Under sterile surgical techniques and positive-pressure respiration, a miniature pressure transducer was inserted into the left ventricular cavity and two pairs of ultrasonic miniature crystals were implanted subendocardially to measure regional wall motion at the left anterior descending artery (LAD) and left circumflex artery (LCX) areas. In the ameroid model, a radiolucent ameroid [6], a Doppler flow probe and a cuff occluder were placed on the left circumflex coronary artery. In case of the repetitive occlusion model, an electromagnetic or a Doppler flow probe and a cuff occluder were placed on the LCX.

Time Course of Collateral Development

Serial changes in regional myocardial shortening during temporary coronary occlusions are shown in two representative cases, one with an ameroid constrictor (Fig. 1a) [16] and the other with repetitive 2-min coronary occlusions (Fig. 1b) [17]. In both models, the level of collateral development was assessed functionally, based on changes in regional wall motion during coronary occlusion. Regional wall motion before coronary occlusion was maintained fairly constant during the entire period in either the ameroid or the repetitive occlusion model; hence, gradual coronary occlusion or repetition of 2-min coronary occlusion did not lead to myocardial damage, such as stunning or hibernation.

As shown in representative changes in the ameroid model, percent shortening of the LCX area during occlusion decreased to around 2% of control and there was no obvious amelioration for 25 days, while there was 5%–8% hypershortening at the LAD area. These responses coincided well with observations noted during coronary occlusion in animals with collateral vessels absent [18]. In the ameroid model, the presence of a lag phase in which the regional wall motion during occlusion was akinetic or diskinetic may be explained by the time needed for progression of coronary constriction to more than 80% stenosis. After the lag, there was progressive recovery of regional hypokinesia associated with reduction in the end-diastolic length (EDL) and finally the regional shortening was unchanged before and after a brief coronary occlusion (Fig. 1a). The duration from the attenuation of regional myocardial hypokinesis to full recovery ranged from 5 to 29 days (14 ± 3 days), while the disappearance of flow signal at the LCX occurred from 11 to 53 days (28 ± 6 days) in 6 dogs.

The time course of collateral development in the repetitive occlusion model was similar to the ameroid one in profile. Two-min occlusions every 30 min were much more efficient than 15-s occlusions every 4 min [15]. The number of

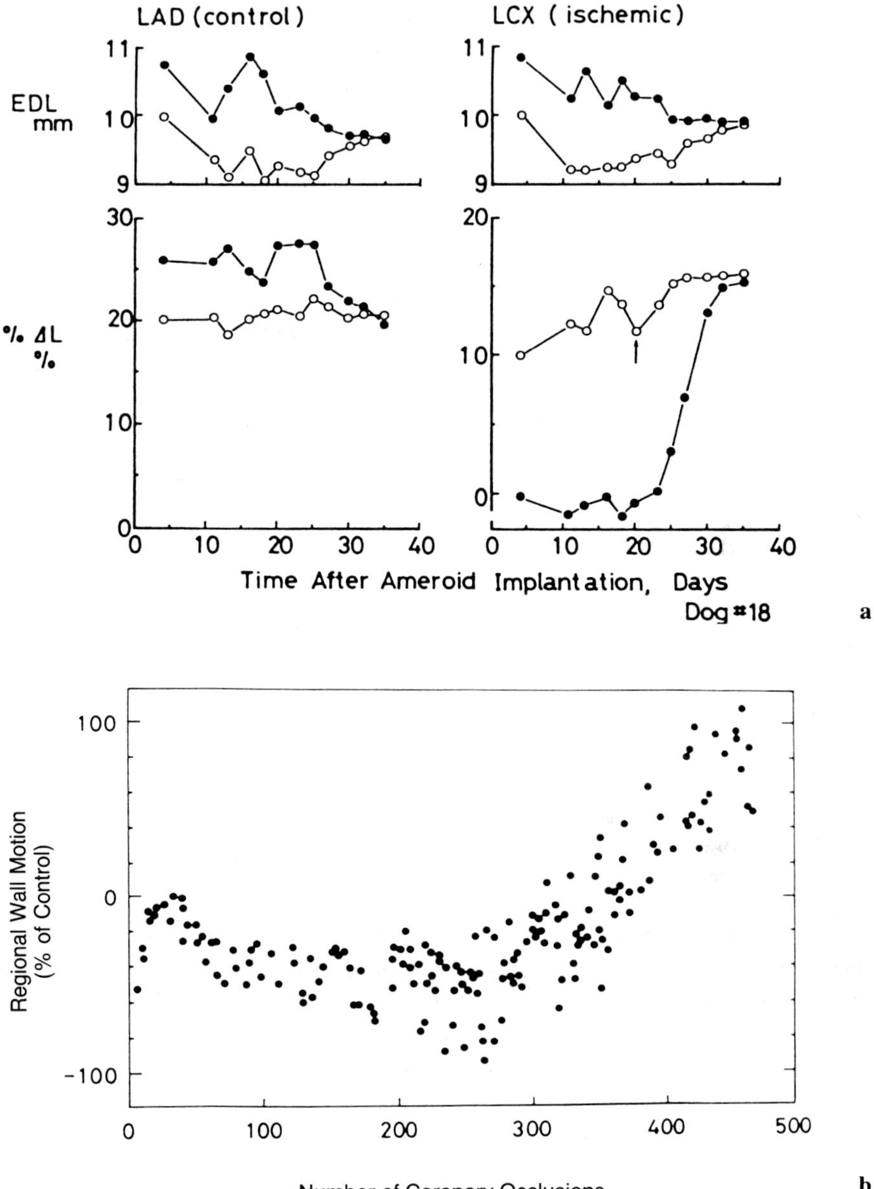

Fig. 1a. Serial changes in end-diastolic length (*EDL*) and % systolic shortening before (*open circles*) and after (*closed circles*) 2-min coronary occlusion (*CO*) in a representative case with an ameroid constriction (data from [16]). *EDL* = end diastolic length; *%ΔL*, percent systolic shortening; *LAD*, left anterior descending artery; *LCX*, left circumflex artery. **b** Time course of collateral development in relation to changes in systolic shortening during 2-min coronary occlusion in a representative case under repetitive coronary occlusions

occlusions or amount of time required for restoration of function due to development of collateral circulation was from 125 to 478 occlusions (265 ± 106) or from 3 to 11 days, respectively, for 11 dogs in the study of Mohri et al. [15]. Mechanisms determining the lag remain unexamined.

Unifying Mechanism in Collateral Growth Among Animal Models

Similarities of functional collateral development between the ameroid and the repetitive coronary occlusion models suggest the importance of blood flow across anastomotic channels. Several mechanical forces have been credited as causes of collateral growth, including the increased wall tension or tangential shear stress due to the presence of flow and/or development of an intravascular pressure gradient. All of these were noted to occur in parallel with the growth of the anastomotic channels [5]. Increase in flow behaves as a positive feedback for collateral vessel development, not only via the dilatation due to endothelium-derived relaxing factor but also via the structural remodeling stimulated by endothelium-derived substances [19].

We noted a big variation among animals in the time necessary for collateral vessels to reach the mature state, in both the ameroid and the repetitive occlusion models. Noma et al. clearly demonstrated the importance of native collaterals for the speed of later development of collateral function in the repetitive occlusion model [20]. As a unifying mechanism common to both the ameroid and repetitive coronary occlusion models, the time course of collateral vessel growth appeared to follow the biological growth curve. Accordingly, serial remodelings of the intraarterial anastomosis may evolve in a cascade of cell-to-blood, cell-to-cell, and cell-to-matrix interactions.

Clinical Implications

It was commonly demonstrated in experimental animals as well as in patients with coronary artery disease that collateral vessels act as an inherent protective mechanism against the evolving myocardial ischemia. Although functionally effective collaterals were reproduced in canine models without significant sacrifice of the myocardium, such situations were not so frequently observed in patients with coronary artery diseases. Collateral development involves, pathophysiologically, dilatation and growth of the anastomotic channels, and angiogenesis. Elucidating factors which promote growth of collaterals toward the ischemic region could allow us explore new horizons in the medical treatment of coronary artery disease.

Acknowledgments. This work was supported in part by Grants-in-Aid for Scientific Research from the Ministry of Education, Science and Culture, Japan.

I thank Prof. Dr. M. Nakamura for critical comments and my co-workers Drs. T. Inou, K. Watanabe, H. Shimokawa, S. Nabeyama, H. Yamamoto, T. Inoue, K. Hisano, M. Mohri, M. Noma, H. Ando, and M. Nagano at the Research Institute of Angiocardiology and Cardiovascular Clinic, Faculty of Medicine, Kyushu University for their participation in numerous experiments; Mr. H. So for machine works; and Ms. M. Sasaki at Yamagata University for secretarial services.

References

1. Martinez-Rios MA, DaCosta BCB, Cecena-Seldner FA, Gensini GG (1970) Normal electrocardiogram in the presence of severe coronary artery disease. Am J Cardiol 25:320–324
2. Hamby RI, Aintablian A, Schwartz A (1976) Reappraisal of the functional significance of the coronary collateral circulation. Am J Cardiol 38:305–309
3. Tomoike H, Franklin D, Kemper WS, McKnown D, Ross J Jr (1981) Functional evaluation of coronary collateral development in conscious dogs. Am J Physiol 241:H519–H524
4. Hill RC, Kleinman LH, Tiller WH Jr (1983) Myocardial blood flow and function during gradual coronary occlusion in awake dog. Am J Physiol 244:H60–H67
5. Schaper W (1971) The collateral circulation of the heart. North-Holland Publishing, Amsterdam
6. Inou T, Tomoike H, Watanabe K, Kikuchi Y, Mizukami M, Kurozumi T, Nakamura M (1980) A newly developed X-ray transparent ameroid constrictor for study on progression of gradual coronary stenosis. Basic Res Cardiol 75:537–543
7. Schaper W, Flameng W, Winkler B, Wüsten B, Türrschmann W, Neugebauer G, Carl M (1976) Quantification of collateral resistance in acute and chronic experimental coronary occlusion in the dog. Circ Res 39:371–377
8. Yamamoto H, Tomoike H, Shimokawa H, Nabeyama S, Nakamura M (1984) Development of collateral function with repetitive coronary occlusion in a canine model reduces myocardial reactive hyperemia in the absence of significant coronary stenosis. Circ Res 55:623–632
9. Sobey CG, Woodman OL (1993) Myocardial ischemia: what happens to the coronary arteries? Trends Pharmacol Sci 14:448–453
10. Bertho E, Gagnon G (1964) A comparative study in three dimensions of the blood supply of the normal interventricular septum in human, canine, bovine, porcine, ovine and equine heart. Dis Chest 46:251–262
11. Schaper W, Jageneau A, Xhonneux R (1967) The development of collateral circulation in the pig and dog heart. Cardiologia 51:321–335
12. Schaper W (1991) Biological and molecular biological aspects of angiogenesis in coronary collateral development. In: Nakamura M, Vanhoutte PM (eds) Coronary circulation in physiological and pathophysiological states. Springer, Berlin Heidelberg New York Tokyo, pp 21–27
13. Franklin D, McKown D, McKown M, Hartley J, Caldwell M (1981) Development and regression of coronary collaterals induced by repeated, reversible ischemia in dogs (abstract). Fed Proc 40:339

14. Chilian WM, Mass HJ, Williams SE, Layne SM, Smith ES, Scheel KW (1990) Microvascular occlusions promote coronary collateral growth. Am J Physiol 258: 1103–1111
15. Mohri M, Tomoike H, Noma M, Inoue T, Hisano K, Nakamura M (1988) Duration of ischemia is vital for collateral development: Repeated brief coronary artery occlusions in conscious dogs. Circ Res 64:287–296
16. Tomoike H, Inou T, Watanabe K, Mizukami M, Kikuchi Y, Nakamura M (1983) Functional significance of collaterals during ameroid-induced coronary stenosis in conscious dogs: Interrelationship among regional shortening, regional flow and grade of coronary stenosis. Circulation 67:1001–1008
17. Tomoike H (1993) Functional aspects of collateral development in animal models. In: Schaper W, Schaper J (eds) Collateral circulation. Kluwer Academic, pp 149–172
18. Theroux P, Ross J Jr, Franklin D, Kemper WS, Sasayama S (1976) Regional myocardial function in the conscious dog during acute coronary occlusion and responses to morphine, propranolol, nitroglycerin, and lidocaine. Circulation 53: 302–314
19. D'Amore PA, Thompson RW (1987) Mechanisms of angiogenesis. Ann Rev Physiol 49:453–464
20. Noma M, Tomoike H, Ando H, Mohri M, Takeshita A, Nakamura M (1994) The rate of functional collateral development following repetitive brief coronary occlusion in conscious dogs is determined by pre-existing collaterals. Jpn Circ J 58:269–277

1.5 Myocardial Ca^{2+} and Na^+ Homeostasis and the Recovery of Postischemic Contractile Function

Martin M. Pike[1], Cameron S. Luo[1], and Masafumi Kitakaze[2]

Summary. Recent measurements from various studies using intact heart models have shown that myocardial free intracellular Ca^{2+} ($[Ca^{2+}]_i$) increases during brief periods of ischemia. To a great extent, this increased $[Ca^{2+}]_i$ during ischemia/reperfusion may be coupled to intracellular Na^+ ($Na^+{}_i$) accumulation, via Na^+/Ca^{2+} exchange. Evidence is presented that Na^+ influx via Na^+/H^+ exchange plays a major role in $Na^+{}_i$ accumulation during ischemia, despite indications that this exchange is a relatively minor mechanism for pH regulation at that time. The recovery of pH during reperfusion is discussed in terms of its potential role in enhancing Na^+ and Ca^{2+} entry at that time. The early reperfusion period may represent a critical period in the metabolic and functional recovery of the heart. During reperfusion, $[Ca^{2+}]_i$ can return to control levels, but its recovery is usually delayed by at least several minutes. Comparison of $[Ca^{2+}]_i$ measurements to measurements of total intracellular Ca^{2+} uptake suggest the presence of a substantial uptake of Ca^{2+} upon reperfusion, which is largely buffered by an unknown mechanism. Postischemic recovery of the myocardium can be improved by interventions which decrease Ca^{2+} accumulation during ischemia and/or reperfusion. These interventions include both direct alterations of Ca^{2+} transport and indirect interventions such as those which decrease myocardial $Na^+{}_i$ accumulation.

Key words: Myocardium—Ischemia—Reperfusion—Calcium—Sodium—pH––Nuclear magnetic resonance

The continuous regulation of the sarcolemmal Ca^{2+} gradient is of great importance to the metabolism and mechanical function of the myocardium.

[1] Division of Cardiovascular Disease, Department of Medicine, 703 S. 19th St., ZRB 308, University of Alabama at Birmingham, Birmingham, AL 35294, USA
[2] Division of Cardiology, First Department of Medicine, Osaka University Medical School, 2-2 Yamadagaoka, Suita, Osaka, 565 Japan

The cytosolic free Ca^{2+} concentration ($[Ca^{2+}]_i$) is a carefully controlled signal which oscillates with each cardiac cycle and regulates successive contraction and relaxation via interaction with the myofibrillar apparatus. The $[Ca^{2+}]_i$ also regulates key enzymes involved in glycogen breakdown and mitochondrial ATP production [1]. Hence $[Ca^{2+}]_i$ has parallel links to both force generation and energy production. However, in addition to these important regulatory roles under normal physiological conditions, alterations in $[Ca^{2+}]_i$ homeostasis may also be involved in ischemic injury mechanisms which cause postischemic contractile dysfunction or cell necrosis. Pathogenic roles related to a $[Ca^{2+}]_i$ overload state could include activation of phospholipases and/or proteases [2], inhibition of mitochondrial function [1,3], or initiation of ventricular fibrillation [4–6]. In this chapter, the validity of a causal relationship between cation homeostasis and ischemic injury will be assessed (1) by examining the evidence that substantial changes in cation homeostasis occur during brief periods of ischemia, and (2) by examining the metabolic and functional results of interventions which alter the timecourse of cation alterations during ischemia/reperfusion. The essential question is whether the alterations in $[Ca^{2+}]_i$ or other intracellular cations can be viewed as simply a result of ischemia and necrosis, or whether such alterations play a significant role in the injury process.

In the evaluation of the timecourse of metabolic changes across ischemia and reperfusion, it is important to choose relevant ischemic models in which coronary flow is a meaningful variable. The cessation of flow, and the accompanying reduction in vascular washout and substrate delivery, is a key component of ischemia which is difficult to mimic appropriately with cells and superfused tissues. Recently, NMR spectroscopy and other modalities have been used to noninvasively monitor cation concentrations in intact tissues. By loading perfused tissues with the fluorinated Ca^{2+} indicator 5F-BAPTA [7], mean time-averaged free $[Ca^{2+}]_i$ levels in the intact perfused heart can be measured with ^{19}F NMR, with a time resolution of approximately 5 min [8]. Cytosolic loading is achieved by perfusing with the membrane-permeable acetoxymethyl ester derivative of the indicator, which is then converted to the nonpermeable Ca^{2+}-sensitive form by nonspecific esterase activity within the cell. Quantitation of the free $[Ca^{2+}]_i$ concentration is obtained by multiplying the K_d (308 nM) [9] times the ratio of the Ca^{2+}-bound and Ca^{2+}-free indicator, obtained from the relative areas of the two resonances observed in the NMR spectrum. ^{19}F NMR spectra from a perfused ferret heart are shown in Fig. 1, from the study of Marban et al. [9]. The spectra indicate an increase in the Ca^{2+}-bound peak during ischemia, and a corresponding decrease in the Ca^{2+}-free peak. From the same study, Fig. 2 indicates mean data obtained from a group of 5F-BAPTA-loaded ferret hearts which were exposed to 20 min of zero-flow ischemia at 30°C, followed by reperfusion. This ischemic model has been previously characterized as being associated with prolonged postischemic contractile dysfunction without the development of necrosis, and as such is a model of "myocardial stunning" [10]. The data clearly indicate that $[Ca^{2+}]_i$

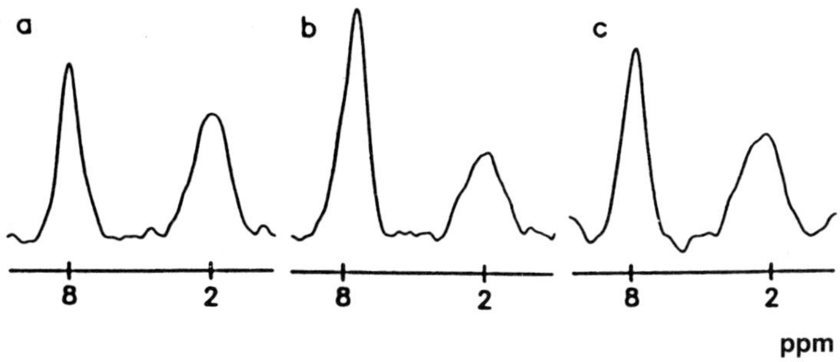

Fig. 1. ^{19}F NMR spectra of a 5F-BAPTA-loaded perfused ferret heart subjected to 20 min of zero-flow ischemia. Each spectrum was acquired in 5 min. The Ca^{2+}-bound resonance is at 8 ppm, and the Ca^{2+} free at 2 ppm, referenced to 6F-tryptophan. Spectrum **a** was acquired during control perfusion, **b** at 12.5 min of ischemia, and **c** after 10 min of reperfusion. (Adapted from [9])

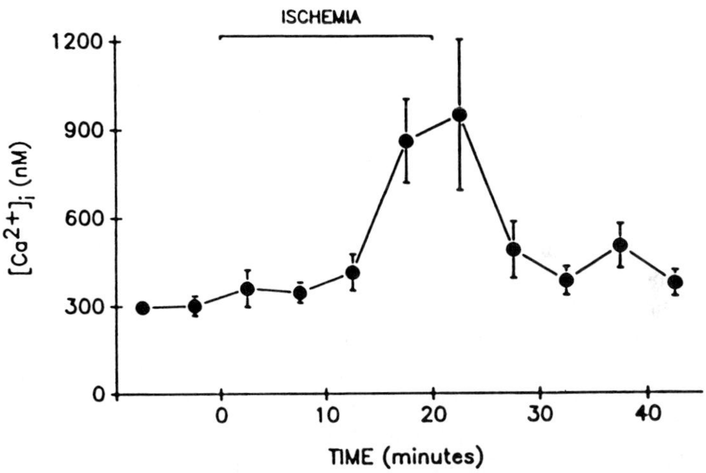

Fig. 2. Mean (±SEM) time-averaged Ca^{2+} levels calculated from a group (n = 11) of 5F-BAPTA loaded ferret hearts exposed to zero-flow ischemia, (20 min, 30°C, 8 mM extracellular Ca^{2+}) and reperfusion. (Adapted from [9])

increases substantially during this brief ischemic period, reaching sustained levels in the range of 1 μM. Importantly, the data also reveal that although the $[Ca^{2+}]_i$ levels do return to normal levels, elevated levels comparable to those at end ischemia are sustained for approximately the first 5 min of reperfusion. The extracellular Ca^{2+} in these experiments was set at 8 mM to offset the Ca^{2+} buffering effect of the 5F-BAPTA loading and the resulting functional attenuation. However, $[Ca^{2+}]_i$ measurements recorded at 2 mM extracellular Ca^{2+} indicated a similar timecourse, with a significant increase during late ischemia which was maintained briefly during reperfusion. The data provide direct evidence that alterations in $[Ca^{2+}]_i$ homeostasis occur early during ischemia and precede necrosis, and are consistent with the hypothesis that such alterations could be involved in ischemic injury mechanisms. The findings are consistent with other ^{19}F NMR studies employing the perfused rat heart model [11–13]. Studies with the fluorescent indicators indo-1 and fura-2 have also indicated increases in $[Ca^{2+}]_i$ during ischemia in the intact heart [14,15]. These indicators are loaded in a similar fashion to that of the ^{19}F NMR indicator, using the esterified permeable derivatives, and $[Ca^{2+}]_i$ is monitored by detecting the relative fluorescence emission at two wavelengths. Absolute quantitation is not feasible due to background fluorescence; the fluorescence ratio is generally reported. However, the methodology has the advantage of rapid time resolution, allowing beat to beat, diastolic, and systolic measurements. A study by Mohabir et al. using indo-1 [14] in the perfused rabbit heart detected a rapid initial rise in $[Ca^{2+}]_i$ during the first several minutes of zero-flow ischemia which slowed but continued steadily upward between 5 and 15 min of ischemia. These changes are consistent with a study using fura-2 in the guinea pig heart [15]. This study included reperfusion $[Ca^{2+}]_i$ measurements, indicating that after 15 min of ischemia, diastolic $[Ca^{2+}]_i$ recovered slowly, and remained elevated above control for 15 min of reperfusion. In another study, Carrozza et al. reported $[Ca^{2+}]_i$ measurements using the bioluminescent protein aequorin, which was macroinjected into intact ferret hearts [16]. This technique provides rapid $[Ca^{2+}]_i$ measurements which can be calibrated and quantitated, and the macroinjection technique minimizes loading into subcellular compartments. The study provided further documentation of increases in diastolic and peak $[Ca^{2+}]_i$ during ischemia, which remained significantly elevated during early reperfusion. The reported timecourses of the $[Ca^{2+}]_i$ changes in the above studies vary somewhat, possibly due to differences in species, methodology, or nonmyocyte indicator loading [17]. Differences exist in the amount of indicator (and additional Ca^{2+} buffering) used in the studies. Importantly, however, all the studies reported that substantial increases in $[Ca^{2+}]_i$ occur during brief, zero-flow ischemia. Those studies reporting reperfusion measurements generally indicated that $[Ca^{2+}]_i$ remained elevated for a period of several minutes or longer.

Studies which have employed direct alterations of Ca^{2+} homeostasis have provided evidence that $[Ca^{2+}]_i$ overload plays a role in ischemic injury. Lopaschuk et al. found that the preischemic treatment with the Ca^{2+} channel blocker diltiazem significantly improved functional recovery of the perfused rat heart, at concentrations which did not alter preischemic function substantially [18]. In another study, ^{19}F NMR spectroscopic measurements indicated that similar concentrations of diltiazem markedly inhibited $[Ca^{2+}]_i$ accumulation during ischemia in that model [19]. The studies suggest that ischemic $[Ca^{2+}]_i$ levels play a role in the postischemic functional recovery, although both reports also indicated that the beneficial effects of diltiazem may also be related to a slowing of energy demand, glycolytic flux, and byproduct accumulation. Other studies have demonstrated that altering the Ca^{2+} flux during the reperfusion period can alter the functional recovery. In a study by Kusuoka et al., ischemic ferret hearts were briefly reperfused with low extracellular Ca^{2+} before Ca^{2+} was gradually restored to normal levels in a stepwise fashion; myocardial stunning was largely ameliorated in the low Ca^{2+} group, with a significant improvement in functional recovery [10]. In the same animal model, a brief exposure to high levels of extracellular Ca^{2+} without any ischemia resulted in depressed left ventricular function which mimicked myocardial stunning [20]. Using the perfused rat heart model, du Toit et al. [21] implemented a range of interventions which alter Ca^{2+} handling, which were carried out during only the first 2 min of reperfusion. Changing the extracellular Ca^{2+} to moderately low levels for that period significantly improved the functional recovery, while increasing the Ca^{2+} had the opposite effect. The use of nisoldipine and other Ca^{2+} channel blockers increased the functional recovery, while interventions thought to increase sarcolemmal Ca^{2+} permeability, such as adding Ca^{2+} ionophores, decreased it. These studies underscore a role for $[Ca^{2+}]_i$ in ischemic injury, and a particular importance for Ca^{2+} handling during reperfusion.

To understand the metabolic context in which alterations in $[Ca^{2+}]_i$ homeostasis occur, it is vital to consider changes in cellular energy and the levels of other ions, such as Na^+ and H^+. Recently, NMR techniques have been developed which enable rapid noninvasive intracellular Na^+ (Na^+_i) measurements in intact tissues [22–24]. Such methodology involves the use of NMR shift reagents, which can be placed in the extracellular compartment and used to selectively shift the frequency of the Na^+ or other cationic NMR sensitive nuclei in that compartment. In this manner, the intra- and extracellular resonances can be resolved, thus enabling studies of cation transport. Using such techniques, Balschi et al. noted a threefold increase in Na^+_i after 28 min of zero-flow ischemia in the perfused rat heart [25]. In the perfused ferret heart, Pike, et al. (1990) [26] recorded a substantial increase in Na^+_i during ischemia, which recovered during reperfusion but nonetheless remained above control levels for the first 8 min of reperfusion. The mechanisms of such Na^+_i accumulation during ischemia and its role in functional recovery were addressed in a study by Pike et al. [27] which employed a specific inhibitor of Na^+/H^+ exchange, 5-(N-ethyl-N-isopropyl)amiloride, (EIPA, 3 μM), with the perfused rat heart model. It was found that infusion of EIPA before 21 min of zero-flow ischemia, greatly enhanced the functional recovery, from 36% of the preischemic developed pressure in untreated hearts, to 104% in EIPA-treated hearts. Insight into the mechanism of this functional improvement was provided by close examination of the measured metabolic variables. In this study, ^{23}Na and ^{31}P spectra were automatically interleaved to obtain measurements of Na^+_i, pH_i, and cellular energy in the same perfused rat heart preparations, using specially designed NMR hardware. This was feasible because the ^{23}Na NMR shift reagent employed for resolution of intra- and extracellular ^{23}Na

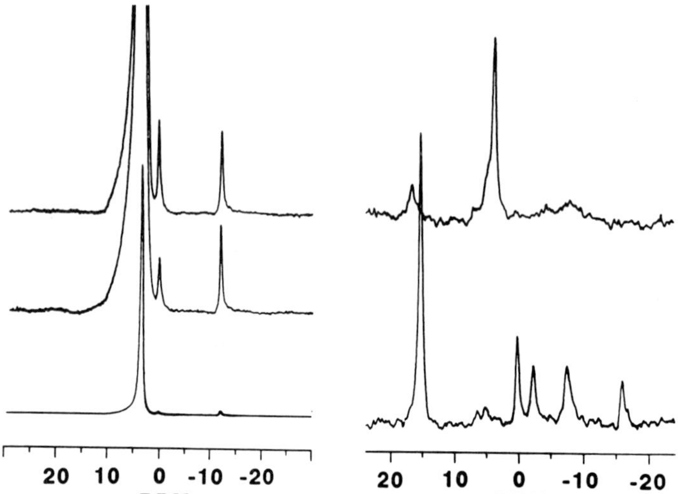

Fig. 3a,b. Interleaved ^{23}Na and ^{31}P spectra of a rat heart perfused with 5 mM $Tm(DOTP)^{5-}$. **a** ^{23}Na NMR spectra: lower and middle spectra are the same (different vertical scales), during control perfusion. Peak assignments: 3 ppm is extracellular and bath Na^+, 0.0 ppm is the unshifted $Na^+{}_i$ resonance, −12 ppm is NaCl reference shifted with $D_y(PPP)^{7-}{}_2$. Top spectrum is after 21 min of ischemia: note the increase in the $Na^+{}_i$ resonance. **b** ^{31}P spectra: resonance at 15 ppm is from 15 mM phenyl phosphonate (PPA) in the perfusate. Other resonances represent P_i (4.9 ppm), PCr (0 ppm), and γ (2.5 ppm), α (7.5 ppm), and β (16 ppm) ATP. Spectrum below is before ischemia, spectrum above is after 21 min of ischemia. (From [27], with permission)

resonances, $Tm(DOTP)^{5-}$ [28], has a relatively low magnetic moment and so has the added advantage of allowing the simultaneous acquisition of excellent ^{31}P spectra. Figure 3 shows interleaved ^{23}Na and ^{31}P NMR rat heart spectra. Those in panel A are the ^{23}Na spectra, before and after 21 minutes of zero-flow ischemia. Note that good resolution of the $Na^+{}_i$ resonance is obtained, even in the presence of the large extracellular/bath Na^+ signal and during control perfusion when $Na^+{}_i$ is low. During ischemia, the $Na^+{}_i$ peak clearly increases in intensity. As shown by the interleaved ^{31}P spectra displayed in Panel B, extensive depletion of high energy phosphates occurs during ischemia. The spectra also show the large resonance from the extracellular pH (pH_e) marker phenyl phosphonate (PPA); decrease in intensity during ischemia occurs due to the removal of bath PPA by flushing with PPA-free perfusate. Figure 4 indicates mean data obtained from the interleaved spectra for two groups of hearts, indicating $Na^+{}_i$, as well as pH_i (obtained from the frequency shift of the P_i peak). One group was untreated, and the other was infused with the Na^+/H^+ exchange inhibitor, EIPA (3 μM), for 15 min before zero-flow ischemia was initiated. In the untreated group, $Na^+{}_i$ increased by approximately 80% during the 20 min ischemic period, and indicated an incomplete recovery during

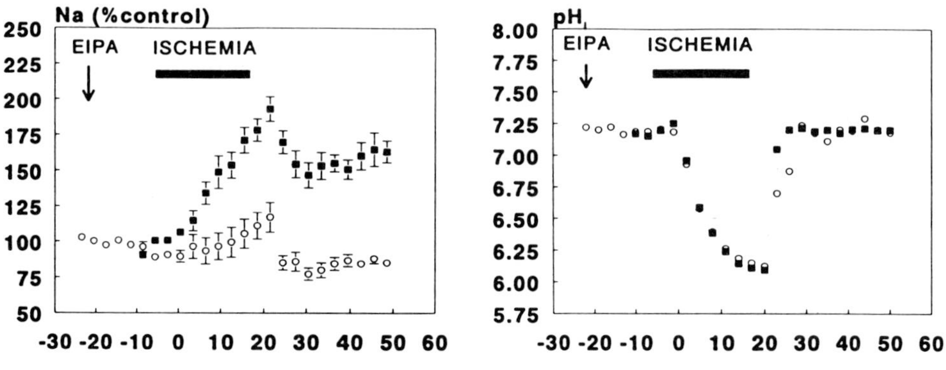

Fig. 4. Measurements of **a** $Na^+{}_i$ levels (±SEM) (in percent of control values before ischemia and EIPA infusion) and **b** pH_i, plotted versus time, during control, 21 min of zero-flow ischemia, and reperfusion, for untreated (n = 6; *solid squares*) and EIPA-treated (3 μM, n = 6; *open circles*) hearts. *Arrow* indicates introduction of EIPA infusion (42 nmoles/min) for EIPA-treated hearts. Error bars omitted for clarity with pH_i data. (Adapted from [27])

reperfusion. In contrast, in the EIPA-treated group, the $Na^+{}_i$ increase during ischemia was completely prevented. This data provides clear evidence that substantial increases in $Na^+{}_i$ occur during brief ischemia, and that Na^+/H^+ exchange is a major mechanism for this increase. Figure 4 indicates that this occurs in the context of severe proton overload, with pH_i decreasing from 7.2 to near 6. This is probably caused by the decrease in vascular washout combined with increased glycolytic energy production and associated proton generation [29]. Data obtained (not shown) from the chemical shift of the PPA in the perfusate indicated that the pH_e tracked the pH_i, showing that an efflux of protons occurred which collapsed the sarcolemmal pH gradient within 5 min of ischemia. Interestingly, however, no differences were observed in the pH_i or pH_e between the untreated and EIPA groups during ischemia. During reperfusion, the pH_i recovery was measurably slowed by EIPA but both groups still recovered rapidly. Hence, despite the substantial $Na^+{}_i$ accumulation resulting from Na^+/H^+ exchange, the data suggest that only a minor portion of the proton extrusion that occurs during ischemia or reperfusion does so by that mechanism. These data are quite consistent with many recent studies with cardiac preparations, which indicate that Na^+/H^+ exchange inhibition has little or no net effect on pH_i during basal control conditions and during ischemia [12,30–33]. Its effects are most easily observed during recovery from a (nonischemic) acid load [30,31]. A study by Vandenberg et al. [33] indicated that lactate-H^+ transport is the dominant H^+ extrusion mechanism upon reperfusion of ischemic myocardium. Ischemia and/or reperfusion may represent a unique

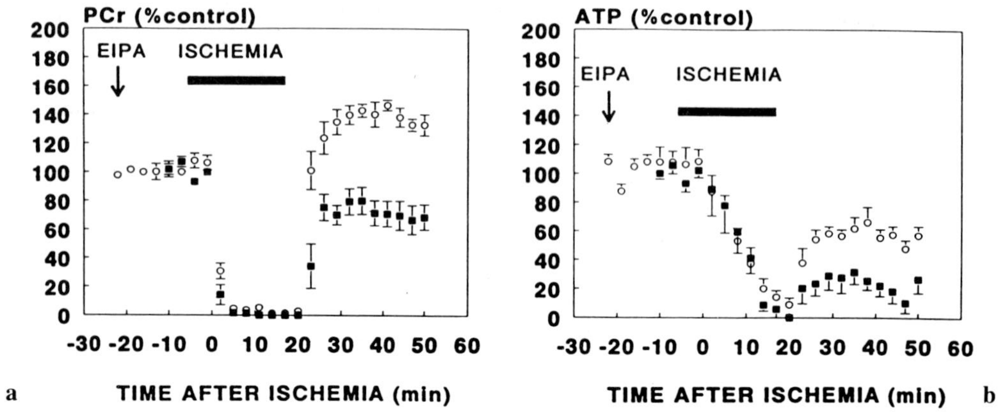

Fig. 5. Measurements of **a** PCr (±SEM) and **b** ATP in percent of control for same groups of hearts as in Fig. 4. *Arrow* indicates introduction of EIPA infusion for EIPA-treated hearts. (Adapted from [27])

situation in which the large production of lactate during ischemia, in the range of 200 μmoles/gram dry weight [34], enables a convenient mechanism for proton extrusion.

While activation of Na^+/H^+ exchange contributes to $Na^+{}_i$ accumulation during ischemia, the accumulation of $Na^+{}_i$ is also likely to be due in part to decreased Na^+ extrusion. Figure 5 shows that the cation alterations were concomitant with a severely depleted energy condition; levels of both ATP and phosphocreatine (PCr) decreased to minimal levels during the ischemic protocol. Such a decrease in energy is likely to decrease Na^+ efflux (and K^+ influx) via the Na^+/K^+ ATPase, the primary Na^+ extrusion mechanism. However, the precise dependence of the enzyme activity on the high energy phosphate concentration is difficult to predict in vivo. The K_m for ATP is reported to be 0.6 mM or below [35], much lower than the approximately 20 mM concentrations normally reported during control perfusion [36]. ATP availability is not the only consideration; if the enzyme is assumed to be at equilibrium, the maximum Na^+ gradient which can be maintained (at a given transmembrane potential) can be directly related to the free energy of ATP hydrolysis [37]. This is closely related to the ATP/ADP ratio, which is in turn greatly affected by the concentration of PCr and creatine kinase activity. While the effect of cellular energy on Na^+ extrusion during ischemia may be substantial, it is perhaps unquantified. Notably, Fig. 5 indicates that both ATP and PCr levels were severely depleted in both untreated and EIPA groups. Despite this, Fig. 4 shows that $Na^+{}_i$ homeostasis can be maintained during the ischemic period if the dominant mechanism for Na^+ entry is inhibited. Hence, it is clear that the $Na^+{}_i$ level during ischemia is not simply controlled by the energy levels and Na^+ pump activity, but is a complicated function of kinetic and thermodynamic factors, likely involving both the activation of Na^+/H^+ exchange due to increased proton loading, and a decrease in Na^+ extrusion via the Na^+/K^+ ATPase.

While only slight differences in cellular energy levels were observed during the ischemic period between the treated and untreated groups, Fig. 5 shows that the energy recovery during reperfusion was markedly different. The Na^+/H^+ exchange inhibition induced a much more rapid and extensive recovery of PCr and ATP. The PCr had completely recovered at 2 min of reperfusion for the EIPA group, compared to a 34% recovery for the untreated. This could be due to incomplete reactivation of energy production in the untreated hearts. Notably, the recovery of Na^+_i was also incomplete in that group. Explanation of changes in these metabolic and functional variables requires consideration of how these variables may relate to $[Ca^{2+}]_i$ homeostasis. The primary sarcolemmal extrusion mechanism for Ca^{2+} in the myocardium is Na^+/Ca^{2+} (3:1) exchange [38]. This mechanism is generally thought to have a very high capacity, much higher than that of the Ca^{2+} ATPase. This effectively couples Ca^{2+} extrusion to the Na^+ gradient, and the stoichiometry dictates that a small Na^+ gradient can drive a very large Ca^{2+} gradient. The electrogenicity of the exchange also provides significant driving force for Ca^{2+} extrusion when the transmembrane potential is at the normal resting potential. This explains why the sarcolemmal Ca^{2+} gradient is approximately 10 000:1, while that of Na^+ is approximately tenfold. However, it also means that the effectiveness of Ca^{2+} extrusion is sensitive to small changes in Na^+_i. Importantly, it is such changes which have the potential to create conditions for $[Ca^{2+}]_i$ overload during myocardial ischemia/reperfusion. An increasing body of evidence indicates that both $[Ca^{2+}]_i$ and Na^+_i increase during brief periods of myocardial ischemia, and is generally consistent with a coupling between them. Hence, in the study outlined above, the direct inhibition of Na^+_i accumulation may have led to an indirect attenuation of $[Ca^{2+}]_i$ accumulation. This could, in turn, have played a role in the dramatically improved functional and energy recovery. Mitochondria are known to sequester large amounts of Ca^{2+} under $[Ca^{2+}]_i$ overload conditions [1,39]. The uptake of sufficient Ca^{2+} by the mitochondria may reduce ATP production [1,3,40] and/or waste ATP by excessive Ca^{2+} cycling at the mitochondrial membrane [41]. Such an effect could help explain the poor recovery of energy levels in the EIPA-treated hearts in the study described above.

An interesting question is when, during ischemia and reperfusion, does an elevated Na^+_i level have the greatest potential to induce Ca^{2+} influx? In the ^{23}Na NMR experiments described above, the EIPA was infused prior to ischemia, and was washed out during reperfusion and presumably had a diminishing effect at that time. However, the prevention of the Na^+_i increase during ischemia also prevents an elevated Na^+_i level upon reperfusion, and so can decrease Ca^{2+} influx at that time as well. Importantly, the modulation of Na^+/Ca^{2+} exchange activity by pH could amplify the importance of the reperfusion Na^+_i level. At low pH, Na^+/Ca^{2+} exchange activity is markedly reduced

[38]. Figure 4 indicates that while Na^+_i increases, pH_i decreases substantially. During ischemia, inhibition of Na^+/Ca^{2+} exchange at the lower pH_i could slow the equilibration of the increased Na^+_i levels to an increased $[Ca^{2+}]_i$. In this regard, the pH decrease could protect the myocardium by slowing Na^+/Ca^{2+} exchange when such exchange is unfavorably balanced towards increased $[Ca^{2+}]_i$. Under such a condition, Ca^{2+} extrusion via the Ca^{2+} ATPase may become important. As shown in Fig. 4 pH_i returns very rapidly towards control levels upon reperfusion, which could have the effect of restoring Na^+/Ca^{2+} activity to maximal levels. Hence an elevated Na^+_i level at that time could be particularly deleterious, having the potential to cause unidirectional Ca^{2+} influx potentially greater than that occurring during ischemia. At the same time, the instantaneous reestablishment of the pH gradient stimulates additional Na^+ influx by Na^+/H^+ exchange [42]. Consistent with this, studies in the ferret and the dog heart have shown that a transient acidosis upon reperfusion prevents myocardial stunning [43,44]. A possible mechanism is that the pH induced depression of Na^+/Ca^{2+} exchange activity during ischemia is prolonged during reperfusion until Na^+_i has an opportunity to recover. As suggested by the study by du Toit et al., the early reperfusion period may be particularly critical for metabolic and functional recovery. Demands on energy production are high as function returns and the restoration of cation homeostasis requires activity of the Na^+/K^+ and sarcolemmal Ca^{2+} ATPases. Potentially important is inhibition of mitochondrial ATP production by $[Ca^{2+}]_i$ overload [39–41]. Such inhibition at this juncture could have the effect of allowing further net Ca^{2+} entry. Upon reperfusion, the reestablishment of energy production needs to be sufficient to quickly extrude the accumulated Na^+_i and $[Ca^{2+}]_i$ while influx of those cations is still increasing. Insufficient extrusion could potentially lead to an irreversible progression towards continued or additional $[Ca^{2+}]_i$ overload and cellular injury. Preservation of a high energy phosphate reserve during ischemia may be important in counteracting cation influx upon reperfusion. This is possibly why after extended low-flow ischemia (with glycolytic substrates present), complete functional recoveries can be observed despite the presence of a substantial degree of net Na^+ influx [27,45]. Recent reports have indicated that glycolytic energy production could play an important role during the reperfusion period, as glycolytic inhibition upon reperfusion has a very deleterious effect on the recovery of $[Ca^{2+}]_i$ homeostasis and left ventricular function in the perfused rabbit heart [46,47].

A study by Murphy et al. indicated that Na^+/H^+ inhibition reduced $[Ca^{2+}]_i$ overload during ischemia and increased postischemic functional recovery, providing evidence that despite the low pH_i, a significant degree of coupling between Na^+_i and $[Ca^{2+}]_i$ does exist during the ischemic period [12]. However, other studies have also indicated that such a Na^+_i-dependent activation of Ca^{2+} influx occurs during reperfusion. Employing extracellular markers, Tani et al. (1989) [34] measured Na^+_i content in (homogenates from) perfused rat hearts, as well as $^{45}Ca^{2+}$ uptake during control perfusion, ischemia, and reperfusion. Interestingly, they found that the $^{45}Ca^{2+}$ uptake increased dramatically during reperfusion to levels 16-fold higher than that found during both control and ischemia. The uptake of $^{45}Ca^{2+}$ during reperfusion correlated very well with the $Na^+{}_i$ level measured at 2 min of reperfusion across a variety of protocols. Both $Na^+{}_i$ accumulation and $^{45}Ca^{2+}$ uptake were reduced by Na^+/H^+ exchange inhibition by amiloride and increased with addition of the Na^+ ionophore, monensin. Importantly, both the reperfusion $Na^+{}_i$ level and the reperfusion $^{45}Ca^{2+}$ uptake correlated very well with the recovery of left ventricular function. It is important to note that measurements of $^{45}Ca^{2+}$ uptake report the size of the pool of exchangeable intracellular Ca^{2+}. It does not necessarily reflect $[Ca^{2+}]_i$, but reflects net changes in total intracellular Ca^{2+}, including Ca^{2+} buffered in the cytosol, as well as SR and mitochondrial Ca^{2+}. The coupling of the large reperfusion Ca^{2+} influx to $Na^+{}_i$ levels suggests that the flux is related to decreased Ca^{2+} extrusion or increased Ca^{2+} entry via Na^+/Ca^{2+} exchange. Unidirectional Ca^{2+} entry can occur by this mechanism when it operates in the reverse mode, which normally occurs during the briefly depolarized transmembrane potentials occurring during normal contraction [38]. This mode may be greatly increased if $Na^+{}_i$ and/or the resting transmembrane electrical potential is persistently elevated, such as may happen during ischemia/reperfusion. The observation in Tani et al. [34] that elevated $Na^+{}_i$ levels persisted well into reperfusion supports this mechanism. This is consistent with the ^{23}Na NMR data presented in Fig. 4, which was also acquired in the rat model, and indicated that $Na^+{}_i$ did not return to control in the untreated hearts. In considering reperfusion $[Ca^{2+}]_i$ homeostasis, it is interesting to compare the timecourse of $^{45}Ca^{2+}$ uptake in this study with various measurements of $[Ca^{2+}]_i$. As discussed earlier, ^{19}F NMR and other data in the ferret and rat have usually indicated an increase in $[Ca^{2+}]_i$ during ischemia. However, this was not reflected in the $^{45}Ca^{2+}$ measurements, which indicated little if any $^{45}Ca^{2+}$ uptake during ischemia. Also, most measurements have indicated a delayed recovery of elevated $[Ca^{2+}]_i$ upon reperfusion, rather than a massive increase at that time, which was shown by the $^{45}Ca^{2+}$ uptake data. An ^{19}F NMR study employing 5F-BAPTA-loaded rat hearts indicated that under a variety of reperfusion conditions, $[Ca^{2+}]_i$ was not observed to increase extensively upon reperfusion [13]. Alteration of the reperfusion conditions did alter the $[Ca^{2+}]_i$ recovery, and poor $[Ca^{2+}]_i$ recoveries were correlated with poor functional recoveries. However, the profile of $[Ca^{2+}]_i$ changes observed in this and other studies is clearly different than that indicated by the $^{45}Ca^{2+}$ uptake data in Tani et al. [34]. Similarly, a study reporting $^{47}Ca^{2+}$ uptake during hypoxia indicates that 45 min of substrate-free hypoxia failed to increase $^{47}Ca^{2+}$ uptake over control, but upon reoxygenation it increased markedly [48]. However, as aequorin measurements have indicated increases in $[Ca^{2+}]_i$ during short periods of hypoxia [49], it does appear unlikely that $[Ca^{2+}]_i$ remained unchanged in the study, which employed a long period of substrate-free hypoxia resulting in severe contracture. The apparent discrepancy may reside in that the total intracellular Ca^{2+} pool in the myocyte is large compared to the $[Ca^{2+}]_i$, and is compartmentalized within different organelles such as the mitochondria and

SR. Hence, it is not surprising that measurements of total intracellular Ca^{2+} differ from that of $[Ca^{2+}]_i$, and that during ischemia, Ca^{2+} uptake measurements do not detect substantial increases. In the case of ischemia the decrease in pH would tend to decrease the Ca^{2+} buffering capacity, and minimize the increase of total Ca^{2+} required to increase $[Ca^{2+}]_i$ [50]. Notably, a study by Quaife et al. [51] measured both $[Ca^{2+}]_i$ and $^{45}Ca^{2+}$ uptake in myocytes, and reported that at the same time that large increases in $^{45}Ca^{2+}$ uptake occurred upon reoxygenation, $[Ca^{2+}]_i$ was gradually decreasing. Hence, the picture that emerges during reperfusion/reoxygenation is that a buffering of $[Ca^{2+}]_i$ occurs while total intracellular Ca^{2+} increases. A likely contributor to the buffering of reperfusion Ca^{2+} uptake is mitochondria. As mentioned above, mitochondria have an enormous capacity to sequester Ca^{2+} under $[Ca^{2+}]_i$ overload conditions [1,39]. This Ca^{2+} uptake, however, is energy-dependent, as it depends on the mitochondrial transmembrane potential. Hence, a possible scenario is that in the presence of high $[Ca^{2+}]_i$ and restored oxygen, the mitochondria are activated as a large Ca^{2+} sink. However, if $Na^+{}_i$ also remains elevated upon reperfusion, Na^+/Ca^{2+} exchange may effect rapid entry of more Ca^{2+} to replace it. In the absence of sufficient Na^+ and/or Ca^{2+} extrusion, intracellular Ca^{2+} loading may continue and mitochondrial energy production could be reduced. In support of this, reperfusion with the mitochondrial Ca^{2+} transport inhibitor ruthenium red has been shown to reduce Ca^{2+} uptake in mitochondria as well as to preserve their ATP-generating capacity [40]. Studies have also shown dramatic improvements in postischemic and/or posthypoxic contractile function with ruthenium red [41,52].

The alteration of cation homeostasis by ventricular fibrillation is a phenomenon which has only recently been studied [4–6,53,54] but also may play a role in ischemia/reperfusion injury. This lethal arrhythmia, characterized by disorganized electrical activity, occurs during low-flow ischemia if excitability remains sufficient [45], or can occur during reperfusion from zero-flow ischemia [55], as is sometimes observed during open-heart surgery [56]. Importantly, it has been shown that during electrically-induced VF in the perfused heart [53], or in VF induced by cardiac glycoside administration [4], $[Ca^{2+}]_i$ rapidly increases. Other studies have provided strong evidence that the initiation of VF is related to a $[Ca^{2+}]_i$ overload state [4–6]. Hence, $[Ca^{2+}]_i$ is thought to play an important role in both the initiation and maintenance of VF. Recently, it has been shown that during VF occurring spontaneously during low-flow ischemia, $Na^+{}_i$ also rapidly increases to high levels upon VF initiation. While the increases in these cations may be related in part to the stimulation of rapid channel activity during VF, it is clear that a large influx of Na^+ will also have an impact on $[Ca^{2+}]_i$ levels because of coupling via Na^+/Ca^{2+} exchange. Hence, even with the occurrence of spontaneous or electrical defibrillation, it is likely that if VF is sustained for any length of time during reperfusion, it will further complicate the ability of the myocardium to recover metabolically and functionally [53]. More studies need to be focused on defining the precise role of this arrhythmia in cation homeostasis during reperfusion.

The ultimate goal of understanding ischemia/reperfusion injury is to design strategies for improving postischemic contractile function. The ability to improve functional recovery by altering reperfusion conditions is important, as in the clinical arena the opportunity for improvement lies solely within that realm. However, the design of reperfusion strategies should carefully consider the complexity of the injury processes. As an example, Tani et al. [36] reported that reperfusion with a low Ca^{2+} perfusate resulted in only minimal improvements in recovery, which is in contrast with other studies [10,21]. In that study, extracellular Ca^{2+} was reduced for 10 min to very low levels, 100 μM, and then was returned the normal level abruptly, instead of in a stepwise manner. The $^{45}Ca^{2+}$ uptake was indeed diminished to minimal levels for the first 10 min, but then increased to very high rates upon the return to normal extracellular Ca^{2+}. This was likely caused by a $Na^+{}_i$ loading effect of the low extracellular Ca^{2+}, which stimulated forward Na^+/Ca^{2+} exchange; unlike with the other experimental groups, the $Na^+{}_i$ levels recovered little during the early reperfusion period. Hence the delay in the $Na^+{}_i$ recovery, followed by the instantaneous return to normal, ultimately resulted in $^{45}Ca^{2+}$ uptake equal or worse than in the control group, essentially negating the earlier attenuation of uptake. This observation demonstrates the importance of considering the complex interplay of Na^+ and Ca^{2+} in the implementation of reperfusion protocols.

Acknowledgments. The authors are grateful to Dr. Eduardo Marban for his important collaborative role in obtaining the indicated ^{19}F NMR $[Ca^{2+}]_i$ data.

References

1. McCormack JG, Halestap AP, Denton RM (1990) Role of calcium ions in regulation of mammalian intra-mitochondrial metabolism. Physiol Rev 70:391–425
2. Reimer KA, Jennings RB (1986) Myocardial ischemia, hypoxia, and infarction. In: Fozzard HA, Haber E, Jennings RB, Katz AM, Morgan HE (eds) The heart and cardiovascular system. Raven, New York, pp 1133–1201
3. Denton RM, McCormack JG (1985) Ca^{2+} transport by mammalian mitochondria and its role in hormone action. Am J Physiol 249:E543–E554
4. Kihara Y, Morgan JP (1991) Intracellular calcium and ventricular fibrillation: studies in the aequorin-loaded isovolumic ferret heart. Circ Res 68:1378–1389
5. Wit AL, Rosen MR (1986) Afterdepolarization and triggered activity. In: Fozzard HA, Haber E, Jennings RB, Katz AM, Morgan HE (eds) The heart and cardiovascular system. Raven, New York, pp 1449–1490
6. Clusin WT, Buchbinder M, Harrison DC (1983) Calcium overload, "injury current", and early ischaemic cardiac arrhythmias-a direct connection. Lancet 1:272–273
7. Smith G, Hesketh RT, Metcalfe JC, Feeney J, Morris PG (1983) Intracellular calcium measurement by ^{19}F NMR of fluorine labeled chelators. PNAS 80:7178–7182

8. Marban E, Kitakaze M, Kusuoka H, Porterfield JK, Yue DT, Chacko VP (1987) Intracellular free calcium concentration measured with ^{19}F NMR spectroscopy in intact ferret hearts. PNAS 84:6005–6009
9. Marban E, Kitakaze M, Koretsune Y, Yue DT, Chacko VP, Pike MM (1990) Quantification of $[Ca^{2+}]_i$ in perfused hearts: critical evaluation of the 5F-BAPTA/NMR method as applied to the study of ischemia and reperfusion. Circ Res 66:1255–1267
10. Kusuoka H, Porterfield JK, Weisman HF, Weisfeldt HF, Weisfeldt ML, Marban E (1987) Pathophysiology and pathogenesis of stunned myocardium, depressed Ca^{2+} activation of contraction as a consequence of reperfusion-induced cellular calcium overload in ferret hearts. J Clin Invest 79:950–961
11. Steenburgen C, Murphy E, Levy L, London RE (1987) Elevation in cytosolic free calcium concentration in myocardial ischemia in perfused rat heart. Circ Res 60:700–707
12. Murphy E, Perlman M, London RE, Steenbergen C (1991) Amiloride delays the ischemia-induced rise in cytosolic free calcium. Circ Res 68:1250–1258
13. Fralix TA, Steenbergen C, London RE, Murphy E (1992) Metabolic substrates can alter post-ischemic recovery in preconditioned ischemic heart. Am J Physiol 262:C17–C23
14. Mohabir R, Lee H, Kurz RW, Clusin WT (1991) Effects of ischemia and hypercarbic acidosis on myocyte calcium transients, contraction, and pH_i in perfused rabbit hearts. Circ Res 69:1525–1537
15. Kato Y, Otani J, Tanaka K, Saito Y, Fukunaka M, Imamura H (1991) Effect of cardioplegic preservation on intracellular calcium transients. Ann Thorac Surg 52:979–986
16. Carrozza JP, Bentivegna LA, Williams CP, Kuntz RE, Grossman W, Morgan JP (1992) Decreased myofilament responsiveness in myocardial stunning follows transient calcium overload during ischemia and reperfusion. Circ Res 71:1334–1340
17. Lorell BH, Apstein CS, Cunningham MJ, Schoen FJ, Weinberg EO, Peeters GA, Barry WH (1990) Contribution of endothelial cells to calcium-dependent fluorescence transients in rabbit hearts loaded with indo-1. Circ Res 67:415–425
18. Lopaschuk GD, Barr R, Wambolt R (1992) Effects of diltiazem on glycolysis and oxidative metabolism in the ischemic and ischemic/reperfusion heart. J Pharmacol Exper Ther 260:1220–1228
19. Watts JA, Norris TA, London RE, Steenbergen C, Murphy E (1990) Effects of diltiazem on lactate, ATP, and cytosolic free calcium levels in ischemic hearts. J Cardiovasc Pharmacol 15:44–49
20. Kitakaze M, Weisman HF, Marban E (1998) Contractile dysfunction and ATP depletion after transient calcium overload in perfused ferret hearts. Circulation 77:685–695
21. du Toit EF, Opie LH (1992) Modulation of severity of reperfusion stunning in the isolated rat heart by agents altering calcium flux at onset of reperfusion. Circ Res 70:960–967
22. Pike MM, Springer CS Jr (1982) Aqueous shift reagents for high-resolution cationic nuclear magnetic resonance. J Magn Reson 46:348–353
23. Gupta RK, Gupta PJ (1982) Direct observation of resolved resonances from intra- and extracellular sodium-23 ions in NMR studies of intact cells and tissues using dysprosium [III]-tripolyphosphate as a paramagnetic shift reagent. J Magn Reson 47:344–350

24. Pike MM, Frazer JC, Dedrick DF, Ingwall IS, Allen PD, Springer CS, Smith TW (1985) ^{23}Na and ^{39}K nuclear magnetic resonance studies of perfused rat hearts. Biophys J 48:159–173
25. Balschi JA, Frazer JC, Fetters JK, Clark K, Springer CS, Smith TW, Ingwall JS (1985) Extra- and intracellular sodium pools in ischemic heart. Circulation 72[II]:1520
26. Pike MM, Kitakaze M, Marban E (1990) ^{23}Na NMR measurement of intracellular Na^{+} in intact perfused ferret hearts during ischemia and reperfusion. Am J Physiol 259:H1767–H1773
27. Pike MM, Luo CS, Clark MD, Kirk KA, Kitakaze M, Madden MC, Cragoe EJ Jr, Pohost GM (1993) NMR measurements of Na^{+} and cellular energy in the ischemic rat heart: role of Na^{+}/H^{+} exchange. Am J Physiol 265:H2017–H2026
28. Buster CD, Castro MMCA, Geraldes CFGC, Malloy CR, Sherry AD (1990) Seimers TC. $Tm(DOTP)^{5-}$: A $^{23}Na^{+}$ shift agent for perfused rat hearts. Magn Reson Med 15:25–32
29. Dennis SC, Gevers W, Opie LH (1991) Protons in ischemia: where do they come from; where do they go to? J Mol Cell Cardiol 23:1077–1086
30. Cingolani HE, Koretsune Y, Marban E (1990) Recovery of contractility and pH_i during respiratory acidosis in ferret hearts: role of Na/H exchange. Am J Physiol 259:H843–H848
31. Imai S, Shi A-Y, Ishibashi T, Nakazawa M (1991) Na^{+}/H^{+} exchange is not operative under low-flow ischemic conditions. J Mol Cell Cardiol 23:505–517
32. Khandoudi N, Bernard M, Cozzone P, Feuvray D (1990) Intracellular pH and role of Na^{+}/H^{+} exchange during ischaemia and reperfusion of normal and diabetic rat hearts. Cardiovasc Res 24:873–878
33. Vandenberg JI, Metcalfe JC, Grace AA (1993) Mechanisms of intracellular pH recovery following global ischemia in the perfused heart. Circ Res 72:993–1003
34. Tani M, Neely JR (1989) Role of intracellular Na^{+} in Ca^{2+} overload and depressed recovery of ventricular function of reperfused ischemic rat hearts: possible involvement of Na^{+}/H^{+} and Na^{+}/Ca^{2+} exchange. Circ Res 65:1045–1056
35. Robinson JD, Flashner MS (1979) The (Na^{+} + K^{+})-activated ATPase; enzymatic and transport properties. Biochim Biophys Acta 549:145–176
36. Tani M, Neely JR (1990) Mechanisms of reduced reperfusion injury by low Ca^{2+} and/or high K^{+}. Am J Physiol 258:H1025–H1031
37. Fiolet JWT, Baartscheer A, Schumacher CA, Coronel R, ter Welle HF (1984) The change of the free energy of ATP hydrolysis during global ischemia and anoxia in the rat heart. J Mol Cell Cardiol 16:1023–1036
38. Sheu S, Blaustein MP (1986) Sodium/calcium exchange and regulation of cell calcium and contractility in cardiac muscle, with a note about vascular smooth muscle. In: Fozzard HA, Haber E, Jennings RB, Katz AM, Morgan HE (eds) The heart and cardiovascular system. Raven, New York, pp 509–535
39. Miyata J, Lakatta EG, Stern MD, Silverman HS (1992) Relation of mitochondrial and cytosolic free calcium to cardiac myocyte recovery after exposure to anoxia. Circ Res 71:605–613
40. Ferrari R, Di Lisa F, Raddino R, Visioli O (1982) The effect of ruthenium red on mitochondrial function during postischemic reperfusion. J Mol Cell Cardiol 14:737–740
41. Benzi RH, Lerch R (1992) Dissociation between contractile function and oxidative metabolism in postischemic myocardium, attenuation by ruthenium red administered during reperfusion. Circ Res 71:567–576

42. Lazdunski M, Frelin C, Vigne P (1985) The sodium/hydrogen exchange system in cardiac cells: its biochemical and pharmacological properties and its role in regulating internal concentrations of sodium and internal pH. J Mol Cell Cardiol 17:1029–1042
43. Kitakaze M, Weisfeldt ML, Marban E (1988) Acidosis during early reperfusion prevents myocardial stunning in perfused ferret hearts. J Clin Invest 82:920–927
44. Hori M, Kitakaze M, Sato M, Iwakura K, Gotoh K, Kusuoka H, Kitabatake A (1989) Transient acidosis by staged reperfusion prevents myocardial stunning. Circulation 80[II]:600
45. Pike MM, Luo SC, Yanagida S, Hageman GR, Anderson PG (1993) Ventricular fibrillation induces rapid changes in cellular energy and Na^+_i in the perfused rat heart: ^{23}Na and ^{31}P NMR studies of normal and hypertrophied myocardium. Proceedings of the 12th annual meeting of the Society of Magnetic Resonance in Medicine, vol 2:1068
46. Jeremy RW, Ambrosio G, Pike MM, Jacobus WJ, Becker LC (1993) The functional recovery of post-ischemic myocardium requires glycolysis during early reperfusion. J Molec Cell Cardiol 25(3):261–276
47. Jeremy RW, Koretsune Y, Marban E, Becker LC (1992) Relation between glycolysis and calcium homeostasis in postischemic myocardium. Circ Res 70:1180–1190
48. Crake T, Poole-Wilson PA (1990) Calcium exchange in rabbit myocardium during and after hypoxia: role of sodium-calcium exchange. J Mol Cel Cardiol 22:1051–1064
49. Kihara Y, Grossman W, Morgan JP (1989) Direct measurement of changes in intracellular Ca^{2+} transients during hypoxia, ischemia, reperfusion of the intact mammalian heart. Circ Res 65:1029
50. Kim D, Smith TW (1987) Altered Ca^{2+} fluxes and contractile state during pH changes in cultured heart cells. Am J Physiol 252:C137–C146
51. Quaife RA, Kohmoto O, Barry WH (1991) Mechanisms of re-oxygenation injury in cultured ventricular myocytes. Circulation 83:566–577
52. Park Y, Bowles DK, Kehrer JP (1990) Protection against hypoxic injury in isolated-perfused rat heart by ruthenium red. J Pharmacol Exper Ther 253:628–635
53. Koretsune Y, Marban E (1989) Cell calcium in the pathophysiology of ventricular fibrillation and in the pathogenesis of post-arrhythmic contractile dysfunction. Circulation 80:369–379
54. Stefenelli T, Wikman-Coffelt J, Shao T, Wu ST, Parmley WW (1992) Intracellular calcium during pacing-induced ventricular fibrillation. J Electrocardiol 25:221–228
55. Robertson E, Hof RP, Zierhut W (1993) Effect of hypertrophy induced by pressure overload or volume overload on reperfusion induced arrhythmias in anaesthetized rats. Cardiovasc Res 27(3):515–519
56. Spadaro J, Bing OHL, Gassch WH, Laraia P, Franklin A, Weintraub RM (1982) Effects of perfusion pressure on myocardial performance, metabolism, wall thickness, and compliance: comparison of the beating and fibrillating heart. J Thorac Cardiovasc Surg 84:398–405

1.6 Mechanism of Early Contractile Failure During Ischemia

HIDEO KUSUOKA[1], YUKIHIRO KORETSUNE[2], MARY C. CORRETTI[3], and EDUARDO MARBAN[4]

Summary. The basis of early ischemic contractile failure was investigated in perfused ferret hearts. Isovolumic left ventricular developed pressure fell by more than 50% within 30 s of the onset of total global ischemia and reached zero by 5 min. Monophasic action potential recordings revealed no decrease in excitability during this period. Phosphorus nuclear magnetic resonance spectra obtained at 30-s resolution showed no significant changes in inorganic phosphate or phosphocreatine during the first 30 s of ischemia. Intracellular pH (pH_i) and ATP changed even more slowly; therefore, none of these metabolites could account for the rapid fall in force. To gauge the contribution of intravascular pressure, we compared ordinary aortic flow occlusion with tissue-level ischemia induced by massive coronary microembolization at the level of the precapillary arterioles. Functional depression developed significantly more slowly in the microembolized hearts, despite accumulation of inorganic phosphate and protons comparable with that in ordinary ischemia. After microembolization, the time course of functional depression reflected much more closely the concomitant inorganic phosphate and pH_i changes. Thus, our results provide novel evidence supporting the importance of vascular collapse in the mechanism of early ischemic contractile failure.

Key words: Excitation–Contraction coupling—Inorganic phosphate—Acidosis—Garden hose effect—Phosphorus NMR spectroscopy—Ischemia—Contractility

[1] Division of Tracer Kinetics, Biomedical Research Center, and [2] First Department of Medicine, Osaka University Medical School, Yamadaoka 2-2, Suita, Osaka, 565 Japan
[3] Division of Cardiology, Department of Medicine, University of Maryland School of Medicine, Baltimore, MD, USA
[4] Division of Cardiology, Department of Medicine, The Johns Hopkins University School of Medicine, Baltimore, MD, USA

Introduction

When coronary flow is interrupted, the force of contraction of the heart plummets. This phenomenon, although recognized as early as 1628 by Harvey [1], still lacks a satisfactory explanation. The multitude of electrical, metabolic, and mechanical changes that are known to occur during acute myocardial ischemia could affect excitation–contraction coupling at virtually any level [2]. Four general classes of mechanisms have been proposed: (1) a fundamental impairment of excitation, such as abbreviation of the action potential by ATP-sensitive potassium channels turned on during ischemia [3–5]; (2) accumulation of metabolites, particularly inorganic phosphate (P_i) and protons (H^+), that inhibit force generation by the contractile proteins [6–9]; (3) depletion of high-energy phosphates [10] sufficient to cause a critical reduction in the free energy that can be derived from ATP hydrolysis [2,11]; and (4) collapse of intravascular pressure, leading to a reduction in the sarcomere length of the myocardial cells that surround the vessels and a consequent fall in tension development via the Frank-Starling effect [12–16]. Although the first, second, and third mechanisms certainly come into play at some point during ischemia, there is reason to doubt whether excitation fails and metabolites change with sufficient rapidity to account for early contractile failure. The fourth idea, which has come to be known as the "garden hose" or "erectile" effect, has been supported only by indirect evidence [12–14] or by exclusion [15].

The experimental challenge of dissecting out any given factor during ischemia has hampered progress. In an attempt to mimic ischemia, hypoxia has been used alone or in combination with glycolytic inhibition. Although such maneuvers are interesting in their own right, they do not accurately reproduce the metabolic or mechanical effects of ischemia. With hypoxia and/or metabolic inhibition in perfused hearts [16–19], there is continual washout of metabolites; if such washout is prevented by working with a restricted extracellular space [20], the putative effects of intravascular pressure remain unassessed. Even in true ischemic models, no simple means have been devised to separate collapse of intravascular pressure from the concomitant changes in excitation and metabolites.

In the present study, we sought to determine the relative roles of these factors in intact Langendorff-perfused ferret hearts. Total global ischemia was induced under hypothermic conditions (27°C) to retard metabolic rundown. Excitability was assessed by monophasic action potential recordings [21]; P_i, intracellular pH (pH_i), phosphocreatine (PCr), and ATP were measured at 30-s resolution by phosphorus nuclear magnetic resonance (NMR) spectroscopy. To assess the contribution of intravascular pressure, we microembolized the coronary circulation [22] at a constant perfusion pressure. This novel strategy produces tissue-level ischemia while maintaining coronary vascular tone. The results provide new and compelling evidence supporting an important role for vascular collapse in the pathogenesis of early ischemic contractile failure.

Materials and Methods

The experimental preparation has been described previously [17]. Briefly, male ferrets (11–14 weeks of age) were anesthetized initially with ether and subsequently with sodium pentobarbital (200 mg i.p. injection; Harvey Laboratories, Philadelphia, Pa., USA) and heparinized. After rapid excision of the heart, the aorta was cannulated rapidly, and retrogradely perfused with a 95% O_2/5% CO_2-bubbled solution of the following composition (mmol/l): NaCl 119, $NaHCO_3$ 24.7, KCI 5.9, $MgCl_2$ 1.2, EDTA 0.5, $CaCl_2$ 2.85, and glucose 16, (pH 7.45). To attenuate the rate of metabolic deterioration during ischemia, we worked at a perfusate temperature of 27°C (maintained by submersion or by a humidified air jacket during ischemia). Coronary flow rate was adjusted such that the initial coronary pressure, measured at the aortic cannula, equalled 80 mmHg; thereafter, flow was kept constant (except during ischemia, which was ordinarily induced by stopping the pump and clamping the perfusion line). A thin latex balloon tied to the end of a polyethylene tube was inserted into the left ventricle and connected to a Statham P23DB pressure transducer (Gould Instruments, Indianapolis, Ind., USA). The balloon was filled with 15 mmol/l magnesium trimetaphosphate for high-energy phosphate measurements by ^{31}P-NMR spectroscopy. The balloon volume was set to achieve an initial end-diastolic pressure of 10–20 mmHg and was kept isovolumic throughout the experiment. Each heart was paced at 1.5 Hz via an agar wick electrode saturated with 3 mole/l KCI.

The data in this paper are derived from experiments in a total of 14 hearts. Nine were used for simultaneous measurements of ^{31}P-NMR spectra and isovolumic pressure; the remaining five were studied outside the magnet for electrical and/or pressure recordings only.

Measurements of Action Potential Duration During Ischemia

Left ventricular epicardial monophasic action potentials were recorded with a contact electrode catheter (model MD-1089-01, Webster Laboratories, Baldwin Park, Calif., USA) [21] in three hearts. Action potential durations were determined as the time from the overshoot to 50% or 90% repolarization. To avoid electrical artifacts, pacing was temporarily discontinued during monophasic action potential recordings. (Because of the discontinuous pacing, results from these three hearts were not included in the pooled data for isovolumic pressure.) After measurements under control conditions, perfusion was completely stopped.

^{31}P-NMR Measurements

In nine hearts, ^{31}P-NMR spectra were acquired at a spectral width of 6 kHz using 34° pulses delivered at 1-s intervals (145.8 MHz for ^{31}P). The spectra were averaged over 30 s and processed as described before [17]. The amounts of P_i, PCr, and ATP in the myocardium were obtained by planimetry of the areas under individual peaks using a digitizer, then normalized by the peak for the magnesium trimetaphosphate standard in the left ventricular balloon, and multiplied by an appropriate scaling factor to derive cytoplasmic concentrations [17]. Intracellular pH was determined from the shift between the P_i and PCr resonances [23].

After five ^{31}P-NMR spectra were obtained under control conditions, hearts were subjected either to total global ischemia ($n = 4$) or to coronary microembolization ($n = 5$). Embolization at the precapillary arteriolar level [22] was accomplished by bolus injection of nonradioactive carbon microspheres (13.7 ± 0.8 μm in diameter, 7×10^5 spheres/ml per min of coronary flow during control; 3M Co., St. Paul, Minn., USA) into the aortic cannula at a coronary perfusion pressure of 80 mmHg. Preliminary experiments showed that maximally effective microembolization (as judged by reduction of coronary flow) was achieved at doses of 6×10^5/ml per min or more. Microspheres were suspended in 0.4–0.6 ml of 10% dextran, agitated for at least 15 minutes in an ultrasonicator (Bransonic 2200, Branson Cleaning Equipment, Shelton, Conn., USA), and stirred by a vortex mixer for at least 1 min. Coronary flow was checked 1 min after microsphere embolization.

Statistical Analysis

All pooled data are presented as mean ± SEM. Statistical analysis was performed by paired or nonpaired *t*-tests or by analysis of variance when indicated [24]. Results were regarded as significant when $P < 0.05$.

Results

Early Ischemic Contractile Failure in Ferret Hearts

Total global ischemia was induced at 27°C. As expected from previous work [25], isovolumic left ventricular pressure decreased rapidly even at this low temperature: the pressure developed by the heart fell by more than 50% in 30 s (e.g., see Fig. 4). Pooled data from six hearts confirm the consistency of the rapid time course of early ischemic contractile failure. Developed pressure fell to 0 by 5 min of ischemia; therefore, we restricted our observations to this brief period. Unlike some previous studies [15], we chose not to subject hearts to repeated episodes of global ischemia to avoid possible cumulative effects such as stunning [26] or preconditioning [27]; the data were all obtained with only one ischemic trial per heart.

Action Potential Duration During Early Ischemic Contractile Failure

Monophasic action potentials were recorded from the left ventricular epicardium during control perfusion and during ischemia. Pooled results from three experiments reveal no signicant changes in overall cardiac excitability during the first 5 min of ischemia. Even though monophasic action potentials do not enable the recording of absolute transmembrane potential [28], they are certainly adequate to exclude the dramatic changes in action potential duration [21] that would have been necessary [29] to produce the rapid functional decay. Thus, these results indicate that a decrease in excitability does not figure in the pathogenesis of early contractile failure under our experimental conditions.

Are Metabolic Changes Well Correlated with Early Contractile Failure During Ischemia?

To ascertain whether or not changes in P_i concentration ($[P_i]$), pH_i, and ATP concentration ([ATP]) parallel those in contraction during ischemia, we compared the time course of the changes in phosphorus NMR spectra with that of the concomitant functional changes. $[P_i]$ and [ATP] are measured directly from the spectra, where they exhibit characteristic peaks (Fig. 1). pH_i can be cal-

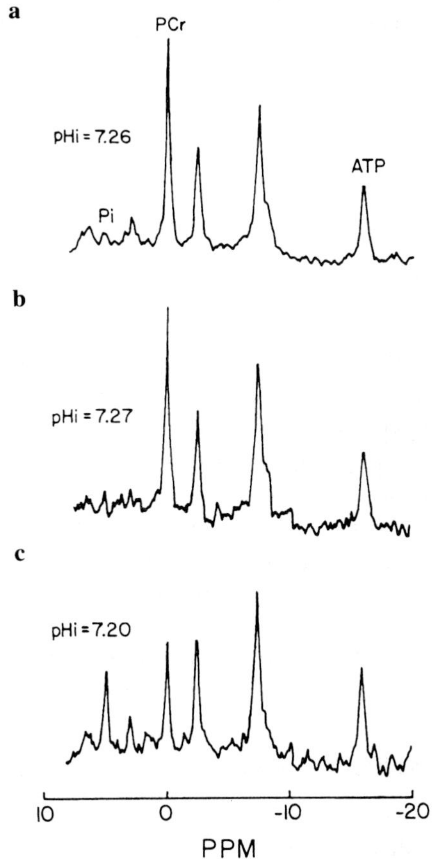

Fig. 1a–c. Representative phosphorus nuclear magnetic resonance spectra from one ferret heart. **a** During control perfusion. **b** 0–30 s of ischemia. **c** 1–1.5 min of ischemia. **a** shows the position of the inorganic phosphate (*P_i*), phosphocreatine (*PCr*), and *ATP* peaks. Intracellular pH (*pH_i*) values shown in each panel are derived from the P_i shift, as explained in the text. *PPM*, parts per million. (From [48], with permission)

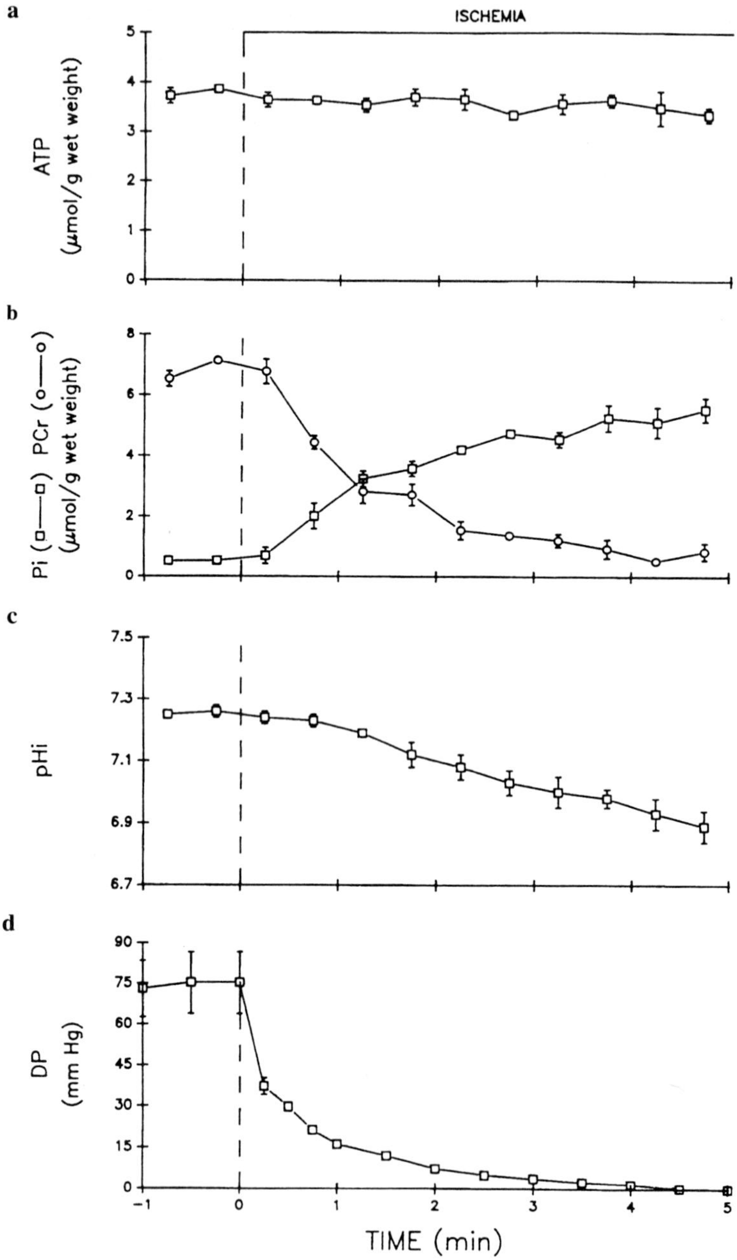

Fig. 2a–d. Graphs showing pooled data from four ferret hearts before and during total global ischemia. **a** ATP. **b** inorganic phosphate (P_i) and phosphocreatine (*PCr*). **c** intracellular pH (pH_i). **d** developed pressure (*DP*). (From [48], with permission)

culated from the P_i resonance, since the protonation of P_i (and its chemical shift) changes measurably in the physiological range of pH_i. Figure 1 shows spectra obtained at various times in a representative experiment. During the initial control period (Fig. 1a), the ^{31}P-NMR spectrum, obtained by sampling over 3 min, reveals a pH_i of 7.21 and an abundance of PCr and ATP. During the first 30 s of ischemia, pH_i, $[P_i]$, and [ATP] did not change (Fig. 1b), despite the fact that early contractile failure was developing most rapidly during that time. P_i was visible increased in the spectra obtained after 1–15 min of ischemia, whereas at this time pH_i still remained equivalent to the control value.

Pooled data from four hearts, shown in Fig. 2, reveal a marked discrepancy of the time course between the metabolic changes (Fig. 2a–c) and the functional depression in the same hearts (Fig. 2d). Although contractile failure was apparent as early as the first 15 s of ischemia, no metabolic changes were evident until more time had elapsed. Neither $[P_i]$ nor [PCr] (Fig. 2b) changed significantly during the first 30 s. pH_i (Fig. 2c) remained steady for 1 min and the gradual downward drift thereafter did not reach statistical significance until after the first 2.5 min. [ATP] (Fig. 2a) stayed quite stable throughout the 5-min period of observation (contrast with Hearse [10]). Thus, the earliest stage of contractile failure, which accounts for more than 50% of the functional decline, cannot be explained by the accumulation of metabolites or by the depletion of high-energy phosphates.

Role of Mechanical Factors in Early Contractile Failure: Coronary Artery Depressurization

Since neither of the two mechanisms considered above can explain the early contractile failure during ischemia, the relative role of the erectile or garden hose effect demands explicit evaluation. We investigated the role of vascular collapse by microembolization at the level of the precapillary arterioles. We reasoned that such a maneuver should produce profound tissue ischemia without depressurization of the coronary arterial tree: distension of the arteries would be maintained by the constant pressure head of 80 mmHg upstream from the arteriolar occlusion.

A maximally effective dose of microspheres (7×10^5/ml per min of control coronary flow) decreased coronary flow from 17 ± 1.2 to 1.2 ± 0.3 ml/min within 1 min of bolus infusion; this dose was used in our experiments. Despite the virtually complete abolition of coronary flow, we ascertained whether the metabolic changes are in fact comparable with those achieved by ordinary occlusion of inflow at the aortic level by comparing the time course of $[P_i]$ and pH_i changes during the two maneuvers. Figure 3 shows that we achieved virtually superimposable (and statistically indistinguishable) metabolic changes with microembolization and standard ischemia. Although not shown here, the changes in PCr concentration ([PCr]) and [ATP] were also comparable in the two groups. Thus, there is good reason to expect that any difference in the

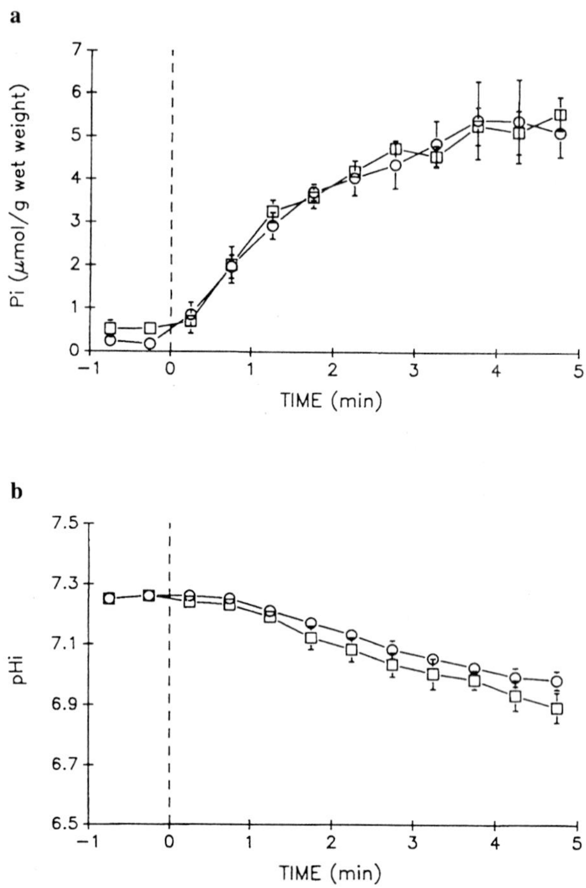

Fig. 3a,b. Graphs showing comparable metabolic accumulation in ordinary global ischemia (*squares*; $n = 4$) and coronary microembolization (*circles*; $n = 5$). **a** Time course of inorganic phosphate (P_i). **b** Time course of intracellular pH (pH_i). (From [48], with permission)

time course of functional decline must be due to the difference in intravascular pressure in the two models.

Figure 4 presents the crucial comparison of the decline in contractile pressure in standard ischemia versus microembolization. Although function declines in both groups, the changes of systolic (Fig. 4a) and developed (Fig. 4c) pressure were considerably slower with microembolization as compared with total global ischemia. For each of these parameters, the difference between the two curves is highly significant ($P < 0.01$ by multivariate analysis of variance). Diastolic pressure changes (Fig. 4b) were comparable in the two groups. The observation of much slower functional decline with microembolization supports the idea that intravascular collapse makes a major contribution to early contractile failure.

If microembolization completely preserves normal intravascular pressure, the functional decline that persists in the microembolized hearts might be due entirely to the superimposed metabolic changes, which, as we have seen, are identical to those in ordinary ischemia. To elucidate the contribution of the

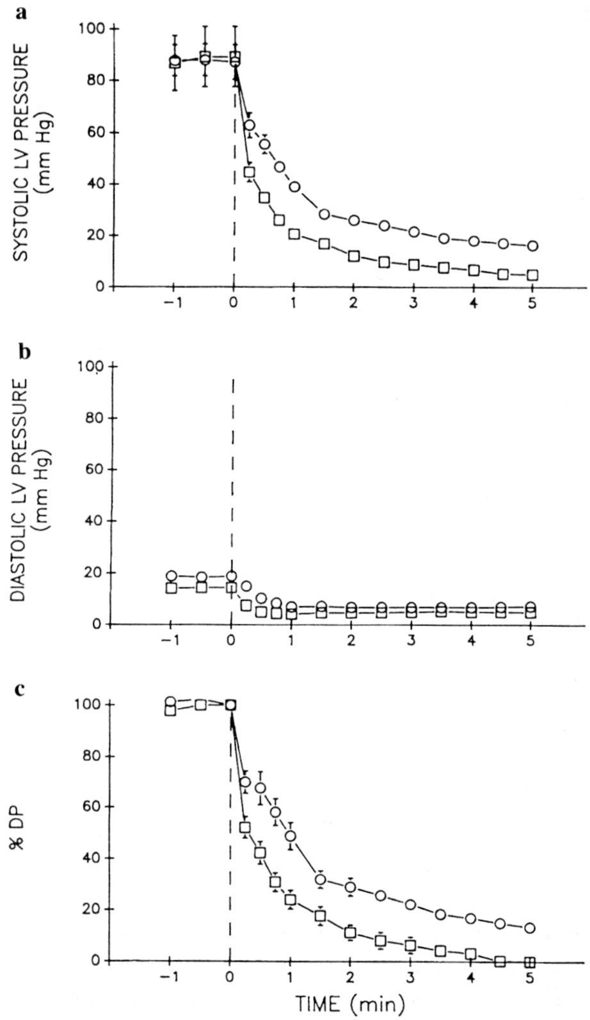

Fig. 4a–c. Graphs showing time course of functional depression in ordinary global ischemia (*squares*) and in microembolization (*circles*). **a** Decline in absolute systolic left ventricular (*LV*) pressure. **b** Decline in absolute diastolic LV pressure. **c** Decline in developed pressure (*DP*), plotted as percent of control. The absolute DP in control was comparable ($P > 0.50$) in the ordinary ischemia (75 ± 13 mmHg) and microembolization (69 ± 6 mmHg) groups. Data are from the same ferret hearts as in Fig. 3. (From [48], with permission)

erectile effect above and beyond that of metabolite accumulation, we compared the observed functional changes in each group with those predicted solely on the basis of the changes in $[P_i]$ and pH_i. From our previous work in which $[P_i]$ and pH_i were altered in the absence of ischemia [23], we estimated the pure effects of these two metabolic factors on developed pressure. The analysis indicates that the ischemia data consistently fall far under the value estimated from $[P_i]/pH_i$; an additional factor must be invoked to explain the contractile failure.

If that additional factor is intravascular pressure, we would expect a much closer correspondence between the microembolization data and the prediction. The analysis confirms that this is indeed the case. The changes in $[P_i]$ and pH_i almost suffice to explain the persistent decline in function when intraarterial pressure is maintained. The agreement would not have been expected to be exact; at best, microembolization preserves only the intraarterial pressure, whereas pressure on the venous side [30], as well as other metabolites not considered here, may well exert additional effects. Nevertheless, the agreement between the observed and predicted data is so close in the microembolized hearts that we conclude other such factors must make only a minor contribution to early contractile failure.

Discussion

We have observed that neither inexcitability nor metabolite accumulation develops with sufficient rapidity to underlie the functional depression during ischemia in ferret hearts at 27°C. Although critical shortening of the action potential certainly occurs at some point during the interruption of coronary flow [25,31–35], Ca^{2+} transients are not decreased in amplitude during ischemic episodes of duration comparable with those used here [36,37]. The fact that the delivery of activator Ca^{2+} remains unimpaired during early ischemia is entirely consistent with the preservation of membrane excitability observed here and elsewhere [37].

Our data argue against an obligatory role for depletion of either ATP or PCr in the pathogenesis of early contractile failure. Figure 2 shows that developed pressure falls by more than 50% in the first 30 s of ischemia, during which time neither [ATP] nor [PCr] changes measurably. The absence of any changes in [P_i], [PCr], and [ATP] within the first 30 s additionally indicates that the free energy that can be derived from ATP hydrolysis [11] is not compromised at this early time. The fall in [ATP] can certainly occur more rapidly under certain ischemic or hypoxic conditions, such as in normothermic rats [10], but the clear dissociation between [ATP] and force observed here and elsewhere [17,23] argues against a simple cause-and-effect relation. After 30–60 s of ischemia, PCr would seem to be a more likely contributor to the contractile failure than ATP, since it falls quickly and dramatically. Indeed, the correlation between the changes in force and [PCr] is as good as the correlation with [P_i]; this is not surprising, since PCr is the main P_i donor during early ischemia or hypoxia [2,17]. Nevertheless, the changes in PCr itself are not likely to play a major role in contractile failure, as emphasized previously [17]. The effect of PCr on the myofilaments is modest, and what effect does occur would be in the wrong direction to explain the observed contractile dysfunction [9].

Previous studies have recognized major discrepancies between the time courses of intracellular acidification and contractile failure. Jacobus and coworkers [15] demonstrated that no fall in pH_i was associated with the earliest stage of functional decline (see also Mohabir et al. [38]). Since then, P_i has also come to be recognized as an important metabolite acting at the level of the myofilaments [9,17]. We find that accumulation of P_i, although faster than that of protons, still occurs too slowly to account for the observed fall in developed pressure during ischemia. The present findings contrast with hypoxia, in which functional depression tracks P_i accumulation faithfully [17]. The difference is understandable, given the recognition of a major role for the erectile effect [14,39,40]: intracoronary pressure is maintained throughout hypoxia, but falls rapidly during global ischemia.

Our results with microembolization demonstrate the primacy of intravascular pressure, rather than coronary flow, in the garden hose phenomenon. In this respect, the results agree with those of others [30,41] who have addressed the question experimentally by producing independent changes in coronary flow and intravascular pressure (but compare with [42] and [43]).

It is important to consider the implications of our observations for ischemic failure in vivo. Although the relative contribution of the erectile effect might be accentuated in crystalloid-perfused hearts, Vogel and coworkers [39] have observed similar "hydraulic" effects of the coronary vasculature in crystalloid- versus blood-perfused hearts. Their observations give good reason to expect that vascular collapse figures prominently in the mechanism of ischemic contractile failure in vivo.

Although our results emphasize the important influence of vascular pressure on myocardial contraction, they leave unresolved the question of precisely how this occurs. The most explicit idea envisions myocytes as being mechanically stretched by the distension of adjacent vascular spaces [12]. Vascular collapse unsplints the myocytes such that they operate at a less favorable end-diastolic length. The fall in force then is simply the result of the Frank-Starling effect [44]. Despite the appeal of this notion, it is supported by little direct evidence. Histological examination of arrested hearts have revealed modest changes in sarcomere length with steady-state alterations in coronary pressure [45], but the conditions were such that extrapolation to intact hearts can only be tentative. The present study was performed under isovolumic loading conditions, so that changes in sarcomere length are inevitably small. Indeed, recent experiments by Kitakaze and Marban [46] give reason to doubt that preload is the sole determinant of changes in force development due to alterations of coronary perfusion. These investigators showed that force generation could increase in response to perfusion pressure even in hearts that had already been stretched to the optimal end-diastolic length. As an alternative to the Frank-Starling effect, it seems equally likely that the vessels themselves, when distended, act as struts that potentiate the strength of myocardial contraction independent of sarcomere length changes. Such uncertainties, coupled with the increasing recognition that endothelial cells can modulate cardiac contraction [47], should prompt thorough reexamination of the cellular mechanism of vasotropic feedback.

Acknowledgment. The authors wish to express appreciation to the American Heart Association, Inc. for permission to use material from Circulation Research [48].

References

1. Harvey W (1628) Anatomical studies on the motion of the heart and blood. Leake CD (translator). Charles C Thomas Publishing, Springfield IL, 1970
2. Allen DG, Orchard CH (1987) Myocardial contractile function during ischemia and hypoxia. Circ Res 60:153–168
3. Weiss JN, Lamp ST (1989) Cardiac ATP-sensitive K^+ channels: Evidence for preferential regulation by glycolysis. J Gen Physiol 94:911–936
4. Stern MD, Silverman HS, Houser SR, Josephson RA, Capogrossi MC, Nichols CG, Lederer WJ, Lakatta EG (1988) Anoxic contractile failure of intracelluar calcium release due to alteration of the action potential. Proc Natl Acad Sci USA 85:6954–6958
5. Lederer WJ, Nichols CG, Smith GL (1989) The mechanism of early contractile failure of isolated rat ventricular myocytes subjected to complete metabolic inhibition. J Physiol (Lond) 413:329–349
6. Katz AM, Hecht HH (1969) The early pump failure of ischemic hearts. Am J Med 47:497–502
7. Kulber W, Katz AM (1977) Mechanism of early pump failure of the ischemic heart: Possible role of adenosine triphosphate depletion and inorganic phosphate accumulation. Am J Cardiol 40:467–471
8. Fabiato A, Fabiato F (1978) Effects of pH on the myofilaments and the sarcoplasmic reticulum of skinned cells from cardiac and skeletal muscle. J Physiol (Lond) 276:233–255
9. Kentish JC (1986) The effects of inorganic phosphate and creatine phosphate on force production in skinned muscles from rat ventricle. J Physiol (Lond) 370: 585–604
10. Hearse DJ (1979) Oxygen deprivation and early myocardial contractile failure: A reassessment of the possible role of adenosine triphosphate. Am J Cardiol 44:1115–1121
11. Kammermier H, Schmidt P, Jungling E (1982) Free energy change of ATP hydrolysis: A causal factor of early hypoxic failure of the myocardium? J Mol Cell Cardiol 14:267–277
12. Arnold G, Losche F, Miessner E, Neitzert A, Lochner W (1968) The importance of the perfusion pressure in the coronary arteries for the contractility and the oxygen consumption of the heart. Pflugers Arch 299:339–356
13. Morgenstern C, Holjes U, Arnold G, Lochner W (1973) The influence of coronary pressure and coronary flow on intracoronary blood volume and geometry of the left ventricle. Pflügers Arch 340:101–111
14. Kleber AG, Riegger CB, Janse MJ (1987) Electrical uncoupling and increase of extracellular resistance after induction of ischemia in isolated, arterially perfused rabbit papillary muscle. Circ Res 61:271–279
15. Jacobus WE, Pores IH, Lucas SK, Kallman CH, Weisfeldt ML, Flaherty JT (1982) The role of intracellular pH in the control of normal and ischemic myocardial contractility: A ^{31}P nuclear magnetic resonance and mass spectrometry study. In: Nuccitelli R, Deamer DW (eds) Intracellular pH: its measurement, regulation, and utilization in cellular function. Liss, New York, pp 537–565
16. Apstein CS, Ahn J, Briggs L, Shapiro HM (1979) Role of decrease in wall thickness in causing acute ischemic cardiac failure (abstract). Clin Res 27:436a

17. Kusuoka H, Weisfeldt ML, Zweier JL, Jacobus WE, Marban E (1986) Mechanism of early contractile failure during hypoxia in intact ferret heart: Evidence for modulation of maximal Ca^{2+}-activated force by inorganic phosphate. Circ Res 59:270–282
18. Eisner DA, Elliot AC, Smith GL (1987) The contribution of intracellular acidosis to the decline of developed pressure in ferret hearts exposed to cyanide. J Physiol (Lond) 391:99–108
19. Ingwall JS (1982) Phosphorus nuclear magnetic resonance spectroscopy of cardiac and skeletal muscles. Am J Physiol 242:H729–H744
20. Allen DG, Lee JA, Smith GL (1989) The consequences of simulated ischemia on intracellular Ca^{2+} and tension in isolate ferret ventricular muscle. J Physiol (Lond) 410:297–323
21. Franz MR, Burkhoff D, Spurgeon H, Weisfeldt ML, Lakatta EG (1986) In vitro validation of a new cardiac catheter technique for recording monophasic action potentials. Eur Heart J 7:34–41
22. Hori M, Inoue M, Kitakaze M, Koretsune Y, Iwai K, Tamai J, Ito H, Kitabatake A, Sato T, Kamada T (1986) Role of adenosine in hyperemic response of coronary blood flow in microembolization. Am J Physiol 250:H509–H518
23. Marban E, Kusuoka H (1987) Maximal Ca^{2+}-activated force and myofilament Ca^{2+} sensitivity in intact mammalian hearts. J Gen Physiol 90:609–623
24. Snedecor GW, Cochran WG (1989) Statistical Methods, edn 8. Iowa State University Press, Ames, Iowa, pp 1–503
25. Shine KI, Douglas AM, Ricchiuti N (1976) Ischemia in isolated interventricular septa: Mechanical events. Am J Physiol 231:1225–1232
26. Stahl LD, Aversano T, Ambrosio G, Becker LC (1987) Effect of repeated episodes of drug-induced ventricular dyskinesia on subsequent regional function in the dog: Comparison with myocardial stunning produced by repeated coronary cclusions. J Am Coll Cardiol 9:1339–1347
27. Mury CE, Jennings RB, Reimer KA (1986) Preconditioning with ischemia: A delay of lethal cell injury in ischemic myocardium. Circulation 74:1124–1136
28. Hoffman BF, Cranefield PF (1976) Electrophysiology of the heart. Futura, Mt Kisco, NY
29. Morad M, Trautwein W (1968) The effect of the duration of the action potential on contraction in the mammalian heart muscle. Pflugers Arch 299:66–82
30. Scharf SM, Bromberger-Barnea B (1973) Influence of coronary flow and pressure on cardiac function and coronary vascular volume. Am J Physiol 224:918–925
31. Russell DC, Smith HJ, Oliver MF (1979) Transmembrane potential changes and ventricular fibrillation during repetitive myocardial ischemia in the dog. Br Heart J 42:88–96
32. Prinzmetal M, Toyoshima H, Ekmekci A, Mizuno Y, Nagaya T (1961) Myocardial ischemia: Nature of ischemic electrocardiographic patterns in the mammalian ventricles as determined by intracellular electrographic and metabolic changes. Am J Cardiol 6:493–503
33. Kardesch M, Hogancamp CE, Bing RJ (1958) The effect of complete ischemia on the intracellular electrical activity of the whole mammalian heart. Circ Res 6:715–720
34. Downar E, Janse MJ, Durrer D (1977) The effect of acute coronary artery occlusion on subepicardial transmembrane potentials in the intact porcine heart. Circulation 56:217–224

35. Gettes LS (1986) Effect of ischemia on cardiac electrophysiology. In: Fozzard HA, Haber E, Jennings RB, Katz AM, Morgan HE (eds) The heart and cardiovascular system. Raven, New York, pp 1317–1341
36. Lee H-C, Mohabir R, Smith N, Franz MR, Clusin WT (1988) Effect of ischemia on calcium-dependent fluorescence transients in rabbit hearts containing indo-1: Correlation with monophasic action potentials and contraction. Circulation 78: 1047–1059
37. Kihara Y, Grossman W, Morgan JP (1989) Direct measurement of changes in intracellular calcium transients during hypoxia, ischemia, and reperfusion of the intact mammalian heart. Circ Res 65:1029–1044
38. Mohabir R, Lee H-C, Clusin WT (1989) Simultaneous recordings of $[Ca^{+}]_i$ and pH_i in perfused rabbit hearts containing indo-1 and BCECF (abstract). Biophys J 55:485a
39. Vogel WM, Apstein CS, Briggs LL, Gaasch WH, Ahn J (1982) Acute alterations in left ventricular diastolic chamber stiffness: Role of the "erectile" effect of coronary arterial pressure and flow in normal and damaged hearts. Circ Res 51:465–478
40. Wexler LF, Weinberg EO, Ingwall JS, Apstein CS (1986) Acute alterations in diastolic left ventricular chamber distensibility: Mechanism differences between hypoxemia and ischemia in isolated perfused rabbit and rat heart. Circ Res 59:515–528
41. Weisfeldt ML, Shock NW (1970) Effect of perfusion pressure on coronary flow and oxygen usage of nonworking heart. Am J Physiol 218:95–101
42. Abel RM, Reis RL (1970) Effects of coronary blood flow and perfusion pressure of left ventricular contractility in dogs. Circ Res 27:961–971
43. Miller WP, Shimamoto N, Nellis SH, Liedtke AJ (1987) Coronary hyperperfusion and myocardial metabolism in isolated and intact hearts. Am J Physiol 253:H1271–H1278
44. Patterson SW, Piper H, Starling EH (1914) The regulation of the heart beat. J Physiol (Lond) 48:456–513
45. Poche R, Arnold G, Gahlen D (1971) The influence of coronary perfusion pressure on metabolism and ultrastructure of the myocardium of the arrested aerobically perfused isolated guinea-pig heart. Virchows Arch [B]8:252–266
46. Kitakaze M, Marban E (1989) Cellular mechanism of the modulation of contractile function by coronary perfusion pressure in ferret hearts. J Physiol (Lond) 414:455–472
47. Brutsaert DL, Meulemans AL, Sipido KR, Sys SU (1988) Effects of damaging the endocardial surface on the mechanical performance of isolated cardiac muscle. Circ Res 62:358–366
48. Koretsune Y, Corretti MC, Kusuoka H, Marban E (1991) Mechanism of early contractile failure: Inexcitability, metabolic accumulation, or vascular collapse? Circ Res 68:255–262

1.7 Cellular Adaptation in Hibernating Myocardium in the Human

J. Ausma[1], F. Ramaekers[1], B. Shivalkar[2], F. Thone[3], W. Flameng[2], and M. Borgers[1,3]

Summary. The aim of this study was to investigate morphologic changes in chronic hibernation. Light and electron microscopy were performed on myocardium derived from the anterior wall of the left ventricle of 165 patients during coronary artery bypass grafting. The changes seen in a substantial part of the cardiomyocytes corresponded to "dedifferentiation" rather than atrophic "degeneration". The affected cardiomyocytes showed a partial to complete loss of sarcomeres, sarcoplasmic reticulum, and T-tubules and presented an abundant amount of glycogen, and lots of small mitochondria. The volume of the cells was similar to that of normal cells. The number of the affected cells was consistently higher in endocardial parts than in epicardial ones. The cell changes occurred in the myocardium of patients both with and without a previous infarction. A significant relationship was found in noninfarcted patients between the presence of affected cells and the amount of connective tissue. It is proposed that myocardial segments in which these structural changes prevail will not recover immediately after revascularization but that they might show a delayed recovery of function, because structural remodeling requires time in order to regain sufficient contractile material and to normalize the amount of connective tissue between the cardiomyocytes.

Key words: Hibernating myocardium—Ultrastructure—PET—Human heart—Molecular cell biology—Differentiation

[1] Department of Molecular Cell Biology and Genetics, Cardiovascular Research Institute, Maastricht, University of Limburg, P.O. Box 616, 6200 MD Maastricht, The Netherlands
[2] Department of Cardiac Surgery, Katholieke Universiteit Leuven, Gashvisberg, Heerestraat, Belgium
[3] Department of Life Sciences, Janssen Research Foundation, Turnhoutseweg 30, 2340 Beerse, Belgium

Definition and Criteria for Identification of Hibernating Myocardium

The term "hibernating myocardium" was coined in 1985 by Rahimtoola [1] to describe a persistent dysfunctional state of human cardiac muscle as a consequence of chronic severe ischemia. The regional wall motion abnormality is reversible after restoration of blood flow, indicating that the blood flow through the original stenosis was sufficient to allow cardiomyocyte viability but insufficient to support normal contractile function. Characteristic features in hibernating myocardium are thus: (1) persistent segmental wall motion abnormality; (2) severely reduced myocardial blood flow regionally; (3) no evidence of myocardial infarction; and (4) reversal of functional abnormality after restoration of blood flow to the area involved.

It is thought that the hibernating response is an act of self-preservation by myocardium endangered by an oxygen supply too low to deliver normal work; in other words, it adapts its functional capacity to the oxygen supply, and hence to the lowered energy availability. An assumption of cardinal importance in the context of hibernation and its reversibility is the presence of viable, although non- or badly functioning, cells. The next important question relates to whether such viable myocardium is structurally normal or not, and whether possible abnormalities in structure contribute to the degree and speed of functional recovery of the myocardium after restoration of blood flow.

In the initial reports [2–5] dealing with regional contractile dysfunction of noninfarcted tissue, before the term "hibernating myocardium" was coined, it was mentioned that since contractile function could resume rather quickly after regional blood flow restoration, the underlying structure of the affected segments should be close to normal. What was meant was that the underlying tissue was not fibrotic as a consequence of infarction. Another argument in favor of this assumption was the immediate response to oxygen-sparing therapy of the left ventricular function [6]. The most convincing observation hitherto made in support of the existence of hibernating viable tissue is the presence of flow-metabolic mismatches in malfunctioning myocardial segments. The methodology *par excellence* is the measurement of regional blood flow with radiolabelled ammonium, and of the metabolic activity of the underlying tissue by measurement of the extraction of labelled fluorodeoxyglucose with Positron Emission Tomography (PET) [7–11].

Subgroups of Hibernating Myocardium

The observation that the hibernating state is quickly reversible after coronary artery bypass grafting (CABG), percutaneous transluminal coronary angioplasty (PTCA), or thrombolytic therapy has been challenged over the years, and not the least by the groups who were initially involved in the recognition of this phenomenon [7,12–16]. These days, one tentatively subdivides hibernating myocardium into (1) acute hibernation, the state in which an almost immediate response in left ventricular function is measured after blood flow restoration, and (2) chronic hibernation, the condition in which the functional response is delayed; i.e., slow (weeks) to very slow (months) after blood flow restoration [14].

Structural Heterogeneity of Chronic Ischemic Myocardium and Its Relation to the Hibernating State

The purpose of studying whether a relation exists between function, metabolism, and structure in hibernating myocardium was to identify a possible structural basis to explain the variable outcome of function after revascularization. To prove a possible relationship between regional wall motion abnormalities of noninfarcted ventricular segments and their underlying histology is not an easy task. The reasons are obvious and concern the limited spatial resolution of the kinetic measurement, on one hand, and the small sample size of the biopsy for histologic examination, on the other. It is clear that one small biopsy might not be representative of the whole dysfunctional segment. However, the biopsy technique offers the only possibility to correlate structure and function in vivo. Undoubtedly, qualitative changes in myocyte structure and connective tissue can be described from biopsy material, but correlations with functional parameters must be addressed by a quantitative approach.

In a first study [17], 61 consecutive patients undergoing CABG procedure, and experiencing wall motion abnormalities and ECG changes, were assessed histologically. The histology of the myocardium was evaluated on transmural biopsies taken at the time of surgery. The patients were divided into three groups. Group I comprised patients with histologic findings associated with severe left anterior descending coronary artery (LAD) stenosis, without abnormal wall motion or ejection fraction. ECG abnormalities were limited to ST changes. Group II comprised patients with severe myocardial cell changes with only modest fibrosis associated with severe LAD stenosis and severely impaired wall motion. The incidence of infarction on the ECG was low. Group III patients had important myocardial cell changes with severe fibrosis associated with severe LAD stenosis, severely depressed wall motion, and significantly impaired ejection fraction. In this group there was a high incidence of infarction apparent on the ECG.

The changes observed in a considerable number of cells of groups II and III involved myolysis and were at that time considered to be degenerative in nature. Indeed, until recently, the described adaptive pattern of structural remodelling after chronic ischemia has been imbued with the notion of degeneration, either atrophic or necrotic. In his extensive review on the matter, Thiedemann [18] described a variety of abnormalities in myocardial cells derived from chronically underperfused segments of patients with chronic obstructive coronary artery disease. These changes included progressive loss of myofilaments, sarcoplasmic reticulum, and mitochondria. In his opinion, the changes described represented stages of damage due to chronic underperfusion. Hence, his viewpoint was that "chronic ischemia" represents a probably slow but progressive process of impairment of myocardial structure and function, rather than a stable condition where the myocardial cells are adapted to a low oxygen environment for a long period of time. In more recently performed analyses of the histology of chronic ischemic myocardium [19–23], comprising a large number of patients (165 in total, of which $\frac{1}{3}$ were documented with PET scans), the original idea that the observed cell changes were degenerative in nature was not retained. In lieu, for reasons mentioned below, it was proposed that the cell changes represent a switch from an actively contractile state to a stable surviving (dormant) state, hence perfectly matching the term hibernation from a morphologic point of view. The detailed structural adaptations under chronic ischemic conditions in these patients are reported next.

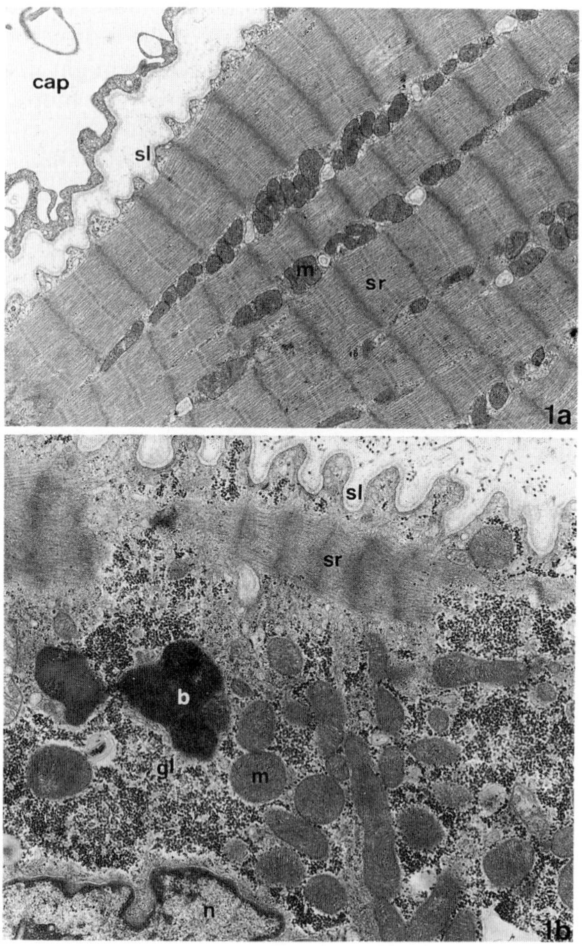

Fig. 1. **a** Electron microscopic (EM) picture of normal human myocardium. Note the regularly structured sarcomeres (*sr*) surrounded by rows of mitochondria (*m*). *sl*, sarcolemma; *cap*, blood capillary (×11 000). **b** EM of a cardiomyocyte from a hibernating myocardial area. A sarcomere row (*sr*) is only seen at the cell periphery. The cytoplasm is occupied by glycogen (*gl*), mitochondria (*m*), and residual bodies (*b*). *n*, nucleus. Note the intact sarcolemma (*sl*) (×15 400)

Ultrastructure of Chronic Hibernating Myocardium

The key observation characterizing cardiomyocytes of hibernating myocardium relates to the progressive loss of contractile material (sarcomeres) without loss of cell volume. This is clearly distinct from atrophic degenerative processes. The depletion of sarcomeres is initially seen at the cell center (perinuclear region) and may extend towards the periphery, involving the whole cytoplasm. In most cases, the space left by the dissolution of the sarcomeres becomes occupied by glycogen (Figs. 1, 2). Quantification of this change is given later.

Another characteristic feature is the presence of numerous small mini-mitochondria (Fig. 2a) in the areas adjacent to the glycogen-rich perinuclear zones. They are often found intermingled with glycogen. In some fortuitous sections the mitochondria are linearly arranged and have an elongated appearance.

A third change concerns the nuclei, which have lost their normal smoothly stretched contour, and instead have a tortuous appearance projecting numerous extensions into the surrounding cytosol. The chromatin is evenly distributed over the nucleoplasm (Fig. 2b). A fourth change involves the loss of the sarcoplasmic reticulum (SR). Organized SR is virtually absent; instead, a network of disorganized profiles of reticular membranes remains present in the myolytic areas. Fragments of rough endoplasmic reticulum (Fig. 2b) are frequently encountered in cells altered like this. In addition, the sarcolemma no longer projects protrusions (T-tubules) into the cytoplasm. Very often, the sarcolemma presents numerous pinocytotic vesicles (Fig. 2c), resembling those

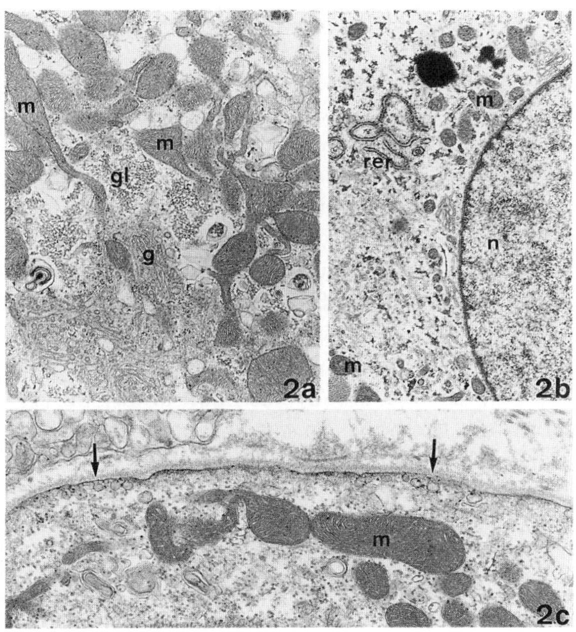

Fig. 2a–c. EM pictures showing characteristic changes in hibernating cells. **a** The cell center shows numerous abnormally shaped but structurally intact mitochondria (*m*), intermingled with clusters of glycogen (*gl*). *g*, Golgi apparatus (×15 400). **b** The round nucleus (*n*) has dispersed chromatin. Rough endoplasmic reticulum (*rer*) and many mini-mitochondria (*m*) are found in its vicinity (×11 500). **c** The cell periphery showing numerous pinocytotic vesicles (*arrows*) associated with the sarcolemma. Note the absence of sarcomeres at the periphery. Mitochondria (*m*) (×24 840)

of endothelial and smooth muscle cells. The number of microperoxisomes in the perinuclear space is also elevated.

Remarkably, typical degenerative changes such as cytoplasmic vacuolization, cytosolic edema, mitochondrial swelling, membrane disruption, accumulation of secondary lysosomes, membrane whorls, and lipid droplets are virtually absent. The general impression is that the substructures present in the cells of such affected segments are perfectly healthy. As far as the intercellular space is concerned, apart from an increased number of collagen fibres, no other striking abnormalities are noticed. Microvascular endothelium, pericytes, and interstitial mesenchymal cells are present in the usual number and display well-preserved substructures. The increase in interstitial collagen and ground substance is substantial and correlates with the degree of myocardial cell change. Obviously, the extracellular compartment may play a significant role in the degree and speed of functional recovery after revascularization.

Morphologic Features Distinguishing Hibernating Cells from Those in Other Pathophysiologic Conditions

The subcellular changes just described are entirely at variance with those seen in stunned myocardium, in acute severe ischemia leading to infarction, and in end-stage cardiomyopathies. The structural alterations of cardiomyocytes in stunned myocardium have not been documented in man, but morphologic features resembling the subtle changes seen in stunned myocardium of animals are frequently encountered in human biopsies prior to and after repeated short ischemic periods when the intermittent aorta cross-clamping procedure is used for CABG (Fig. 3).

In animals, stunning resulted in a characteristic change: the loss of intramatricial granules in mitochondria and the occurrence of clumped mitochondrial cristae, a picture never seen in normal or hibernating myocardium. Clumping of cristae was the earliest sign of deterioration noticed and was shown to be accompanied by activation of proton-translocating ATPase and the intramitochondrial formation of harmful oxygen species [24]. As the structural equivalent of stunned myocardium is unknown in humans, it is impossible to say whether the stunned myocardium is more or less vulnerable to structural deterioration, for example in states of acute ischemia during cardiac surgery.

The detail morphology of acute myocardial infarction and healed infarction (scar or fibrotic tissue) has been amply described before and can be retrieved from any textbook on cardiac pathology. A picture demonstrating a necrotic cell in the acute phase of infarction is seen in Fig. 4. An interesting aspect, however, which is not well documented, concerns the immediate surroundings of a healed infarction. Cells that border the fibrotic scar are often of the "hibernating" type.

A more complex picture of structural changes is seen in cardiomyopathic myocardium. In a significant number of the biopsies obtained from cardiomyo-

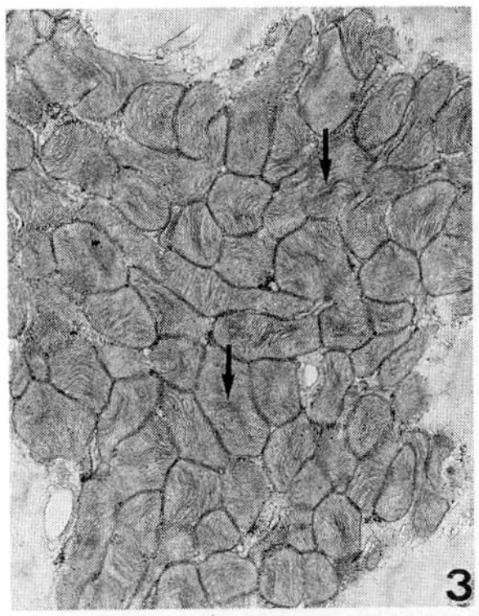

Fig. 3. EM of stunned myocardium. Mitochondria, although normally shaped, are devoid of intramatrix granules and possess clumped cristae (*arrows*). These are the only changes which are at variance with normal myocardial cells (×11 750)

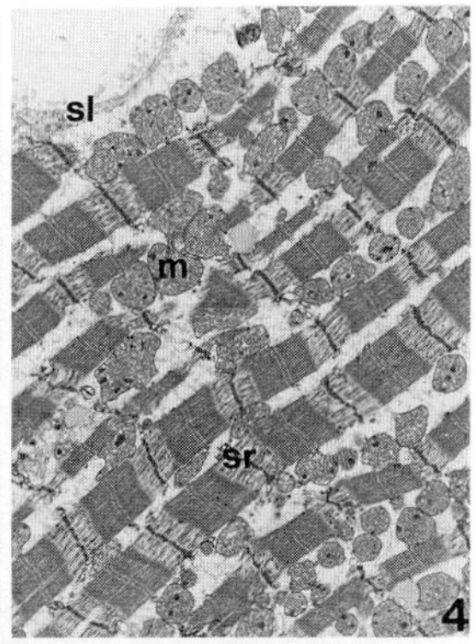

Fig. 4. EM of an acutely infarcted area. Note the irreversibly degenerated structures such as mitochondria (*m*), sarcomeres (*sr*) in an edematous cytosol. The sarcolemma (*sl*) is barely recognizable (×5700)

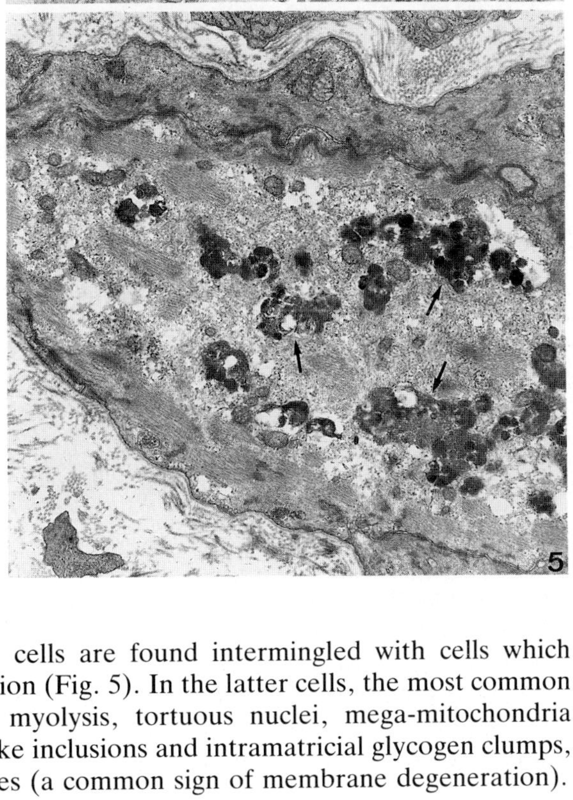

Fig. 5. EM of cardiomyopathic degeneration. The center of this myolytic cell is, in contrast to hibernating cells, filled with necrotic remnants (*arrows*) (×13 300)

pathic patients, "hibernating" cells are found intermingled with cells which clearly show signs of degeneration (Fig. 5). In the latter cells, the most common morphologic changes include myolysis, tortuous nuclei, mega-mitochondria (the size of nuclei) with lipid-like inclusions and intramatricial glycogen clumps, and whorl-like myelin structures (a common sign of membrane degeneration).

Glycogen Storage and Altered Metabolism in Hibernating Myocardium

Quantitative Aspects of Cell Change in Hibernating Myocardium

Since glycogen accumulation was the hallmark of the myocardial cell change, the degree of myocardial change was quantitatively evaluated in light micros-

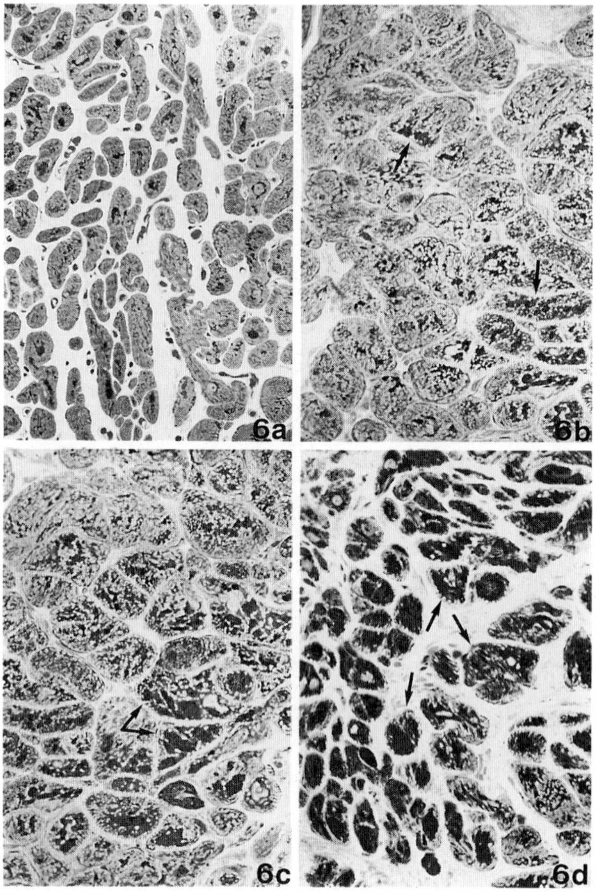

Fig. 6a–d. Light microscopy of different degrees of cell change in chronic ischemic myocardium. The sections are stained with periodic acid Schiff (PAS), a stain for glycogen (*dark areas*). **a** Section through a nonaffected area, showing absence of PAS stain (×265). **b** A minority of cells are PAS positive (*arrows*) (×265). **c** A significant number of otherwise normally shaped cells stain for glycogen (*arrows*) (×265). **d** The large majority of cells are darkly stained, due to the accumulation of huge amounts of glycogen (*arrows*) (×265)

copic sections stained with periodic acid Schiff (PAS), a reagent that specifically interacts with glycogen (Fig. 6). In each cell where the nucleus was visible, the amount of glycogen was planimetrically scored. The glycogen content varied from slight deposition to huge accumulation of glycogen in severely myolytic cells, in which only a few sarcomeres remained at the periphery of the cell. Figure 7 shows the number of affected cells and degree of cell change in a total of 165 patients. The percent glycogen per total cell volume ranged between 5% and 44%, meaning that up to 44% of the total cell mass in noninfarcted areas was occupied by glycogen. In individual cells the amount of glycogen ranged from 0% to 100% (all sarcomeres replaced by glycogen). Figure 7 shows that 88% of the patients had cells with more than 10% glycogen, and at the other extreme, 9% of the patients contained cells with 90% glycogen. The amount of glycogen was higher in the subendocardial than in the subepicardial cells.

The number of affected cells in the endocardium was found to be related to local wall motion abnormalities and to the degree of stenosis [23]. In this study,

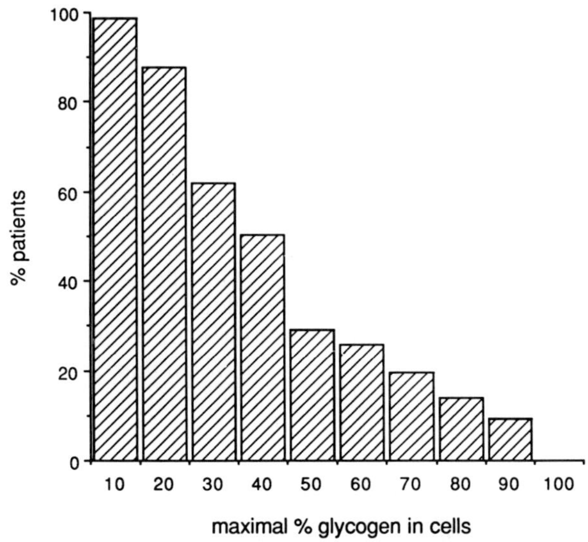

Fig. 7. Histogram representing the distribution of cells containing various amounts of glycogen in myocardial samples obtained from 165 patients

cells were considered as affected when myolysis (i.e., glycogen content) occupied more than 10% of the total cell volume.

Relation between Glycogen and Switch of Metabolic Substrate in Hibernating Cells

A point needing a more in-depth discussion is the accumulation of glycogen in relation to the possible alteration of preference of metabolic substrate by hibernating cells. With Positron Emission Tomography (PET), it is well documented that a normal to enhanced glucose extraction often takes place in underperfused myocardial segments [8,22]. It may be speculated that, subsequent to the lowered oxygen availability, glucose is preferred over fatty acids as an energy source, and the high amounts of glycogen observed may reflect such enhanced uptake of glucose by the hibernation cells. It is not clear why glucose would be stored as glycogen. Storage of glycogen may represent the metabolic excess of glucose utilization, or the consequence of impaired catabolism of glycogen due to a defective phosphorylase activity following a decrease in catecholamines [25]. So far, the catecholamine content has not been determined in hibernating myocardium.

In a limited number of patients an attempt has been made to correlate histologic change, in particular glycogen accumulation, with glucose extraction, by use of PET imaging [19,21,22]. Although not proven, because of the low number of cases studied, the data strongly suggest a direct relation between the existence of hibernating cells loaded with glycogen and a supranormal glucose extraction pattern. On the other hand, since glycogen storage is seen in embryonic (not well-differentiated) heart cells which have a preference for glucose over triglycerides as an energy source [26], glycogen accumulation in hibernating cells can be interpreted as a characteristic of "dedifferentiation." This hypothesis will be elaborated on next.

Hibernating Cells —A Phenotypic Change Akin to Dedifferentiation?

Before addressing this important question, we have to consider first a number of criteria that allow us to exclude changes of another nature. We have already argued that the changes in hibernating cells were not of the degenerative type. Moreover, there are observations that indicate that these cells are actively metabolizing and possess a number of characteristics that classify them as healthy:

1. Cytochrome oxidase activity can be demonstrated in their mitochondria, despite the fact that they are morphologically altered (Fig. 8). There is no sign of uncoupling of mitochondria because proton translocating ATPase is absent (Borgers, unpublished data).
2. The integrity of cellular calcium homeostasis is suggested by the absence of cytochemically demonstrable calcium overload (Fig. 9). The phospholipid-

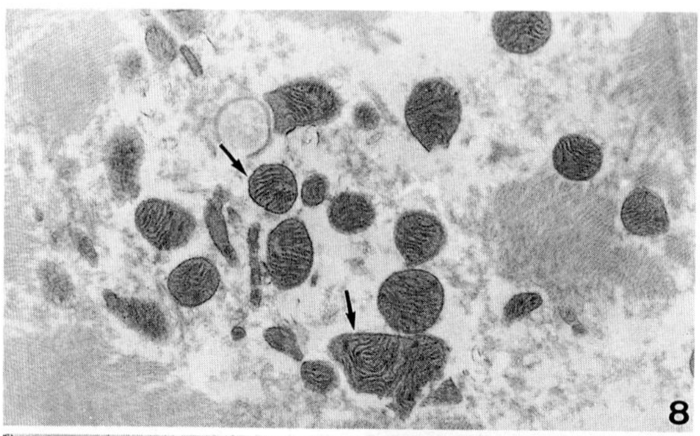

Fig. 8. EM picture of cytochrome c oxidase activity present in the abnormally shaped mitochondria of hibernating cells. The activity is seen as dark precipitate confined to the mitochondrial cristae (*arrows*) (×15 730)

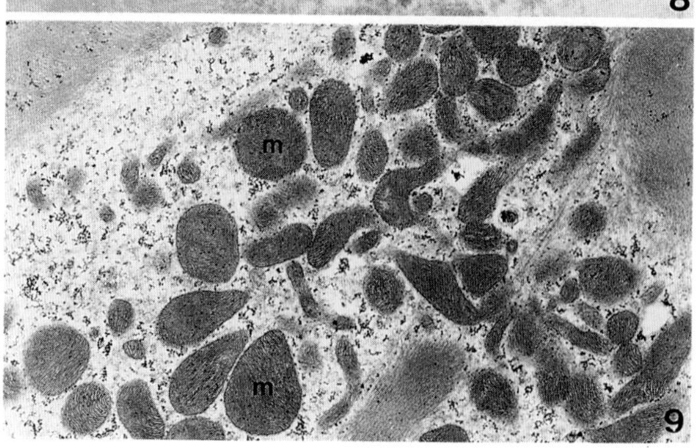

Fig. 9. EM picture of calcium localization in mitochondria (*m*) of a hibernating cell. Unlike the mitochondria of normally structured cells (not shown), the mitochondria of this cell are virtually devoid of calcium precipitate (×16 150)

bound fraction of calcium is preserved at the plasma membrane of hibernating cells and mitochondria are virtually devoid of calcium-precipitate [27].

3. Hibernating cells are less susceptible to acute ischemia than their neighboring normally structured cells [28]. Examination of biopsies from hibernating myocardium taken at the end of CABG reveals that "hibernating" cells are much less susceptible to acute ischemia than are the adjacent cells which have a normal ultrastructure. The most pronounced differences between these are seen at the level of mitochondria, nuclei, and the sarcolemma-glycocalyx complex [28]. After CABG, the mini-mitochondria of hibernating cells are not or only slightly swollen, whereas in adjacent normally structured cells, mitochondria show a more marked clarification of the matrix. The latter mitochondria show a lot more calcium deposits than those of the hibernating cells.

Most of the adaptive changes that "hibernating" cells undergo during chronic ischemia are changes that are reminiscent of dedifferentiation. Hence, the question can be asked whether hibernating cells are of an embryonic or fetal differentiation phenotype. The changes corresponding to structural features of embryonic or neonatal myocardial cells are (1) depletion of contractile filaments, (2) accumulation of glycogen, (3) presence of altered nuclei with peculiar distribution of chromatin, (4) strong decrease in the amount of sarcoplasmic reticulum, (5) presence of rough endoplasmic reticulum, (6) virtual absence of T-tubuli, and (7) vesicularization of the sarcolemma.

In the developing heart, as well as in adult cardiomyocytes after a prolonged stay in culture, sarcomeres are much less abundant than in adult cells. In embryonic cells, glycogen also accumulates around the nucleus [29] and glucose is preferred over fatty acids are energy source. However, the amount of glycogen in "hibernating" cells sometimes greatly exceeds the amount visualized in embryonic cells. The nuclei of embryonic cells are characterized by an even distribution of the heterochromatin, in contrast to adult cells where the heterochromatin is clustered towards the nuclear membrane. Moreover, a structural feature typical for embryonic and fetal heart cells is the presence of rough endoplasmic reticulum, which may be considered a sign of actively synthesizing cells. The smooth sarcoplasmic reticulum is not extensively developed and lacks organization in both embryonic and hibernating cells. Although the morphologic resemblance between hibernating cells and embryonic or fetal cells is striking, it is necessary to perform a number of studies to make a firm case for a "dedifferentiation" hypothesis for hibernating myocardium.

Perspectives and Outlook

Before it can be concluded that hibernating cells are of a "dedifferentiated" phenotype, specific differentiation markers need to be assessed. The expression and organization patterns of contractile and cytoskeletal molecules such as actin, α-actinin, α- and β-myosin heavy chains, embryonic and adult myosin subtypes, titin, tubulin, and tropomyosin with molecular probes have to be evaluated on biopsies of patients with chronic hibernating myocardium. It will be essential to compare the expression, organization, and assembly of these markers of cardiac cell development in hibernating and embryonic hearts [30–33]. In addition, the assessment of factors involved in transcriptional regulation in normal and hibernating myocardium may be of interest [34].

Identification of factors that trigger myolysis and/or myofribrillogenesis is of great importance in relation to potential reversibility of the change. In a recent article, Borisov [35] presented evidence that cardiomyocytes at early, intermediate, and terminal stages of differentiation are capable of adaptive remodelling of the contractile system and show significant plasticity of their structure. The author furthermore states that adaptive remodelling of cell structure and activation of myofribrillogenesis can occur even in the absence of hemodynamic load, e.g., in cell culture, but that factors inherent in the organism that regulate hemodynamic loading, neurohumoral responses, and blood supply are determinants of cardiac growth.

Conclusions

A number of aspects related to the underlying causes of the hibernating response remain to be elucidated. In the first place, as put forward in a recent paper by Vanoverschelde et al. [22], it is not certain whether hibernation is the consequence of a "persistent" low-flow ischemia or is brought on by repetitive periods of transient ischemia, hence making the distinction between hibernating and stunned myocardium less obvious. Hibernation would then be a state of long-term stunning in which normalization of function is not brought about, because each new episode of ischemia would trigger a stunning response before the previous one had gone, i.e., the individual periods of stunning would overlap.

Another unanswered question, however, relates to the reversibility of "dedifferentiated" state of cells after restoration of blood flow. If these cells could redifferentiate in time, they might be held responsible for the recovery of function (although delayed) after revascularization, as seen in a subset of patients with hibernating myocardium. Indeed, it is conceivable that if the structural changes in the affected cardiomyocytes are reversible, it may take at least weeks to months before cells can rebuild a normal contractile machinery, hence contributing to a delayed recovery of ventricular function.

Most important, however, is that we think hibernating myocardium will remain a controversial issue until a reproducible animal model becomes available, in which the various clinical aspects of the chronic hibernating state in man are mimicked. As it stands right now, a low-flow ischemic model for acute hibernation has been described in the dog [36], but a model for chronic hibernating myocardium without concomitant focal infarctions is still lacking in animals. Until such a model exists, basic questions related to substrate preference, dedifferentiation, and the eventual reversibility of cellular changes, will be difficult to answer.

References

1. Rahimtoola SH (1985) A perspective on the three large multicenter randomized clinical trials of coronary bypass surgery for chronic stable angina. Circulation (Suppl V) 72:123–135
2. Horn HR, Teichholz LE, Cohn PF, Herman MV, Gorlin R (1974) Augmentation of left ventricular contraction pattern in coronary artery disease by an inotropic catecholamine. Circulation 49:1063–1071
3. Bodenheimer MM, Banka VS, Hermann GA, Trout RG, Pasdar H, Helfant RH (1976) Reversible asynergy. Histopathologic and electrographic correlations in patients with coronary artery disease. Circulation 53:792–796
4. Stinson EB, Billingham ME (1977) Correlative study of regional left ventricular histology and contractile function. Am J Cardiol 39:378–383
5. Walter P, Schwarz F, Becker V, Schaper J, Flameng W, Hehrlein F (1980) Morphology of poorly contracting ventricle in patients with coronary artery disease. Thorac Cardiovasc Surgeon 28:177–183
6. Rahimtoola SH (1982) Coronary bypass surgery for chronic angina. A perspective. Circulation 65:225–241
7. Schelbert HR (1991) Positron emission tomography for the assessment of myocardial viability. Circulation (Suppl I) 84:I-122–I131
8. Schelbert HR (1991) Myocardial scar or hibernating myocardium? The role of positron emission tomography. In: Bulla N (ed) LV function in stunned and hibernating myocardium. Proc Symp 13th Congress European Society of Cardiology, Amsterdam, Excerpta Medica, pp 56–68
9. Takeishi Y, Tono-oka I, Kubota I, Ikeda K, Masakane I, Chiba J, Abe S, Tsuiki K, Komatani A, Yamaguchi, I, Washio M (1991) Functional recovery of hibernating myocardium after coronary bypass surgery: Does it coincide with improvement in perfusion? Am Heart J 122:665–670
10. Brunken R, Tillisch J, Schwaiger M, Child JS, Marshall R, Mandelkern M, Phelps ME, Schelbert HR (1986) Regional perfusion glucose metabolism and wall motion in chronic electrocardiographic Q-wave infarctions. Evidence for persistence of viable tissue in some infarct regions by positron emission tomography. Circulation 73:951–963
11. Tillisch J, Brunken R, Marshall R, Schwaiger M, Mandelkern M, Phelps M, Schelbert HR (1986) Prediction of cardiac wall motion abnormalities predicted by using positron tomography. N Engl J Med 36:1995–1999
12. Rahimtoola Sh (1989) The hibernating myocardium. Am Heart J 117:211–221
13. Ross JJ (1991) Myocardial perfusion-contraction matching. Implications for coronary heart disease and hibernation. Circulation 83:1076–1083
14. Tubau JF, Rahimtoola SH (1992) Hibernating myocardium: a historical perspective. Cardiovasc Drugs Ther 267–271
15. Braunwald E, Rutherford JD (1986) Reversible ischemic left ventricular dysfunction: evidence for the "hibernating myocardium." J Am Coll Cardiol 8:1467–1470
16. Kloner RA, Przyklenk K, Patel B (1989) Altered myocardial states. Am J Med [Suppl A] 86:14–22

17. Flameng W, Wouters L, Sergeant P, Lewi P, Borgers M, Thoné F, Suy R (1984) Multivariate analysis of angiographic, histologic, and electrocardiographic data in patients with coronary heart disease. Circulation 70:7–17
18. Thiedemann KU (1979) Ultrastructure in chronic ischemia. Studies in human hearts. In: Schaper W (ed) The pathophysiology of myocardial perfusion. Elsevier/North Holland Biomedical Press, Amsterdam, pp 675–716
19. Depré C, Melin JA, Essamri B, Grandin C, Wijns W, Borgers M (1991) Ultrastructural correlates of flow–metabolism mismatch pattern on positron emission tomography. Circulation 84[Suppl II]:II-90
20. Borgers M, Flameng W (1992) Morphologic identification of chronic hibernating myocardium in man. Circulation 86[Suppl I]:I-438
21. Shivalkar B, Mortelmans L, Schiepers C, Borgers M, Nuyts J, Bormans G, Flameng W (1992) Glycogen storage in chronically hypoperfused myocardium associated with maintained FDG uptake. Circulation 86[Suppl I]:I-417
22. Vanoverschelde JLJ, Wijns W, Depré C, Essamri B, Hendrickx R, Borgers M, Bol A, Melin J (1993) Mechanisms of chronic regional postischemic dysfunction in humans: New insights from the study on non-infarcted collateral dependent myocardium. Circulation 87:1513–1523
23. Borgers M, Thoné F, Wouters L, Ausma J, Shivalkar B, Flameng W (1993) Structural correlates of regional myocardial dysfunction in patients with critically coronary artery stenosis: chronic hibernation? Cardiovasc Pathol 2:237–245
24. Vandeplassche G, Hermans C, Thoné F, Borgers M (1991) Stunned myocardium has increased mitochondrial NADH oxidase and ATPase activities. Cardioscience 2:47–53
25. Stull JT, Mayer SE (1979) Biochemical mechanisms of adrenegic and cholinergic regulation of myocardial contractility. In: Berne RM et al (eds) Handbook of physiology, sect 2: the cardiovascular system. American Physiological Society, Bethesda, Maryland, vol I, pp 741–774
26. Harary I (1979) Biochemistry of cardiac development: in vivo and in vitro studies. In: Berne RM et al (eds) Handbook of physiology, sect 2: the cardiovascular system. American Physiological Society, Bethesda, vol I, pp 43–60
27. Borgers M, De Nollin S, Thoné F, Wouters L, Van Vaeck L, Flameng W (1993) Distribution of calcium in a subset of chronic hibernating myocardium in man. Histochem J 25:312–318
28. Borgers M, Flameng W (1993) Morphology of the acute and chronic ischemic myocardium in man. In: Piper HM, Preusse CJ (eds) Ischemia-reperfusion in cardiac surgery. Kluwer Academic, pp 353–375
29. Manasek FJ (1968) Mitosis in developing cardiac muscle. J Cell Biol 37:191–196
30. Van der Loop FTL, Schaart G, Langmann W, Ramaekers FCS, Viebahn Ch (1992) Expression and organization of muscle specific proteins during the early development stages of the rabbit heart. Anat Embryol 185:439–450
31. Schaart G, Viebahn Ch, Langmann W, Ramaekers F (1989) Desmin and titin expression in early postimplantation mouse embryos. Development 107:585–596
32. Schaart G, Pieper FR, Kuijpers HJH, Bloemendal H, Ramaekers FCS (1991) Baby hamster kidney (BHK-21/C13) cells can express striated muscle type proteins. Differentiation 46:105–115
33. Fischman DA (1986) Myofibrillogenesis and the morphogenesis of skeletal muscle. In: Engel AG, Banker BQ (eds) Myology: basic and clinical. McGraw-Hill, New York, pp 5–30

34. Chien KR, Zhu H, Knowlton KU, Miller-Hance W, Van Bilsen M, O'Brien TX, Evans SM (1993) Transcriptional regulation during cardiac growth and development. Annu Rev Physiol 55:77–95
35. Borisov AB (1991) Myofibrillogenesis and reversible disassembly of myofibrils as adaptive reactions of cardiac muscle cells. Acta Physiol Scand S559:71–80
36. Marban E (1991) Myocardial stunning and hibernation. The physiology behind the colloquialism. Circulation 83:681–688

1.8 Alterations in Membrane Phospholipids During Ischemia and Reperfusion

GER J. VAN DER VUSSE, MARC VAN BILSEN, and ROBERT S. RENEMAN[1]

Summary. Loss of cellular integrity in the cardiomyocyte is most probably caused by overt rupture of cellular membranes, in particular the sarcolemma enclosing the cytoplasmic space. A variety of mechanisms may underlie the process of destabilization of the sarcolemma, which occurs prior to irreversible disintegration of the semipermeable barrier between the extra- and intracellular environment. The factors thought to provoke membrane instability are chemical (hydrolysis and synthesis of membrane phospholipids), physicochemical (including loss of phospholipid asymmetry, phase transition of membrane phospholipids, and extrusion of lipid material from the membrane), and ultrastructural (detachment of cytoskeleton and sarcolemma, and impaired anchoring of basement membrane to sarcolemma). During the acute phase of reperfusion, production of oxygen free-radicals, enhanced cytoplasmic levels of Ca^{2+}, osmotic load, and resumption of contractile activity may cause directly or indirectly overt rupture of the cellular membrane, weakened during the preceding ischemic insult.

Key words: Heart—Ischemia—Reperfusion—Membranes—Phospholipids—Arachidonic acid

Introduction

Impaired perfusion (ischemia) of cardiac tissue ultimately results in loss of cellular viability [1]. Due to the lack of molecular oxygen, cellular energy conversion becomes impaired, cytoplasmic phosphocreatine and ATP levels fall, and energy-requiring processes, such as myofibrillar contraction and transport of ions, become hampered. When the duration of ischemia is prolonged,

[1]Cardiovascular Research Institute Maastricht, Department of Physiology, University of Limburg, P.O. Box 616, 6200 MD Maastricht, The Netherlands

cellular functions become severely depressed and loss of cellular integrity is readily seen. The latter phenomenon is characterized by massive loss of macromolecules from the cytoplasm into the extracellular space and the invasion of extracellular components into the intracellular compartment. Since the sarcolemma, the membrane enclosing the cytoplasmic space of the cardiomyocyte, plays a critical role in maintaining cellular integrity, it has been hypothesized that alterations in sarcolemmal function are responsible for the loss of cell viability [1].

Timely restoration of flow (reperfusion) to the ischemic myocardium prevents the cardiac cells from lethal damage. Recent studies suggest that reperfusion per se might inflict damage upon cells weakened by the preceding ischemic insult [2]. This type of damage is characterized by an accelerated loss of cytoplasmic enzymes indicating breakdown of the sarcolemma as the semipermeable barrier between the intra- and extracellular compartment.

Although it is generally accepted that ischemia- and reperfusion-induced damage is a multifactorial process, chemical and physical alterations in cellular membranes are most probably a critical step in the chain of events leading to irreversible loss of cellular integrity. In the present chapter, attention will be paid to the structure and function of normal cardiac membranes and perturbations thereof observed in the ischemic and reperfused hearts. Current ideas on mechanisms underlying loss of cell membrane integrity during prolonged ischemia and during restoration of blood flow will be discussed.

Membranes Enclosing Cardiac Cells—Normoxic Situation

Like all living cells, cardiomyocytes are enclosed in a plasma membrane or sarcolemma. Internal membranes surround the organelles localized inside the cardiac cells. The major constituents of cellular membranes are phospholipids, cholesterol, and proteins. The sarcolemma represents on the order of 5%–10% of the total cardiac membrane mass [3]. The majority of cellular phospholipids is incorporated in the mitochondrial membranes.

Phospholipids consist of a hydrophobic part and a hydrophilic headgroup connected to a glycerol backbone. Since the chemical nature of both the hydrophobic tail, generally composed of two long-chain fatty acids, and the hydrophilic headgroup varies, phospholipids are present in a variety of molecular species. The hydrophilic headgroup is composed of an alcohol molecule bound to the third (Sn_3) carbon atom of the glycerol backbone of the phospholipid molecule via a phosphate group (Fig. 1) [4]. In cardiac cells, the most common alcohols incorporated in the phospholipid molecule are choline, ethanolamine, serine, inositol and glycerol. The latter alcohol is predominantly present in diphosphatidylglycerol (cardiolipin), which is an important constituent of mitochondrial membranes.

The hydrophobic part of the phospholipid molecule is in general composed of two aliphatic chains covalently bound to the carbon atoms at the Sn_1 and Sn_2

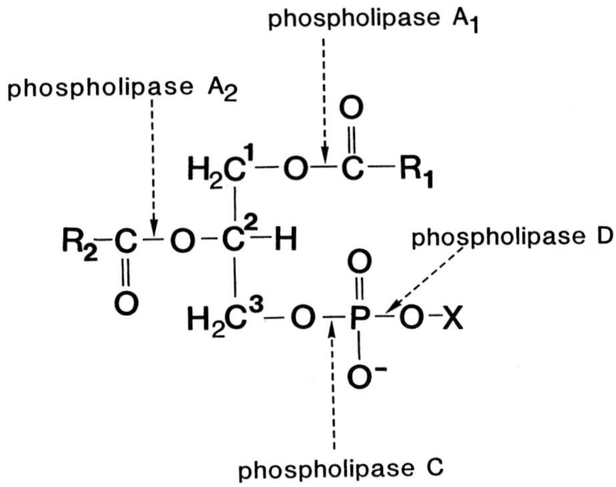

Fig. 1. Schematic representation of the chemical structures of diacylglycerol phospholipids. R_1 and R_2 refer to fatty acyl chains. *X* is commonly choline, ethanolamine, serine, inositol, or glycerol. The specific sites of hydrolytic action of various phospholipases are indicated by *arrows*. The numbers *1*, *2*, and *3* refer to position Sn_1, Sn_2, and Sn_3 on the glycerol backbone. (Modified from [4], with permission)

position of the glycerol backbone. The aliphatic chains are commonly derived from long chain fatty acids, ranging in chain length from 12 to 24 and in number of unsaturated bonds from zero to 6. The relative composition of the fatty acid molecules varies considerably among the phospholipid species. Where the aliphatic chain at position Sn_1 is a vinyl ether linkage instead of an ester bond, the phospholipid is present in the plasmalogen form. In some animal species, up to 40% of the total cardiac phospholipid pool consists of plasmalogens [1]. In addition to phospholipids, sphingomyelin is present in cellular membranes. The backbone in this compound is sphingosine, to the amino group of which a fatty acid moiety is linked.

Because phospholipids readily form bilayers, cellular membranes are composed of two leaflets. The hydrophilic head groups of the inner leaflet of the sarcolemma point toward the cytoplasmic space and the hydrophilic moieties of the phospholipids in the outer leaflet face the extracellular environment. The hydrophobic aliphatic chains are buried in the core of the lipid bilayer. Interestingly, the distribution of the various phospholipid species is asymmetric over the inner and outer surface of the lipid bilayer. Phosphatidylethanolamine, phosphatidylserine, and phosphatidylinositol are the main constituents of the inner leaflet. The outer surface contains a high proportion of sphingomyelin. Phosphatidylcholine is almost equally distributed over the inner and outer leaflet [5]. The asymmetric distribution of phospholipids and sphingomyelin over the inner and outer leaflet creates a selective enrichment of negatively charged phospholipids in the inner leaflet and a difference in fluidity between the two leaflets. To compensate for this difference in fluidity, the outer leaflet is relatively enriched in cholesterol.

Normal cellular performance requires proper functioning of sarcolemma and internal membranes. Since membranes are structurally and functionally asymmetric, membranes are able to create microenvironments in the cell and its organelles with optimal conditions to maintain specific chemical and physiological processes. Basically, membranes are impermeable for macromolecules and polar substances. To ensure transport across the lipid bilayer of compounds that are vital for cellular functioning, proteins are present in the membrane that specifically regulate transport of molecules across the membrane. Like phospholipids, most proteins are asymmetrically distributed over the inner and outer surface of the membrane. In addition to protein-mediated transport, macromolecules can pass the barrier formed by the phospholipid bilayer by processes such as endo- and exocytosis. Furthermore, some small solutes can pass the lipid bilayer by passive diffusion, depending on charge and polarity of the substances to be transported.

The phospholipid molecules in membranes are subjected to a turnover process. Studies with radiolabeled fatty acids and such compounds as ethanolamine and choline have shown that both the fatty acyl moieties and the polar head groups are continuously removed from the glycerol backbone and replaced by new molecules [6]. This turnover cycle enables the cardiomyocyte to synthesize any required phospholipid and to control the fatty acyl compositions of the phospholipids and, hence, the overall chemical and physical properties of the membranes surrounding the cytoplasmic space and the intracellular organelles.

A variety of enzymes is present in the cardiac cells to hydrolyze phospholipids [6]. As indicated in Fig. 1, phospholipase A_1 catalyzes the cleavage of the ester linkage between the fatty acyl moiety and the carbon atom of glycerol at position Sn_1. Phospholipase A_2 removes acyl moieties from the Sn_2 glycerol position. Phospholipase C breaks the binding between the polar head group and the carbon atom of glycerol at position Sn_3. Phospholipase D cleaves the connection between phosphate and the alcohol moiety that form together the polar head group. The end products of phospholipase A_1 and A_2 activity are lysophospholipids and fatty acids. The remaining fatty acyl chain in lysophospholipids can be removed by the action of lysophospholipase. Recently, enzymes specifically hydrolyzing either the vinylether bond or the acyl ester bond in plasmalogens were identifed in cardiac tissue [7,8]. These enzymes are called plasmalogenase and plasmalogen-specific phospholipase A_2. In general, enzymes with phospholipid-hydrolyzing properties are localized both in the cytoplasmic space and bound to the sarcolemma and internal membranes. Phospholipase A_2 activity has been detected in the soluble cytoplasm, in mitochondrial membranes, and in sarcoplasmic reticulum. Phospholipase A_2 has been found to be attached to the sarcolemma as well. These enzymes show their maximal activity at mildly alkaline conditions. In contrast, lysosomal phospholipase A_1 and A_2 show their highest activity at a pH varying from 4 to 5 [6]. Most cardiac phospholipases A_2 were found to be stimulated by relatively high levels of calcium ions. Interestingly, plasmalogen-specific phospholipase A_2 appears to be Ca^{2+} insensitive [8].

While most phospholipases A_2 are present in the cell in a low molecular weight form (14 kDa), recent investigations have disclosed the presence of a novel type of phospholipase A_2 ranging in molecular weight from 60 to 110 kDA

[9]. The latter enzyme can be recovered from the cytosolic fraction of a variety of cell types including kidney cells, macrophages, and platelets. The high molecular weight phospholipase A_2 shows an interesting response towards increasing Ca^{2+}-concentrations within the physiological range. Upon exposure to Ca^{2+} the enzymes shift from the aqueous space to the membranes to execute their phospholipid-hydrolyzing activity [9]. Moreover, they are thought to play a role in arachidonic acid mediated signal transduction. At present, the occurrence of this high molecular weight enzyme in cells of cardiac origin remains to be established.

Lysophospholipases are present in the sarcoplasmic space, and in subcellular structures like mitochondria, sarcoplasmic reticulum, and lysosomes [6]. Phospholipase C is predominantly present in the soluble cytoplasm, whereas activity of the enzyme has also been recovered in mitochondrial, microsomal, and sarcolemmal membrane fractions of rabbit hearts [10]. The activity of phospholipase D has also been identified in cardiac structures [11].

The sarcoplasmic reticulum has been identified as the site of phospholipid synthesis [6]. When phospholipids are subjected to the deacylation-reacylation cycle (pathway I in Fig. 2), lysophospholipids serve as substrate for the lysophospholipid acyl transferase catalyzed reincorporation of fatty acyl moieties in phospolipids. Alternatively, phospholipids can be synthetized de novo from diacylglycerol and phosphorylcholine or phosphorylethanolamine. The latter two compounds are activated to cytidine diphospho (CDP-)choline and CDP-ethanolamine, respectively, prior to condensation with diacylglycerol to yield choline- and ethanolamine-containing phospholipids (Fig. 2, pathway II).

The newly synthetized phospholipid molecules are probably transported through the cytoplasm from the production site to their final destinations, i.e., one of the (sub)cellular membranes, by the use of specific phospholipid-binding proteins [12].

When the cardiac cell is in a steady state, resynthesis of membrane phospholipids is quantitatively in equilibration with phospholipase mediated hydrolysis. At present, the nature of the factors controlling degradation and resynthesis of membrane phospholipids is incompletely elucidated. Choy and coworkers [7,13–17] have extensively investigated the process of phospholipid synthesis in cardiac tissue. They concluded that de novo synthesis of phosphatidyl choline may be regulated at at least four different levels: (1) the cellular uptake and metabolic conversion of choline into phosphocholine; (2) the cellular cytidine triphosphate (CTP) concentration; (3) the activity of the enzyme, catalyzing the rate-limiting step in the overall pathway of phosphatidylcholine biosynthesis, i.e., CTP: phosphocholine cytidylyl transferase; and (4) the availability and selection of molecular species of diacylglycerol. The activity of cytidylyl transferase is most likely to be the critical step in the overall rate of phospholipid synthesis, since stearic acid-induced stimulation of phosphatidyl production is accompanied by a severalfold enhancement of the activity of CTP: phosphocholine cytidylyl transferase in the endoplasmic reticulum [18]. Phospholipid hydrolysis is regulated by a variety of enzymes and chemical compounds and by the physicochemical characteristics of the cellular membranes. Theoretically, the following factors may be involved:

(1) synthesis and post-translational modification of phospholipases;
(2) intracellular levels of Ca^{2+};
(3) the content of vitamin E in the cardiac cells;
(4) the energy status of the cardiomyocytes;
(5) the presence of nonenzymatic proteins with affinity for membrane phospholipids;
(6) hormonal activation;
(7) feedback inhibition by products released during phospholipid degradation;
(8) physicochemical alterations in membranes, including phospholipid peroxidation, phase transition of membrane lipids, and extrusion or blebbing of lipid material. Each of these issues will be discussed later.

Soluble pancreatic phospholipase A_2 can be activated by the chemical conversion of a biologically inactive form (zymogen) into a protein with hydrolyzing activity towards phospholipids. This mechanism of controlling phospholipase A_2 activity is probably also operative in parenchymal cells, such as hepatocytes, and in platelets. However, no evidence is available that this process occurs in cardiac tissue.

With the exception of lysosomal phospholipases and plasmalogen-specific phospholipase A_2, most cardiac phospholipases are sensitive to Ca^{2+} [6]. It is still a matter of debate whether intracellular fluctuations in Ca^{2+} within the physiological ranges (i.e., from 0.1 to $1.0\,\mu M$) will have a great impact on endogenous phospholipase activity. In vitro studies have shown that Ca^{2+} has to vary over a broader range (up to mmolar levels of Ca^{2+}) to provoke a biologically significant enhancement of phospholipid-hydrolyzing activity [19]. However, it is uncertain whether in vitro findings can be extrapolated to the intracellular conditions of the heart in vivo. In addition, it cannot be excluded that due to compartmentalization of Ca^{2+}-ions inside the cardiac cells, conditions are created which are favorable for Ca^{2+}-mediated alterations in phospholipase activity.

Choy and coworkers [20,21] have observed that the vitamin E status of the cardiac cell regulates both phospholipid degradation and biosynthesis. Vitamin E was found to inhibit in a noncompetitive manner the activity of cardiac phospholipase A_1 and A_2 indicating that vitamin E may partake in the control mechanism of cardiac phospholipid turnover.

The presence of nonenzymatic proteins interfering with phospholipid metabolism has attracted considerable attention during recent years, because these factors may constitute important control mechanisms in degradation and resynthesis of cardiac phospholipids [6,19]. On the one hand, fatty acid binding protein (FABP), abundantly present in the cytoplasmic space of the cardiomyocyte, may regulate phospholipid formation by enhancing the flux of fatty acyl moieties to the site of phospholipid biosynthesis; on the other hand, FABP might be involved in the regulation of the rate of phospholipid hydrolysis by removing fatty acyl moieties from the site of production, thereby mitigating the proposed feedback inhibition of fatty acids on phospholipid-hydrolyzing activity [6,22]. Another class of nonenzymatic proteins, that might be involved in phospholipid homeostasis, is the family of annexins. Members of this family show high affinity to negatively charged phospholipids, that are predominantly present in the inner leaflet of the plasmalemma. Ca^{2+} was found to be involved in the interaction between annexins and membrane phospholipids. In vitro studies have indicated that one member of the family, annexin V, mitigates Ca^{2+} induced phospholipid hydrolysis [19]. This annexin, which is present in cardiac tissue, might play a role in the regulation of the turnover of cardiac membrane phospholipids. The precise mode of action, however, remains to be elucidated. It is unknown whether the heart contains nonenzymatic proteins, which are directly involved in the stimulation of phospholipid degradation. The presence of a recently discovered protein, referred to as phospholipase-activating protein (PLAP) [23], that is functionally related to mellitin and which possesses phospholipase A_2 activating properties, remains to be established in the heart.

The energy status of the cell obviously plays a role in the maintenance of cardiac phospholipid homeostasis. Low cellular ATP levels will hamper the ATP-dependent conversion of fatty acids into fatty acyl CoA, a reaction catalyzed by acyl CoA synthetase. Fatty acyl CoA serves as the intermediate for the incorporation of fatty acyl moieties into phospholipids. In the normoxic cell, endogenous ATP levels are appreciably higher than the affinity constant of acyl CoA synthetase for ATP [6,24]. Hence, it is very unlikely that ATP will modulate the rate of phospholipid synthesis in normal conditions. This situation may dramatically change in ischemic cells (see later). Recent studies performed by Gross and coworkers [8,25] have revealed the presence of a plasmalogen-specific phospholipase A_2 in cardiac structures. This cytoplasmic Ca^{2+}-independent phospholipid-hydrolyzing enzyme was found to be highly sensitive to ATP, suggesting a potential role of the energy state of the cell in modulating the fatty acyl composition of plasmalogen phospholipids and, hence, the chemical and physical properties of the cellular membrane.

Hormones such as norepinephrine and glucagon, when included in the perfusion medium, enhance the release of lysophospholipids from isolated rat hearts [6]. Bradykinin was found to stimulate the release of arachidonic acid, a fatty acid predominantly localized at the Sn_2 position of membrane phospholipids [6]. These findings indicate that hormonal regulation of phospholipid hydrolysis in cardiac structures has to be considered. The mechanism underlying hormone-induced degradation of phospholipids has not been completely elucidated. Cytoplasmic cAMP might play an intermediary role. This second messenger is supposed to promote direct phosphorylation of phospholipases or of a cellular protein with phospholipase-activating properties. Cyclic AMP may also enhance the cytoplasmic concentration of Ca^{2+} and, hence, the rate of phospholipid degradation. These hypothetical explanations await further experimental proof.

Feedback inhibition of phospholipases by high levels of fatty acids has been proposed to be a regulatory mechanism in the turnover of the cardiac phospholipid pool. Since under normal conditions, tissue fatty acid levels are extremely low (30–50 nmol/g wet weight in dog hearts in situ) [26], it remains uncertain whether this type of regulation contributes significantly to overall phospholipid turnover. The finding that phospholipid hydrolysis in freeze-thawed tissue kept under anoxic conditions was not inhibited, while the fatty acid content increased to 10 µmol/g wet weight [27], also argues against feedback inhibition of phospholipases by high levels of endogenous fatty acids.

Physicochemical alterations in cellular membranes may render the phospholipid components more or less vulnerable to the attack of phospholipid-hydrolyzing enzymes. The nature of these alterations may be multiple: changes in fluidity and packing of lipid building blocks in the membrane, phase separation (the coexistence of liquid and solid phases), and accumulation of biological detergents. In addition, peroxidation of long chain polyunsaturated fatty acyl chains by oxygen free radicals may create conditions favorable for enhanced degradation of membrane phospholipids.

It should be kept in mind that the aforementioned potential regulating factors and mechanisms will result in an equilibration between phospholipid degradation and resynthesis in the normal heart. Under pathophysiological conditions, such as ischemia and reperfusion, the imbalance between breakdown and resynthesis might play a critical role in the sequela of events resulting in the loss of cell viability.

Phospholipid Homeostasis in the Ischemic and Reperfused Heart

Impaired perfusion of the coronary system causes an insufficient supply of molecular oxygen to cardiac cells to maintain energy conversion at an appropriate level, and accumulation of waste products in the affected cells. Shortage of oxygen forces cardiac metabolism to shift from aerobic to anaerobic metabolism. Lactate is produced in appreciable amounts and phosphocreatine levels fall dramatically, followed by a gradual decline in tissue ATP. Ion balances become disturbed and macromolecules start to leak from the cytoplasmic space into the extracellular compartment. Most investigators consider leakage of macromolecules (soluble proteins from the cytoplasm) as the definitive sign of loss of cellular viability, although some loss of proteins from reversibly damaged cells cannot be excluded. Interestingly, there exists a notable cell-to-cell difference with respect to the time interval between the onset of ischemia and the loss of cytoplasmic proteins. In general, significant numbers of cardiomyocytes start to lose their viability after 30 min of severe ischemia [6]. Irreversible cellular injury is thought to be associated with seriously damaged cellular membranes. Since cellular membranes are composed of phospholipids, cholesterol and proteins, alterations in membrane phospholipids or their loss might be a critical event in the onset of cell death. Both chemical and physical perturbations, separately or in concert, in membrane phospholipid homeostasis might lead to loss of the semipermeable properties of the membranes.

Loss of phospholipids from cellular membranes is caused by either extrusion of lipid material from the affected membrane or by an imbalance between phospholipid hydrolysis and resynthesis. Possible alterations in the activity of enzymes involved in hydrolysis and resynthesis in the ischemic/reperfused heart will be discussed later, since it is assumed that disturbed phospholipid turnover might play a critical role in the loss of cell membrane integrity.

Loss of Membrane Phospholipids in the Ischemic and Reperfused Heart

Evidence is accumulating that degradation of membrane phospholipids occurs in ischemic tissue [6]. In addition, the release of degradation products of phospholipid hydrolysis correlated very closely with the time course of the development of loss of cellular viability of the ischemic cell [28].

Pioneering studies of Weglicki and colleagues [29] showed that significant amounts of arachidonic acid, a sensitive indicator of phospholipid hydrolysis, are released from isolated blood-perfused dog hearts, rendered ischemic for 30 min. Later studies indicated that this fatty acid accumulates predominantly in the most severely affected area of the ischemic left ventricle, i.e., the subendocardial layers [26,30]. Arachidonic acid starts to accumulate approximately 20–30 min after the onset of ischemia [24,31]. Enhanced levels of other degradation products of phospholipid hydrolysis, such as lysophospholipids, have also been observed in flow-deprived tissue [24,32,33]. In a variety of studies the total phospholipid pool was found to be decreased [6]. The latter observation was made in long-term ischemic tissue and appeared to be confined to phosphatidylcholine and phosphatidylethanolamine [31,34].

Information on the specific (intra)cellular site of membrane phospholipid hydrolysis and accumulation of degradation products is scarce. Loss of phospholipid material from mitochondria in ischemic regions of the heart has been reported by Yanagishita and colleagues [35] and Kajiyama and associates [36]. The phospholipid content of the sarcoplasmic reticulum was also found to be decreased. Interestingly, Suyatna and coworkers [37] failed to detect a change in the phospholipid and lysophospholipid content in sarcolemmal preparations obtained from rat heart rendered ischemic for 60 min.

Experimental findings suggest that restoration of flow to the ischemic heart results in additional damage inflicted upon cells weakened during the preceding period of flow deprivation [2]. A variety of studies indicate that restoration of flow is accompanied by (further) loss of tissue phospholipids [38,39]. Investigations performed in our laboratory on dog and rat hearts [24,40] revealed a significant additional accumulation of arachidonic acid in the previously ischemic myocardium after the onset of reperfusion. In isolated rat heart preparations, post-ischemic arachidonic accumulation correlated with the release of the cytoplasmic enzyme lactate dehydrogenase [24]. The (sub)-cellular site of phospholipid degradation and arachidonic accumulation is uncertain. The phospholipid content in a sarcolemmal preparation isolated from rat hearts rendered ischemic for 60 min followed by 30 min of reperfusion, did not change [41]. Mitochondrial phospholipid content was only affected in hearts suffering from fibrillation during the reperfusion period following 15 min of ischemia [42].

These findings lead to at least two fundamental questions. First, which mechanisms underlie ischemia- and reperfusion-induced loss of membrane phospholipids? Second, is phospholipid degradation the critical step in the transition from reversible to irreversible damage? As discussed in the next section, these questions are closely related.

Putative Mechanisms Underlying Ischemia- and Reperfusion-Induced Alterations of Membrane Phospholipids

Net loss of membrane phospholipids can be caused by either enhanced hydrolysis of phospholipids or impaired resynthesis of these building blocks of cellular membranes, or both. As indicated in Fig. 2, synthesis of phospholipids may occur via reacylation of lysophospholipids or de novo synthesis of phospholipids with diacylglycerol as intermediate. Both pathways are energy-dependent. De novo synthesis of phospholipids requires, among others CTP, a high-energy phosphate compound, the concentration of which is probably reduced during prolonged ischemia [6]. Indeed, recent studies performed on isolated hypoxic rat hearts indicated that the de novo synthesis of phosphatidylcholine was impaired [43]. Reacylation of lysophospholipids requires ATP for the conversion of fatty acids into acyl CoA moieties. It is rather unlikely that the decline of cellular ATP, readily observed in ischemic cardiac tissue and preceding the accumulation of arachidonic acid, is the sole cause of impaired reacylation of phospholipids, since the affinity of acyl CoA synthetase for ATP is relatively high. Accumulation of ATP degradation products such as AMP and adenosine might be more important factors in depressing reacylation of lysophospholipids, as they were found to be potent inhibitors of acyl CoA synthetase [6,24]. In this regard, the finding that loss of ATP is not a decisive factor in net degradation of membrane phospholipids in neonatal cardiomyocytes is worthy to note [44].

The activity of one of the key enzymes in the reacylation pathway, i.e., lysophosphatidylcholine acyl transferase, was found to be depressed in tissue preparations made from ischemic pig heart [39,45]. This finding supports the notion that in the ischemic heart (part of) the loss of phospholipids can be explained by disturbed resynthesis of these compounds, and strongly suggests that either the configuration and, hence, the activity of the enzyme is permanently modified during the ischemic attack, or an endogenous inhibitor

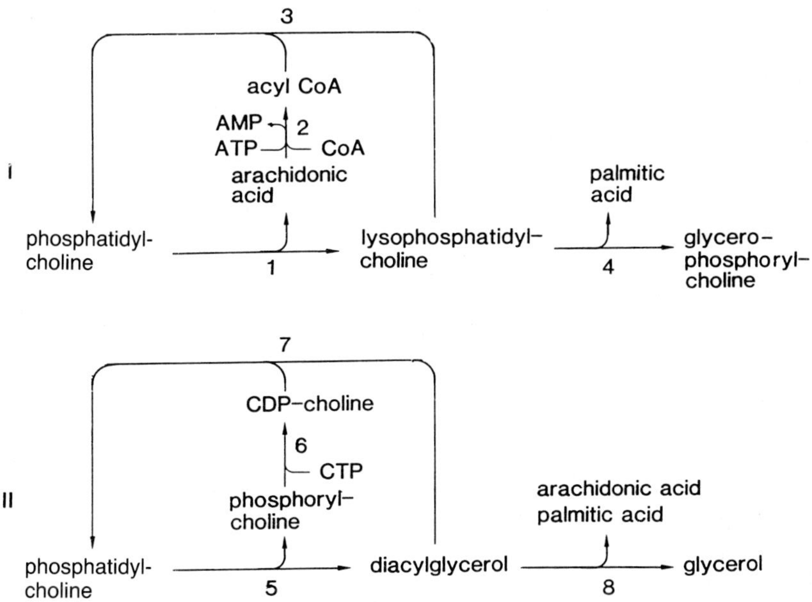

Fig. 2. Schematic representation of degradation and synthesis of phosphatidylcholine. Pathway I: deacylation-reacylation pathway; pathway II: turnover of the hydrophilic headgroup phosphorylcholine. Numbers refer to enzymes involved: *1*, phospholipase A_2; *2*, acyl-CoA synthetase; *3*, lysophosphatidylcholine acyltransferase; *4*, lyosphospholipase; *5*, phospholipase C; *6*, CTD: phosphocholine cytidylyltransferase; *7*, phosphocholine transferase; *8*, diacylglycerol, monoacylglycerol lipases. (From [6], with permission)

is not removed by the homogenization procedure. Because this enzyme is sulfydryl-sensitive, loss of activity may be related to the oxidative conversion of glutathione into glutathione disulfide during the ischemic insult [36]. It is uncertain whether, during reperfusion, ATP and its degradation products, AMP and adenosine, negatively influence the capacity of the heart to convert fatty acids to acyl CoA, a critical step in the reacylation pathway. In general, tissue ATP levels increase and the cellular content of AMP and adenosine falls after reinstallation of flow [46].

Net loss of phospholipids and accumulation of hydrolytic products such as lysophospholipids and arachidonic acid in flow-deprived cardiac tissue, can also be caused by enhanced hydrolysis of phospholipids. Antibodies raised against phospholipase A_2 were found to be effective in preventing ischemia- and reperfusion-induced damage in isolated rat hearts [47]. Besides, a host of drugs with putative antiphospholipase A_2 blocking properties were able to prevent phospholipid degradation and the accumulation of arachidonic acid in ischemic and reperfused hearts [48]. These studies provide circumstantial evidence that phospholipase activity is involved in the loss of phospholipids in flow-deprived and reperfused cardiac structures.

No definitive explanation is yet available for the mechanism(s) underlying ischemia- and reperfusion-induced hydrolysis of cardiac membrane phospholipids. To understand the increased hydrolysis of membrane phospholipids, all aspects of cardiac phospholipid homeostasis have to be included. As pointed out earlier, beside differences in phospholipid composition of cellular and intracellular membranes, a variety of endogenous enzymes with phospholipid-hydrolyzing properties have been identified in the cardiac cell. In vitro studies have provided some clues as to how the hydrolytic activity of these enzymes might be regulated. It is basically unknown whether test tube results can be extrapolated to the ischemic and reperfused myocardium without introducing heuristic errors.

Attempts to provide evidence that the activity of endogenous phospholipases is increased in flow-deprived tissue and reperfused tissue have led to conflicting observations [6]. The activity of phospholipase A_2 was found to be depressed in homogenates and subcellular fractions of ischemic rat hearts [49], indicating the presence of intrinsic measures to protect the heart against endogenous phospholipase activity. Comparable findings were reported on phospholipase C [50]. Enhanced activity of phospholipase A_2 was obtained in membrane fractions harvested from ischemic and reperfused pig myocardium [39]. Recently, a plasmalogen-specific phospholipase A_2 was identified in cardiac tissue [51]. The activity of this Ca^{2+}-insensitive enzyme was found to be enhanced in heart tissue preparations within 2 min after the onset of ischemia. Interestingly, the enzymatic activity returned to normal values after restoration of flow. At present it is unknown which factors are responsible for the change in enzymatic activity that persists after preparing subcellular fractions of the affected hearts. In addition to permanent changes in the activity of the enzymes, changes in the microenvironment of the proteins with hydrolytic activity have to be considered.

Changes in the microenvironment of phospholipases, eventually resulting in a higher rate of phospholipid hydrolysis, may be multiple. On the one hand those changes may directly affect the enzyme-protein. On the other hand, alterations in the chemical and physical properties of the phospholipid membranes may render the membranes more sensitive to attack by phospholipid-hydrolyzing enzymes. Increased intracellular levels of cations such as H^+ and Ca^{2+} may activate endogenous phospholipases. In particular, lysosomal lipases were found to be highly sensitive to a decrease in intracellular pH, whereas part of the cardiac phospholipase activity is Ca^{2+}-sensitive. It is still a matter of debate whether the increase in intracellular Ca^{2+} in a reversibly damaged cell is sufficiently high to provoke a substantial rise in phospholipase activity. The decline in ATP levels in tissue subjected to prolonged ischemia probably counteracts in situ the rise of plasmalogen-specific phospholipase A_2, as observed in subcellular preparations [25], because the activity of this type of phospholipase A_2 is highly dependent on ATP.

Upon reperfusion of previously ischemic hearts, intracellular conditions may dramatically change, resulting in activation of endogenous phospholipase activity. On the one hand, intracellular Ca^{2+} overload may trigger some types of phospholipases to attack membrane phospholipids more vigorously [6], while peroxidation of fatty acyl chains in membrane phospholipids may make these and/or neighboring phospholipids a target for endogenous phospholipases [52]. According to the "free radical-triggered lipolysis by phospholipases" theory, membrane phospholipids are peroxidized by highly active oxygen free radicals, abundantly generated in cardiac tissue affter restoration of flow.

In addition to peroxidative alterations of membrane phospholipids, physical changes in cardiac membranes may render the phospholipid building blocks more susceptible to the activity of endogenous phospholipases. Typical ultrastructural changes in membrane structures in ischemic cardiac tissue have been reported. Short-term ischemia (up to 30 min of oxygen depletion) results in the reorganization of mitochondrial membranes [53,54]. Membrane vesicles were formed and electron-dense bands of stacked cristae became evident. When the duration of ischemia was prolonged to 60 min, the reorganization of mitochondrial membranes resulted in multilamellar vesicles and the sarcolemma-glycocalyx complex started to disrupt. In addition, intramembrane particles were aggregating, the sarcolemma appeared to separate from the cytoskeleton, and lipid-containing blebs were extruded from the sarcolemma [54]. Ultrastructural changes in the sarcolemma were also observed in reperfused cardiac tissue [53]. The formation of multilamellar vesicles in the sarcolemma was generally enhanced when flow was restored in rabbit hearts rendered ischemic for 60 min [53].

The typical ultrastructural changes in cardiac membranes may be caused by a variety of factors. First, loss of phospholipid asymmetry may destabilize both mitochondrial membranes and sarcolemma. Since asymmetry is maintained by the activity of an ATP-dependent phospholipid translocase, low cytoplasmic ATP levels may cause scrambling of phospholipids over the inner and outer leaflets of the lipid bilayer. Second, there may be separation of cytoskeleton and plasmalemma due to either enzymatic degradation of protein components of the cytoskeleton or reduced capability of the membrane phospholipids or membrane protein to interact with the cytoskeleton. Third, enhanced intracellular levels of H^+ and Ca^{2+} may cause phase transition of phosphatidylethanolamine (PE) moieties in the sarcolemma [55]. PE molecules tend to adopt hexagonal structures. Under physiological conditions, this tendency is suppressed by the presence of other phospholipid moieties in biological membranes, resulting in the formation of lipid bilayers. However, acidification of the intracellular compartment (ischemia) and enhanced levels of Ca^{2+} (ischemia and in particular during reperfusion) will readily lead to a lateral phase transition in biological membranes and to the formation of hexagonal structures [55]. These ultrastructural changes may add to membrane destabilization, and ultimately to irreversible loss of cellular integrity [6,55]. Although definite proof is lacking, it is tempting to state that lateral phase transition, extrusion of lipid material from membranes, and the formation of multilamellar vesicles will render the membrane phospholipids more susceptible to hydrolysis by endogenous phospholipases.

Although it is evident that phospholipid degradation is a hallmark of myocardial ischemia and reperfusion, it is still a matter of debate whether enzymatic hydrolysis of membrane phospholipids is a key event in the transition from reversible to irreversible cellular damage [56]. Earlier-mentioned studies performed with antibodies against phospholipase A_2 [46] strongly suggest that phospholipase A_2-mediated degradation of membrane phospholipids sets the stage for irrepairable loss of cellular integrity. Other studies [57] indicate that phospholipid hydrolysis is a late phenomenon, probably reflecting enzymatic digestion of membrane fragments of severely injured cells. Experiments performed in our laboratory support the notion that accumulation of arachidonic acid (a measure of phospholipid hydrolysis) occurs in a small number of heavily damaged cardiomyocytes [24]. More detailed experimental studies are necessary to provide a definite answer to the question as to the precise role of enzymatic phospholipid degradation in ischemia- and reperfusion-induced damage of cardiac tissue.

Acknowledgments. This study was supported by grants from the Netherlands Heart Foundation (NHS grant no. 89.213) and the Netherlands Organization for Scientific Research (NWO grant no. 900.516.126). The authors are greatly indebted to Mrs. Claire Bollen and Emmy van Roosmalen for their invaluable help in preparing the manuscript.

References

1. Van der Vusse GJ, van Bilsen M, Sonderkamp T, Reneman RS (1990) Hydrolysis of phospholipids and cellular integrity. In: Piper HM (ed) Pathophysiology of severe ischemic myocardial injury. Dordrecht, Kluwer, pp 167–193
2. Kloner RA, Przyklenk K (1992) Reperfusion injury to the heart. Is it a phenomenon? In: Acosta D Jr (ed) Cardiovascular toxicology. Raven, New York, pp 131–140
3. Anversa P, Olivetti G, Melissari M, Lound AV (1980) Sterological measurements of cellular and subcellular hypertrophy and hyperplasia in the papillary muscle of adult rat. J Mol Cell Cardiol 12:781–795
4. Achari A, Scott D, Garlow P, Vidal JC, Otwinowski A, Brunie S, Sigler PB (1987) Facing up to membranes: structure/function relationship in phospholipases. Cold Spring Harbor Symp. Quant Biol 52:441–452
5. Post JA, Langer GA, Op den Kamp JAF, Verkleij AJ (1988) Phospholipid asymmetry in cardiac sarcolemma. Analysis of intact cells and gas-dissected membranes. Biochim Biophys Acta 943:256–266
6. Van der Vusse GJ, Glatz JFC, Stam HCG, Reneman RS (1992) Fatty acid homeostasis in the normoxic and ischemic heart. Physiol Rev 72:881–940

7. Arthur G, Covic L, Wientzek M, Choy PC (1985) Plasmalogenase in hamster heart. Biochim Biophys Acta 833:189–195
8. Hazen SL, Ford DA, Gross RW (1991) Activation of a membrane associated phospholipase A_2 during rabbit myocardial ischemia which is highly selective for plasmalogen substrate. J Biol Chem 266:5629–5633
9. Chanon JY, Leslie CC (1990) A calcium-dependent mechanism for associating a soluble arachidonoyl-hydrolyzing phospholipase A_2 with membrane in the macrophage cell line RAW 264.7. J Biol Chem 265:5409–5413
10. Wolf RA (1989) Cardiolipin-sensitive phospholipase C in subcellular fractions of rabbit myocardium. Am J Physiol 257:C926–C935
11. Lindmar RR, Löffelholz K, Sandman J (1988) On the mechanism of muscarinic hydrolysis of choline phospholipids in the heart. Biochem Pharmacol 37:4689–4695
12. Wirtz KWA, Gadella TWJ (1990) Properties and modes of action of specific and non-specific phospholipid transfer proteins. Experientia 46:592–599
13. Arthur G, Choy PC (1984) Acyl specificity of hamster heart CDPcholine: 1,2-diacylglycerol phosphocholine transferase in phosphatidylcholine biosynthesis. Biochim Biophys Acta 795:221–229
14. Arthur G, Mock T, Zaborniak C, Choy PC (1985) The distribution and acyl composition of plasmalogens in guinea pig heart. Lipids 20:693–698
15. Arthur G, Page L, Mock T, Choy PC (1986) The catabolism of plasmenylcholine in guinea pig heart. Biochem J 236:475–480
16. Arthur G, Page L, Zaborniak C, Choy PC (1987) The acylation of lysophosphatidylglycerocholines in guinea pig heart mitochondria. Biochem J 242:171–175
17. Choy PC, Man RYK, Chan AC (1989) Phosphatidyl-choline metabolism in isolated rat heart: modulation by ethanol and vitamin E. Biochim Biophys Acta 1005:225–232
18. Mock T, Slater TL, Arthur G, Chan AC, Choy PC (1986) Effects of fatty acids on phosphatidylcholine biosynthesis in isolated hamster heart. Biochem Cell Biol 64: 413–417
19. Van Bilsen M, Reutelingsperger CPM, Willemsen PHM, Reneman RS, van der Vusse GJ (1992) Annexins in cardiac tissue: cellular localization and effect on phospholipase activity. Mol Cell Biochem 116:95–101
20. Chan AC, Fragiskos B, Douglas CE, Choy PC (1985) Increased arachidonate incorporation in perfused heart phospholipids from vitamin E-deficient rats. Lipids 20:328–330
21. Chien KR, Han A, Sen A, Buja LM, Willerson TJ (1984) Accumulation of unesterified arachidonic acid in ischemic canine myocardium. Circ Res 54:313–322
21. Hatch GM, Owaga K, Choy PC (1989) Regulation of phosphatidylcholine metabolism in mammalian hearts. Biochem Cell Biol 67:67–77
22. Glatz JFC, van der Vusse GJ (1990) Cellular fatty acid-binding proteins: current concepts and future directions. Mol Cell Biochem 98:247–251
23. Clark MA, Conway TM, Shorr RGL, Crooke ST (1987) Identification and isolation of a mammalian protein which is antigenically and functionally related to the phospholipase A_2 stimulatory peptide mellitin. J Biol Chem 262:4402–4406
24. Van Bilsen M, van der Vusse GJ, Willemsen PHM, Coumans WA, van der Vusse GJ, Reneman RS (1989) Lipid alterations in isolated, working rat hearts during ischemia and reperfusion: Its relation to myocardial damage. Circ Res 64:304–314
25. Hazen SL, Gross RW (1991) ATP-dependent regulation of rabbit myocardial cytosolic calcium-independent phospholipase A_2. J Biol Chem 266:14526–14534

26. Van der Vusse GJ, Roemen THM, Prinzen FW, Coumans WA, Reneman RS (1982) Uptake and tissue content of fatty acids in dog myocardium under normoxic and ischemic conditions. Circ Res 50:538–546
27. Van der Vusse GJ, de Groot MJM, Willemsen PHM, van Bilsen M, Schrijvers AHGJ, Reneman RS (1989) Degradation of phospholipids and triacylglycerol, and accumulation of fatty acids in anoxic myocardial tissue, disrupted by freeze-thawing. Mol Cell Biochem 88:83–90
28. Chien KR, Engler R (1990) Calcium and ischemic myocardial injury. In: Langer GA (ed) Calcium and the heart. Raven, New York, pp 333–354
29. Weglicki WB, Owens K, Urschel CW, Serur JR, Sonnenblick EH (1973) Hydrolysis of myocardial lipids during acidosis and ischemia. Rec Adv Stud Cardiac Struct Metab 3:781–793
30. Prinzen FW, van der Vusse GJ, Arts T, Roemen THM, Coumans WA, Reneman RS (1984) Accumulation of nonesterified fatty acids in ischemic canine myocardium. Am J Physiol 247:H264–H272
32. Corr PB, Yamada KA, Creer MH, Sharma AD, Sobel BE (1987) Lysophosphoglycerides and ventricular fibrillation early after onset of ischemia. J Mol Cell Cardiol 19[Suppl V]:45–53
33. Shaikh NA, Downar E (1981) Time course of changes in porcine myocardial phospholipid levels during ischemia. Circ Res 49:316–325
34. Chien KR, Reeves JP, Buja LM, Parkey RW, Willerson JT (1981) Phospholipid alterations in canine ischemic myocardium. Circ Res 48:711–719
35. Yanagishita T, Konno N, Goshi E, Katagiri T (1987) Alterations in phospholipids in acute ischemic myocardium. Jpn Circ J 5:41–50
36. Kajiyama KJ, Pauly DF, Hughes H, Yoon SB, Entman ML, McMillin-Wood JB (1987) Protection by verapamil of mitochondrial glutathione equilibrium and phospholipid changes during reperfusion of ischemic canine myocardium. Circ Res 61:301–310
37. Suyatna FD, van Veldhoven PP, Borgers M, Mannaerts GP (1988) Phospholipid composition and amphiphile content of isolated sarcolemma from normal and autolytic rat myocardium. J Mol Cell Cardiol 20:47–62
38. Burton KP, Buja LM, Sen A, Willerson JT, Chien KR (1986) Accumulation of arachidonate in triacylglycerols and unesterified fatty acids during ischemia and reflow in the isolated rat heart. Correlation with the loss of contractile function and the development of calcium overload. Am J Pathol 124:238–245
39. Das DK, Engelman RM, Rousou JA, Breyer RH, Otani H, Lemeshow S (1986) Role of membrane phospholipids in myocardial injury induced by ischemia and reperfusion. Am J Physiol 251:H71–H79
40. Van der Vusse GJ, Prinzen FW, Reneman RS (1987) Disturbances in myocardial lipid homeostasis during ischemia and reperfusion. In: Sideman S, Beyar R (eds) Activation, metabolism and reperfusion of the heart. Simulation and experimental models. M Nijhoff, Dordrecht, pp 665–682
41. Bester R, Lochner A (1988) Sarcolemmal phospholipid fatty acid composition and permeability. Biochim Biophys Acta 941:176–186
42. Hattori M, Owaga K, Satake T, Sugiyama S, Ozawa T (1985) Depletion of membrane phospholipid and mitochondrial dysfunction associated with coronary reperfusion. Basic Res Cardiol 80:241–250
43. Lochner A, De Villiers M (1989) Phosphatidylcholine biosynthesis in myocardial ischaemia. J Mol Cell Cardiol 21:151–163

44. Jones RL, Miller JC, Hagler HK, Chien KR, Willerson JT, Buja LM (1989) Association between inhibition of arachidonic acid release and prevention of calcium loading during ATP depletion in cultured rat cardiac myocytes. Am J Pathol 135:541–556
45. Otani H, Engelman RM, Breyer RH, Rousou JA, Lemeshow S (1986) Mepacrine, a phospholipase inhibitor. J Thorac Cardiovasc Surg 92:247–254
46. Van Bilsen M, van der Vusse GJ, Coumans WA, de Groot MJM, Willemsen PHM, Reneman RS (1989) Degradation of adenine nucleotides in ischemic and reperfused rat heart. Am J Physiol 257:H47–H54
47. Prasad RM, Popescu LM, Moraru II, Liu X, Maity S, Engelman RM, Das DP (1991) Role of phospholipases A_2 and C in myocardial ischemic reperfusion injury. Am J Physiol 260:H877–H883
48. Van der Vusse GJ, Reneman RS (1992) Protection of the ischemic heart: a possible role for phospholipase inhibitors? Circ Control 13:357–372
49. Bentham JM, Higgins AJ, Woodward B (1987) The effects of ischaemia, lysophosphatidylcholine and palmitoylcarnitine on rat heart phospholipase A_2 activity. Basic Res Cardiol 82[Suppl II]:127–137
50. Schwertz D, Halverson J, Isaacson T, Feinberg H, Palmer JW (1987) Alterations in phospholipid metabolism in the globally ischemic rat heart: emphasis on phosphoinositide specific phospholipase C activity. J Mol Cell Cardiol 19:685–697
51. Gross RW (1992) Myocardial phospholipases A_2 and their membrane substrates. Trends Cardiovasc Med 2:115–121
52. Weglicki WB, Low MG (1987) Phospholipases of the myocardium. Basic Res Cardiol 82[Suppl I]:107–112
53. Schrijvers AHGJ, de Groot MJM, Heynen VVTh, van der Vusse GJ, Frederik PM, Reneman RS (1990) Ischemia and reperfusion induced multilamellar vesicles in isolated rabbit hearts: Time correlation between morphometric data and metabolic alterations. J Mol Cell Cardiol 22:653–665
54. Musters RJ Ph, Post JA, Verkleij AJ (1991) The isolated neonatal rat cardiomyocyte used in an in vitro model for ischemia. I. A morphological study. Biochim Biophys Acta 1091:270–277
55. Verkleij AJ, Post JA (1987) Physico-chemical properties and organization of lipids in membranes: their possible role in myocardial injury. Basic Res Cardiol 82[Suppl I]:85–91
56. Van der Vusse GJ, van Bilsen M, Reneman RS (1989) Is phospholipid degradation a critical event in ischemia- and reperfusion-induced damage? News Physiol Sci 4:49–53
57. Steenbergen C, Jennings RB (1984) Relationship between lysophospholipid accumulation and plasma membrane injury during total in vitro ischemia in dog heart. J Mol Cell Cardiol 16:605–621

1.9 Reperfusion Injury in Patients with Acute Myocardial Infarction

Plasma Free-Radical Scavenger Activity Is a Factor Involved in Reducing the Infarct Size Following Successful Reperfusion

Kazuhisa Kodama and Atsushi Hirayama[1]

Summary. It has been shown in the clinical situation that the infarct size varies in patients with acute myocardial infarction after successful reperfusion, even if the factors determining the infarct size, i.e., area at risk, time from onset to reperfusion, or collaterals at the onset, were the same. The reasons for this variability remain unknown. In this study, we attempted to clarify one such reason. A group of 68 patients with first anterior acute myocardial infarction with successful reperfusion was divided into three subgroups according to the infarct size in proportion to time from the onset to reperfusion: the "large" group (n = 24), the "standard" group (n = 18), and the "small" group (n = 26). There were no significant differences among the three groups in patients' characteristics, the area at risk, time from onset to reperfusion, and collateral grade at the initial angiography. The infarct size (mean ± SE) determined by thallium-201 single photon emission computed tomography (SPECT) of the large group (1479 ± 106 units) was significantly greater than that of both the small group (323 ± 74 units) and the standard group (735 ± 117). Significant difference was observed among the three groups in the plasma free-radical scavenger activity, one of the factors involved in determining the infarct size: the plasma free-radical scavenger activity in the large group (24.1 ± 0.7 NU/l) was significantly lower than that of both the standard group (27.0 ± 1.0 NU/l) and the small group (29.9 ± 1.3 NU/l). These results suggested that the biological free-radical scavenger system prevented the myocardial reperfusion injury caused by the free-radical generation at the time of reperfusion, thereby reducing the infarct size. The variations in infarct size in the clinical situation might reflect the individual differences in the free-radical scavenger activities.

Key words: Acute myocardial infarction—Infarct size—Reperfusion injury—Free radical—Reperfusion therapy

---

[1] Cardiovascular Division, Osaka Police Hospital, 10-31 Kitayama-cho, Tennoji-ku, Osaka, 543 Japan

Introduction

Reperfusion of the occluded coronary artery by either thrombolysis or percutaneous coronary angioplasty in the early period of myocardial infarction has been shown to reduce the infarct size and preserve left ventricular function [1–5]. There is also evidence to suggest that this beneficial effect might be blunted because reperfusion, while terminating ischemia, may also cause further damage to jeopatdized cells [6–8]. This adverse effect of reperfusion, known as myocardial reperfusion injury, has been shown to be prevented by the administration of agents having free-radical scavenging activity [9,10] or by preventing the generation of free radicals [11,12] in animal models. These experimental results suggested that free radicals generated at the time of reperfusion played the major role in myocardial reperfusion injury [8]. However, myocardial reperfusion injury has not been demonstrated in patients receiving reperfusion therapy [13]. One of the major problems leading to the failure to demonstrate myocardial reperfusion injury is the difficulty in the standardization of the major factors believed to influence the infarct size; for example, the area at risk of myocardial infarction [14], collaterals present at the onset of infarction [15,16], time to reperfusion from onset [17], and so on. Furthermore, our previous study [18] showed that plasma free-radical scavenger activity was one of the factors affecting the infarct size, and was independent from the other factors.

In this study, we selected patients so as to standardize the area at risk, the time to reperfusion from onset, and collaterals. There was still some variation in the infarct size among the patients after standardizing these factors. With this group of patients, we studied the relation between plasma free-radical scavenger activity and infarct size and discussed the significance of this relation for patients receiving reperfusion therapy.

Materials and Methods

Patient Selection

Patients were selected from 121 consecutive patients who were admitted to the coronary care unit of the Osaka Police Hospital during an 8-year period with acute myocardial infarction less than 6 h from onset. Inclusion criteria were: (1) the presence of persistent ST segment elevation of 0.2 mV or greater in two or more leads on the standard 12-lead electrocardiogram, and severe chest pain lasting more than 30 min; (2) under 80 years of age; (3) no prior history of myocardial infarction; and (4) absence of cardiomyopathy, severe valvular disease, ventricular septal defect, or cardiogenic shock (systolic pressure <80 mmHg). Patients with the following conditions were excluded: severe untreated hypertension; perfusion state of the infarct-related artery exceeded thrombolysis in myocardial infarction (TIMI) grade 1 at the initial angiography performed during the study; extension of infarction observed during the study; and finally, reocclusion of the infarct-related vessel demonstrated by angiography performed during the chronic phase. Ultimately, 68 patients were admitted to the study.

Cardiac Catheterization

After obtaining informed consent, coronary angiography was performed by the Judkins technique [19]. After baseline hemodynamic measurement, right and left coronary angiograms were recorded. Subsequently, thrombolysis with urokinase or tissue plasminogen activator according to the method described previously was attempted. If the occluded infarct-related vessel was recanalized with a perfusion status over TIMI grade 2, the procedure was judged successful. Patients with a perfusion status less than TIMI grade 2 at the completion of thrombolysis received coronary angioplasty. Finally, reperfusion of the infarct-related vessel was obtained in 68 patients. All patients were reexamined angiographically during the chronic phase (35 $\pm$ 28 days after onset; range 21–73 days; median 32 days).

Assessment of Left Ventriculography

Left ventriculography was performed with the patients in 30° right anterior oblique position using a power injection. The endocardial contours of the left ventricle at end-diastole and end-systole in left ventriculograms, obtained about one month after symptom onset, were traced by an observer who was unaware of clinical and coronary angiographic data on each patient. In 27 patients, left ventriculography was also performed after the completion of reperfusion therapy and analyzed by the procedure used in the chronic phase. Left ventricular volume was calculated by the area–length method [20] and was used to determine the ejection fraction. Regional wall motion was calculated by the centerline method [21], of which details were described previously [22]. Abnormality in wall motion was calculated by two approaches. First, the severity of hypokinesis in the infarct site was calculated as the mean of the chord lying in the hypokinetic area, and expressed as SD/chord. Second, the circumferential extent of hypokinesis was calculated as the set of contiguous chords whose motion was depressed more than 2 SD below the normal mean, and expressed as a percentage of the endocardial contour length.

Estimation of Infarct Size by Thallium-201 Single Photon Emission Computed Tomography (SPECT)

Myocardial tomograms were obtained about four weeks after the onset of myocardial infarction. SPECT was performed with a large field of view, rotating, single-crystal gamma camera (ZLC 7500, Shimadzu, Kyoto, Japan) equipped with a low-energy, high-resolution collimator and interfaced to the computer (Scintipack 70A, Shimadzu, Kyoto, Japan). Image acquisition commenced in the 30 × right anterior oblique projection approximately 3h after the injection of 5 mCi thallium-201. Thirty-two sequential images separated by 5.6° intervals were acquired over 180°. Data were stored on a 64 × 64 matrix for subsequent analysis. The size of myocardial infarct (defect volume) was assessed by the method previously described [22]. Briefly, the images of the left ventricle were sliced into six layers at equidistant intervals perpendicular to its long axis. The circumferential curve at each slice from a patient was compared with the corresponding slice from that of the normal data obtained previously from 60 subjects. Mean defect severity at each slice was determined by the area under the circumferential curve less than 2 standard deviations (SD) below normal. Defect volume was defined as the summation of the mean severity of the defect of each slice, and expressed in arbitrary units, representing the extent of damaged myocardium in the total left ventricle.

Subgroups

The patients were classified into three groups according to defect volume in proportion to the time to reperfusion from onset of myocardial infarction. There was a significant correlation between defect volume and time to reperfusion from the onset ($r^2 = 0.344$, $P = 0.0001$) as shown in Fig. 1 [23]. In Fig.

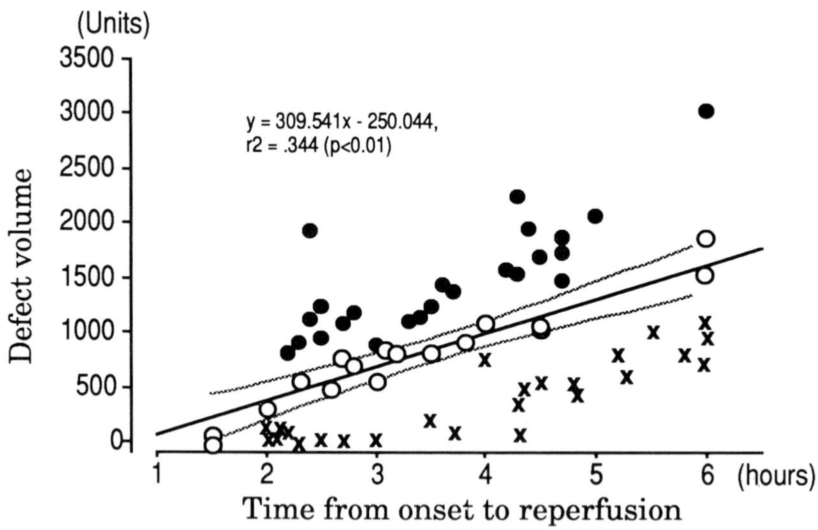

Fig. 1. Linear regression analysis of the relationship between the infarct size (*defect volume*) and time from onset to reperfusion. *Dotted line*, the 90% confidence range of the linear regression line. *Closed circles* located *above the upper dotted line* were classified as the "large" group. *Crosses* located *below the lower dotted line* were classified as the "small" group. *Open circles* located *between the dotted lines* were classified as the "standard" group

1, 24 patients located above the 90% confidence range of the linear regression line were classified as the "large" group; that is, their infarct size was great in proportion to the time to reperfusion from the onset. In contrast, 26 patients located below the 90% confidence range of the linear regression line were classified as the "small" group; that is, their infarct size was small in proportion to the time to reperfusion from the onset. Eighteen patients located within the 90% confidence range of the linear regression line formed the "standard" group; that is, their infarct size was proportional to the time to reperfusion from the onset.

Measurement of Plasma Free-Radical Scavenger Activity

A blood sample was taken into a tube containing heparin and then the plasma was separated by centrifugation. After recentrifugation was performed to remove red blood cells completely, the supernatant was mixed with Sepharose beads coated with anti superoxide dismutase monoclonal antibody, and centrifuged. After confirming that the concentration of superoxide dismutase in the supernatant was less than 0.1 pg/l, the supernatant was used for the measurement of plasma free radical scavenger activity. Plasma free-radical scavenger activity was measured by the modified nitrate method [24,25]. Briefly, the superoxide anion generated by xanthine and xanthine oxidase was measured by the nitrate. The serial dilution of plasma which inhibited the control reaction by 50% was used to define the plasma free-radical scavenger activity. The accuracy and reproducibility of this assay have already been demonstrated in the previous study [18].

Statistical Analysis

Data were expressed as the mean ± SE. Multiple comparisons among groups were performed by one-way analysis of variance combined with Scheffe's test. The chi-squared test or Fisher's exact test was used for analyzing categoric variables. Correlations were performed by linear regression analysis, computed by the least squares method. Results were considered significant at a probability value less than 0.05.

Results

Patient Characteristics

Table 1 shows that there were no significant differences between groups in age, gender, extent of coronary artery disease, the degree of collateral development at the inital angiographic examination, and the incidence of acute coronary angioplasty. The times to reperfusion from the onset in the large, standard, and small groups were 3.6 ± 0.2, 3.3 ± 0.3, and 3.6 ± 0.3 h, respectively, and

Table 1. Clinical and angiographic characterization of 68 patients according to infarct size.

Group	Small group	Standard group	Large group
Number of patients	26	18	24
Age (mean)	60	57	58
Gender (% male)	83	83	92
Time to reperfusion*	3.6 ± 0.3	3.3 ± 0.3	3.6 ± 0.2
Collateral (% good collateral)	15.4	16.7	8.3
Acute angioplasty (%)	19.2	16.7	33.3
Stenosis of the infarct-related vessel during the chronic phase	69 ± 6	69 ± 9	58 ± 7

* Interval from onset of chest pain to reperfusion (mean ± SE)

there were no significant differences among them. Hemodynamic variables on admission as well as in the chronic phase were comparable among the three groups (data not shown). The perfusion state of the infarct-related vessel was TIMI grade 3 in the three groups, and the degree of stenosis of the infarct-related vessel in the three groups did not significantly differ (Table 1).

In 27 patients, left ventriculography was performed during the acute stage: 8 patients in the small group, 9 patients in the standard group, and 10 patients in the large group. There were no significant differences in the clinical and angiographic characteristics between patients with and without paired left ventriculography (data not shown). The severity of the hypokinesis in the infarcted site during the acute phase in the large, the standard, and the small group was −4.19 ± 0.24, −4.28 ± 0.32, and −4.22 ± 0.14, respectively, and not significantly different. The circumferential extents of hypokinesis during the acute phase among the three groups were not significantly different (50% ± 2% in the large group, 51% ± 2% in the standard group, and 47% ± 3% in the small group).

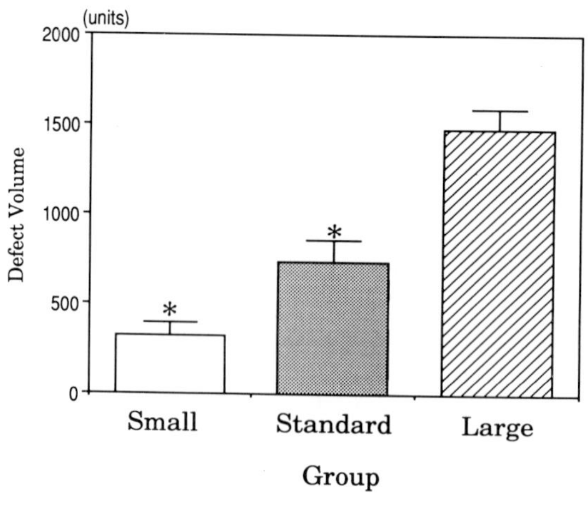

Fig. 2. Comparison of the defect volume among the small, the standard, and the large group. *, $P < 0.05$ *vs* the large group

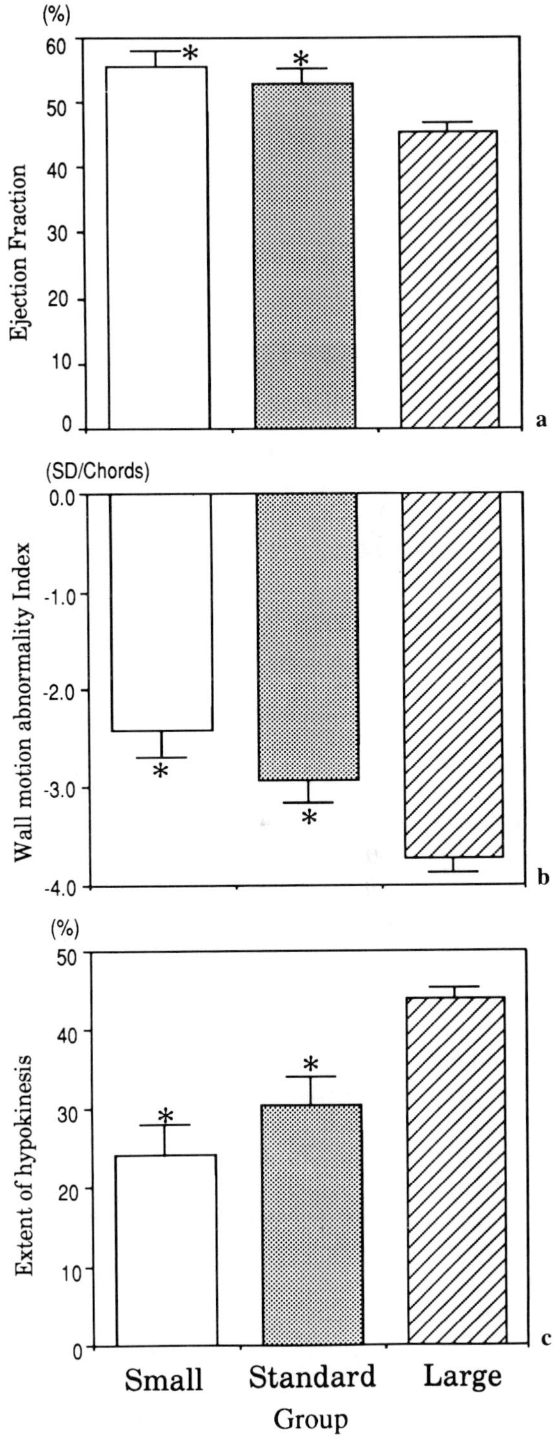

Fig. 3a–c. Comparison of the left ventricular function among the small, the standard, and the large groups. **a** Global ejection fraction; **b** wall motion abnormality index; **c** extent of hypokinesis. *, $P < 0.05$ *vs* the large group

Table 2. Clinical and angiographic characterization of patients, with or without measurement of plasma free-radical scavenger activity, according to infarct size.

Group	Small group		Standard group		Large group	
	With	Without	With	Wthout	With	Without
Number of patients	12	14	9	9	12	12
Age (mean)	58	60	56	60	54	58
Gender (% male)	83	86	78	89	92	75
Time to reperfusion*	3.7 ± 0.4	3.5 ± 0.4	3.1 ± 0.1	3.4 ± 0.6	3.8 ± 0.3	3.5 ± 0.4
Collateral (% good collateral)	12	14	22	11	8	8

* Interval from onset of chest pain to reperfusion (mean ± SE)

Infarct Size and Left Ventricular Function During the Chronic Phase

As shown in Fig. 2, the defect volume in the large group was 1479 ± 106 units and significantly larger than that of both the small group (735 ± 117 units) and the standard group (323 ± 74 units). The global ejection fraction (EF) in the large group (46% ± 1%) was inferior to that of both the standard group (53% ± 2%) and the small group (55% ± 2%), as shown in Fig. 3a. The same relations were observed in both of the severity of hypokinesis in the infarcted site (−3.73 ± 0.14 in the large group, −2.94 ± 0.22 in the standard group, and −2.42 ± 0.26 in the small group) and the circumferential extent of hypokinesis (44% ± 1% in the large group, 30% ± 4% in the standard group, and 24% ± 4% in the small group) (Figs. 3b,c).

Infarct Size and Plasma Free-Radical Scavenger Activity

Plasma free-radical scavenger activities were measured in 33 patients (12 patients in the large group, 9 patients in the standard group, 12 patients in the small group). Age, gender, time to reperfusion from onset of myocardial infarction, the degree of collateral development at the initial angiographic examination, and defect volume, between the patients with and without measurement of plasma free-radical scavenger activity in each group, were all similar (Table 2). As shown in Fig. 4, plasma free-radical scavenger activity in the large group (24.1 ± 0.7 NU/l) was significantly lower than that of both the small group (29.9 ± 1.3 NU/l) and the standard group (27.0 ± 1.0 NU/l). There was a significant inverse correlation between plasma free-radical scavenger activities and defect volume in patients with known plasma free-radical scavenger activities ($r^2 = 0.24$, $P = 0.0028$), as shown in Fig. 5.

Discussion

In this study, we attempted to clarify the relationship between the reperfusion injury and the reasons why the infarct size was different among the patients,

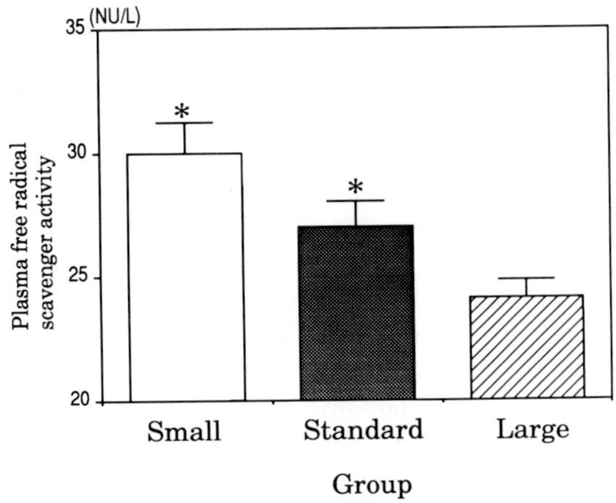

Fig. 4. Comparison of the plasma free-radical scavenger activity among the small, the standard, and the large group. *, $P < 0.05$ *vs* the large group

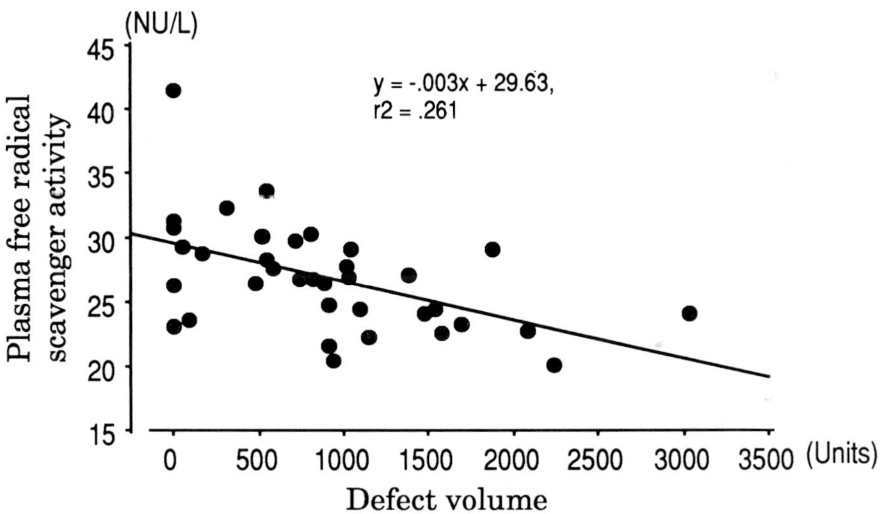

Fig. 5. Correlation between the plasma free-radical scavenger activity and defect volume

even if the various factors influencing the infarct size, such as the area at risk of myocardial infarction [14], time to reperfusion from onset [17], and presence of collaterals at the onset [15,16], were standardized.

First of all, we selected patients with first anterior infarction in which the proximal protion of left anterior infarction was totally occluded at the initial angiography, to standardize the risk area. Second, defect volume, determined by thallium-201 SPECT, was used as the index of the infarct size, because it was not influenced by perfusion state [22]. Third, the patients whose time to reperfusion from the onset was known, and who had not experienced cardiac events after reperfusion, were selected. In this clinical situation, there was a significant linear correlation between the infarct size and time to reperfusion from the onset, as shown in Fig. 1. The linear regression between the infarct size and time to reperfusion was the same as the results previously obtained in animal [17] and clinical studies [26]. The relation also showed that there were great variations in the infarct size even if the time to reperfusion from onset was similar. We divided these patients into three groups according to the infarct size in proportion to time to reperfusion from onset: these were the large, standard, and small groups. The patients' characteristics, time to reperfusion from onset, area at risk determined by left ventriculography during the acute stage, and the grade of the collaterals at the initial angiographic examination, were similar among the three groups. The major factors influencing the infarct size were similar among the three groups; however, the infarct size as well as the left ventricular function were significantly different between the large group and the small group (Fig. 3).

The plasma free-radical scavenger activity in the small group was higher than that in the large group. Plasma free-radical scavenger acitivity was not measured in all patients; however, the clinical characteristics and infarct size between patients with and without measurement of the free-radical scavenger activity were similar in each group. Furthermore, multivariate analysis, performed with multiple regression to determine the infarct size, showed that the elapsed time and plasma free-radical scavenger activity were related to the infarct size in 33 patients with known plasma free-radical scavenger activity. These findings suggested that the plasma free-radical scavenger activity might be one of the factors influencing infarct size in the clinical situation. In our previous study [18], plasma free-radical scavenger activity was inversely correlated with the infarct size and was independent of other factors determining the infarct size. The same relation was also shown in this study (Fig. 5). As previously discussed, the reasons for the differences in the plasma free-radical scavenger activity among patients are not known. A repetitive ischemic episode might enhance the free-radical scavenger activity in patients, since Hoshida et al. [27] demonstrated that preconditioning altered myocardial antioxidant activity in the canine model. Another explanation might be that plasma free-radical scavenger activity is genetically determined [18]. The finding obtained in this study—that is, plasma free-radical scavenger activity in patients was related to the infarct size—indicated that plasma free-radical scavengers reduce the size of the myocardial infarct. The plasma free-radical scavenger activity might reflect the intracellular radical scavenger activity [25]. Intracellular free-radical scavengers protect the ischemic myocardium from injury induced by free radicals generated at the time of the reperfusion, whatever the source of the free radicals. Thus, these results suggest that the variety of infarct size among patients reflected the degree of the reperfusion injury caused by the free radicals, and also implied that it might be possible to limit infarct size by supplementing the intracellular free-radical scavenger activity before reperfusion.

Acknowledgments. We acknowledge the contributions of Shinsuke Nanto, MD, Masayoshi Mishima, MD, Masashi Naka, MD, and Yasushi Matsumura, MD in the collection of the clinical data; Jirou Sasaki for his technical assistance; and Hideo Kusuoka, MD, of the First Department of Medicine, Osaka University Medical School for his excellent advice.

References

1. Simoons ML, Serruys PW, Van den Brand M, Res J, Verheugt FWA, Krauss XH, Remme WJ, Bar F, de Zwaan C, van der Laarse A, Vermeer F, Lubsen J (1986) Early thrombolysis in acute myocardial infarction: limitation of infarct size and improved survival. J Am Coll Cardiol 7:717–728
2. Sheehan FH, Doerr R, Schmidt WG, Bolson EL, Uebis R, von Essen R, Effert S, Dodge HT (1988) Early recovery of left ventricular function after thrombolytic therapy for acute myocardial infarction: an important determinant of survival. J Am Coll Cardiol 12:289–300
3. Van der Werf, Arnold AER (1988) Intravenous plasminogen activator and size of infarct, left ventricular function and survival in acute myocardial infarction. Br Med J 297:1374–1379
4. O'Rourke M, Baron D, Keog A, Kelly R, Nelson G, Barnes C, Raftos J, Graham K, Hillman K, Newman H, Healey J, Woolridge J, Riverrs J, White H, Whitlock R, Norris R (1988) Limitation of myocardial infarction by early infusion of recombinant tissue-type plasminogen activator. Circulation 77:1311–1315
5. Pepine CJ, Prida X, Hill JA, Feldman RL, Conti R (1984) Percutaneous transluminal coronary angioplasty in acute myocardial infarction. Am Heart J 107:820–822
6. Hearse DJ (1977) Reperfusion of the ischemic myocardium. J Mol Cell Cardiol 9:605–616
7. Braunwald E, Kloner A (1985) Myocardial reperfusion: a double-edged sword? J Clin Invest 76:1713–1719
8. Hammond B, Hess ML (1985) The oxygen free radical system: potential mediator of myocardial injury. J Am Coll Cardiol 6:215–218
9. Jolly SR, Kane WJ, Bailie MB, Abrams GD, Lucchesi BR (1984) Canine myocardial reperfusion injury. Its reduction by the combined administration of superoxide dismutase and catalase. Circ Res 54:277–284
10. Werns SW, Shea MJ, Driscoll EM, Cohen C, Abrams GD, Pitt B, Lucchesi (1985) The independent effects of oxygen radical scavengers on canine infarct size. Reduction by superoxide dismutase but not catalase. Circ Res 56:895–898
11. Chambers DE, Parks DA, Patterson G, Roy R, McCord JM, Yoshida S, Parmley LF, Downey JM (1985) Xanthine oxidase as a source of free radical damage in myocardial ischemia. J Mol Cell Cardiol 17:145–152
12. Romson JL, Hook BG, Kunkel SL, Abrams GD, Schort MA, Lucchesi BR (1983) Reduction of the extent of ischemic myocardial injury by neutrophil depletion in the dog. Circulation 67:1016–1023
13. Werns SW, Brinker J, Gruber J, Rothbaum D, Heuser R, George B, Burwell L, Kereiakes D, Mancini GBJ, Flaherty A (1989) A randomized, double-blind trial of recombinant human superoxide dismutase (SOD) in patients undergoing PTCA for acute MI. Circulation 80[Suppl II]:II-213

14. Reimer KA, Jennings RB (1979) The "wave front phenomenon" of myocardial ischemic cell death. II. Transmural progression of necrosis within the framework of ischemic bed size (myocardium at risk) and collateral flow. Lab Invest 40:633–644
15. Jennings RB, Reimer KA (1983) Factors involved in salvaging ischemic myocardium: Effect of reperfusion of arterial blood. Circulation 68[Suppl. I]:I-25
16. Reimer KA, Lowe JE, Rasmussen MM, Jennings R (1977) The wave front phenomenon of ischemic cell death. I. Myocardial infarct size vs duration of coronary occlusion in dogs. Circulation 56:786–794
17. Saito Y, Yasuno M, Ishida M, Suzuki K, Matoba Y, Emura M, Takahashi M (1985) Importance of coronary collaterals for restoration of left ventricular function after intracoronary thrombolysis. Am J Cardiol 55:1259–1263
18. Kodama K, Hirayama A, Komamura K (1989) Human plasma superoxide dismutase (SOD) activity on reperfusion injury with successful thrombolysis in acute myocardial infarction. Jpn J Med 28:202–206
19. Judkins MP (1967) Selective coronary angiography: a percutaneous transfemoral technique. Radiology 89:815–824
20. Dodge HT, Sandler H, Baxley WA, Hawley RR (1966) Usefulness and limitation of radiographic methods for determining left ventricular volume. Am J Cardiol 18:10–24
21. Sheehan FH, Bolson EL, Dodge HT, Mathey DG, Schofer J, Woo HW (1986) Advantages and applications of the centerline method for characterizing regional ventricular function. Circulation 74:293–305
22. Hirayama A, Adachi T, Asada S, Mishima M, Nanto S, Kusuoka H, Yamamoto K, Matsumura Y, Hori M, Inoue M, Kodama K (1993) Late reperfusion for acute myocardial infarction limits the dilatation of left ventricle without the reduction of infarct size. Circulation 88:2565–2574
23. Hirayama A, Mishima M, Nishida K, Kodama K (1993) Preangina and plasma radical scavenger activity limit the size of infarct in patients with successful thrombolysis. Jpn Circ J 57[Suppl IV]:1352–1355
24. Elstner EF, Heupel A (1976) Inhibition of nitrate formation from hydroxylamine-chloride: Simple assay for superoxide dismutase. Arch Biochem 70:616–620
25. Kono Y (1978) Generation of superoxide radical during autoxidation of hydroxylamine and an assay for superoxide dismutase. Arch Biochem Biophys 186:189–195
26. Tiefenbrunn AJ, Sobel BE (1992) Timing of coronary recanalization: Paradigm, paradoxes, and pertinence. Circulation 85:1259–1263
27. Hoshida S, Kuzuya T, Fuji H, Yamashita N, Oe H, Hori M, Suzuki K, Taniguchi N, Tada M (1993) Sublethal ischemica alters myocardial antioxidant activity in the canine heart. Am J Physiol 264:H33–H39

Cardioprotection from Ischemia and Reperfusion

1.10 Beneficial Role of Interaction Between Alpha-Adrenoceptor Activity and Adenosine in Myocardial Ischemic and Reperfusion Injury

Masatsugu Hori[1], Masafumi Kitakaze[1], Toshimazu Morioka[1], Tetsuo Minamino[1], Seiji Takashima[1], Hiroshi Sato[1], Koichi Node[1], Michitoshi Inoue[2], and Takenobu Kamada[1]

Summary. One of the major cardiovascular effects of alpha-adrenoceptor stimulation in the heart is coronary vasoconstriction, which predominantly restricts epicardial coronary flow and maintains endocardial coronary flow during exercise and ischemia. Recently, our laboratory has revealed the phenomenon that alpha-adrenoceptor activity is closely related to production and effect of adenosine: $alpha_1$-adrenoceptor stimulation enhances the release of adenosine through activation of 5′-nucleotidase, and $alpha_2$-adrenoceptor stimulation increases the sensitivity of the effects of adenosine. The interactions between alpha-adrenoceptor activation and adenosine may contribute to attenuation of ischemic and reperfusion injury. Indeed, $alpha_1$-adrenoceptor stimulation during 15 min of ischemia and subsequent reperfusion attenuated the severity of myocardial contractile dysfunction via enhanced release of adenosine. Furthermore, we found that activation of 5′-nucleotidase activity plays a crucial role for attenuation of infarct size. Ischemic preconditioning, which markedly limits infarct size, increased 5′-nucleotidase activity through activation of $alpha_1$-adrenoceptor stimulation, because prazosin blunted activation of 5′-nucleotidase and thereby attenuated the infarct size limiting effect. Transient exposures of methoxamine increased 5′-nucleotidase and mimicked the infarct size limiting effect. Taking these results together, we propose potential mechanisms for cardioprotection attributable to the interaction between alpha-adrenoceptor activity and adenosine. Further basic and clinical studies are necessary to test the proposed mechanisms.

[1] The First Department of Medicine, 2-2 Yamadagaoka, Suita, Osaka University School of Medicine, Osaka, 565 Japan
[2] Department of Medical Information Sciences, Osaka University Hospital, Osaka, Japan

Key words: Alpha-adrenoceptor—Adenosine—5′-nucleotidase—Ischemia—Reperfusion injury—Cardioprotection

Introduction

During myocardial ischemia, norepinephrine is released from the sympathetic nerve terminals and stimulates both alpha- and beta-adrenergic receptors in the heart [1–4]. The release of norepinephrine during myocardial ischemia may modulate the severity of ischemia; beta-adrenergic stimulation may increase myocardial contractility and oxygen demand, which may deteriorate myocardial ischemia. Alpha-adrenergic stimulation may cause vasoconstriction, which may limit oxygen supply to myocardium and worsen ischemia. However, the effects of alpha-adrenoceptor stimulation are worthy of study because of the multiplicity of its cardiovascular effects. In addition to the direct coronary vasoactive effect [5–7], alpha-adrenoceptor stimulation increases the sensitivity of adenosine receptors in coronary arteries and augments the capacity for adenosine production [8–12]. Since adenosine is a cardioprotective substance in the heart, there is no clear consensus whether the net effects caused by alpha-adrenoceptor stimulation are beneficial or deleterious to ischemic and reperfusion injury. Here, we will discuss the individual and overall effects of alpha-adrenoceptor activity on myocardial ischemia and reperfusion and clarify a crucial role of the interaction between alpha-adrenoceptor activation and adenosine.

Norepinephrine Release in the Ischemic Heart

Myocardial ischemia is believed to be a potent trigger of norepinephrine release from the sympathetic nerve terminals [3,4,13]. Deleterious events such as fetal arrhythmias [14,15] and myocardial cell damage [16,17], which are recognized as catecholamine injury, have been attributable to the excessive stimulation of both alpha- and beta-adrenergic receptors of myocardium and coronary arteries. Release of norepinephrine is predominantly enhanced at the local nerve endings in the ischemic myocardium, which is not influenced by the central sympathetic nerve activity [3]. Indeed, Schömig et al. [3] demonstrated that a large amount of norepinephrine is released during ischemia in the Langendorff preparation of rat hearts, and showed that the amount of the released norepinephrine is increased as the ischemic period is prolonged. They also reported that the release of catecholamine occurs within 10 min after the onset of ischemia. Furthermore, Wollenberger and Shaab [1] observed in rabbit isolated hearts that 3–4 min of ischemia causes the overflow of a large amount of norepinephrine. Similarly, in in vivo dog hearts, a coronary arterial occlusion of 2.5 min also results in a net overflow of norepinephrine [18]. These consistency of the time course of norepinephrine release in the isolated and in vivo hearts may support the idea that the ischemia-induced norepinephrine release is regulated by local factors rather than by central nervous regulation.

Coronary Vasoactive Responses to Norepinephrine

Norepinephrine is known to activate both alpha- and beta-adrenoceptors [19]. Alpha-adrenoceptor stimulation contracts the isolated coronary arteries [5–7], while beta-adrenoceptor stimulation mediates coronary vasorelaxation. Zuberbuhler and Bohr [5] showed that an exposure to norepinephrine under beta-adrenoceptor blockade exerts potent contraction of the canine isolated coronary artery, and concluded that alpha-adrenoceptor stimulation mediates coronary vasoconstriction. The vasoconstrictive action caused by alpha-adrenoceptor stimulation is more potent in the larger coronary arteries than in the smaller coronary arteries [5]. Vatner and coworkers [6,7] confirmed in the conscious dog that alpha-adrenoceptor stimulation caused by exogenous and endogenous norepinephrine causes potent vasoconstriction of large epicardial coronary arteries; they directly measured coronary arterial diameters using an ultrasonic dimension gauge. On the other hand, Kelley and Feigl [20] reported that increases in coronary vascular resistance during an exposure of norepinephrine are due to the vasoconstriction in both large and small coronary arteries (Fig. 1). Indeed, Chillian et al. [21] directly observed that 100–300 μm of small coronary arteries respond well to alpha-adrenoceptor stimulation. The contribution of small coronary arteries to the increase in coronary vascular resistance during alpha-adrenoceptor stimulation is reported to be approximately 40% [20]. These studies show that small coronary arteries as well as large coronary arteries participate in the regulation of coronary blood flow when alpha-adrenergic receptors are stimulated. This aspect of alpha-adrenoceptor-mediated vasoconstriction may enable the appropriate distribution of intramyocardial flow, since it is reported that alpha-adrenoceptor

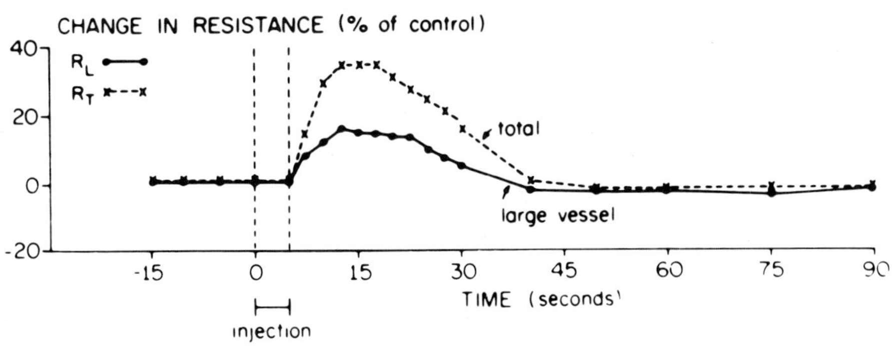

Fig. 1. Changes in coronary vascular resistance due to large (R^L) and small (R^T) coronary vessels during an infusion of norepinephrine (From [20], with permission)

stimulation favors an increase in endocardial flow at the expense of epicardial flow reduction during exercise and coronary hypoperfusion [22,23].

Interactions Between Alpha-Adrenoceptor Activity and Vasoactive Substances

When we discuss the role of alpha-adrenoceptor activity on the coronary vascular tone, we need to separate the vasoactive effects due to chemical vasoactive substances mediated by alpha-adrenoceptor activity, and direct vasoconstriction. There are several substances which are mediated by alpha-

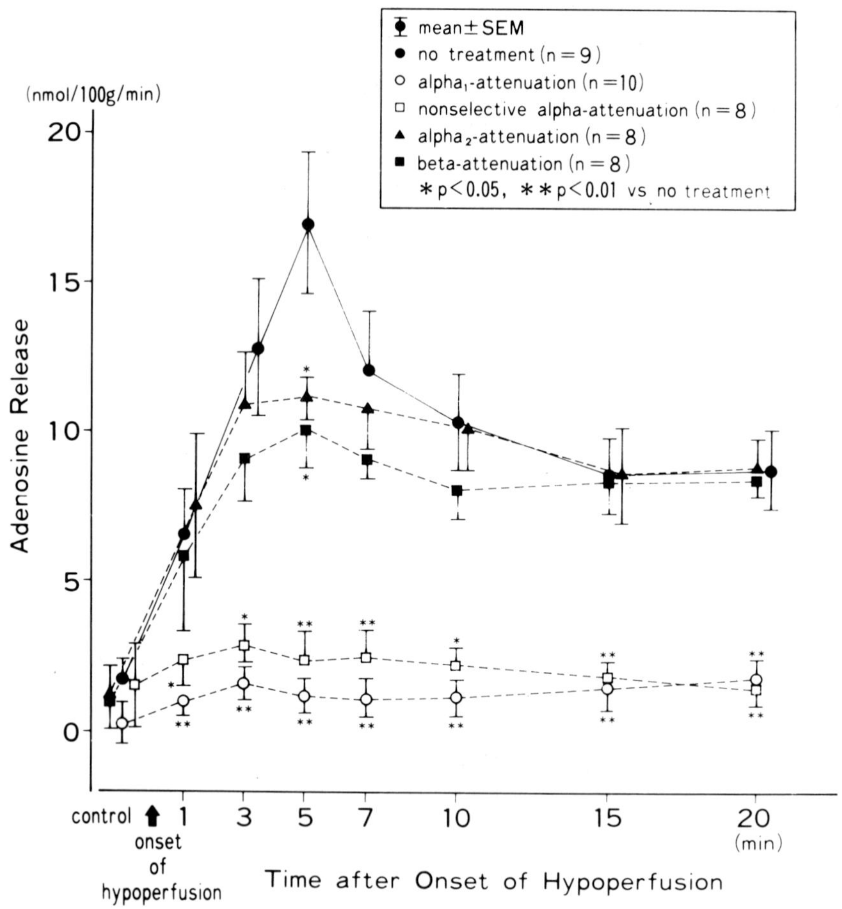

Fig. 2. Adenosine release during coronary hypoperfusion under alpha$_1$- (prazosin), alpha$_2$- (yohimbine + propranolol), nonselective alpha- (phentolamine + propranolol), and beta-adrenoceptor (propranolol) attenuations. Note that both prazosin and phentolamine markedly reduced release of adenosine (From [8], with permission)

adrenoceptor stimulation. Alpha$_2$-adrenoceptor stimulation enhances the release of endothelial-derived relaxing factor (EDRF) from endothelial cells [25] and inhibits the norepinephrine release from the sympathetic nerve endings [26], resulting in a decrease in the coronary arterial tone. It is also known that alpha$_2$-adrenoceptor stimulation releases histamine in the skeletal muscle [27]. If histamine is released by alpha$_2$-adrenoceptor stimulation in the heart, this substance may increase coronary blood flow.

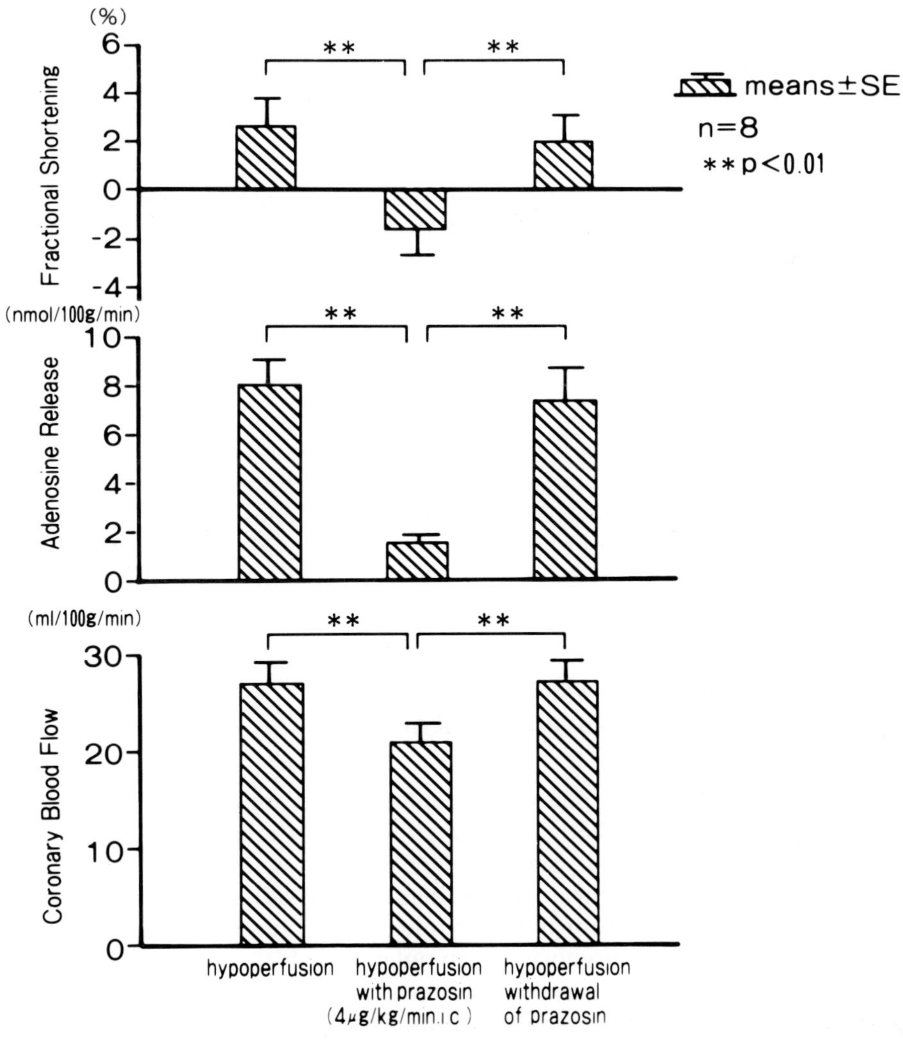

Fig. 3. Changes in coronary hemodynamics, myocardial metabolism, and adenosine release after onset and withdrawal of alpha$_1$-adrenoceptor attenuation during hypoperfusion (From [8], with permission)

On the other hand, $alpha_1$-adrenoceptor stimulation augments the release of adenosine in ischemic myocardium. Figure 2 depicts the effects of alpha- and beta-adrenoceptor activities on adenosine release from the canine ischemic myocardium. Administration of a low dose of prazosin, which does not affect the basal coronary blood flow, reduced both adenosine release and coronary blood flow (Fig. 3, [8]). The results obtained in the ischemic myocardium [8,28] contrast well to those in the nonischemic myocardium [29]. In rat isolated cardiomyocytes, intracellular adenosine is increased during hypoxia by $alpha_1$-adrenoceptor stimulation. The production of adenosine is also increased by phorbol 12-myristate 13-acetate (PMA), a stimulator of protein kinase C, and is inhibited by H-7, an inhibitor of protein kinase C, indicating that activity of protein kinase C plays a crucial role for adenosine production in the ischemic heart [30]. These results suggest that protein kinase C may affect the enzymes responsible for adenosine production and degradation, or production of 5′-AMP. It should be noted, however, that enhanced release of adenosine by $alpha_1$-adrenoceptor stimulation is observed only during ischemia. Thus, the underlying mechanism for this phenomenon may be different from that of adenosine release when beta-adrenoceptors are stimulated.

There is an interaction between alpha-adrenoceptor activity and the vasodilatory action of adenosine. Recently, our laboratory reported that $alpha_2$-adrenoceptor stimulation increases the coronary vasodilatory effects of adenosine [9,10]. Adenosine is known to be an endogenous substance released during exercise and ischemia, and it increases coronary blood flow [31]. We revealed that yohimbine, an $alpha_2$-adrenoceptor antagonist, attenuates adenosine-induced coronary vasodilation in open chest dogs. Clonidine, an $alpha_2$-adrenoceptor agonist, adversely enhances adenosine-induced coronary vasodilation [11]. These observations are consonant with the results of Nayler et al. [32].

Effects of Alpha-Adrenoceptor Activity and Adenosine on Myocardial Ischemia

Considering the effects of alpha-adrenoceptor activity on myocardial and coronary vascular functions, whether alpha-adrenoceptor stimulation is beneficial or deleterious to myocardial ischemia is a complex question. When the circulating level of norepinephrine is not high, $alpha_2$-adrenoceptor stimulation provides a beneficial effect for ischemic injury [11]. During coronary hypoperfusion, moderate $alpha_2$-adrenoceptor stimulation, which does not cause direct coronary vasoconstriction, increases coronary blood flow in the ischemic area and restores myocardial contractile function. We also observed beneficial effects of clonidine even in denervated hearts, showing that the attenuation of release of norepinephrine by $alpha_2$-adrenoceptor stimulation is not involved. It is of interest that the beneficial effects of $alpha_2$-adrenoceptor on myocardial ischemia are abolished by treatment with 8-phenyltheophylline, an antagonist of adenosine receptors. Therefore, we hypothesize that adenosine-induced coronary vasodilation is primarily involved in the beneficial effects of alpha$_2$-adrenoceptor stimulation. However, if the dose of clonidine is high, ischemia may be worsened because high doses of clonidine adversely blunt the adenosine-induced coronary vasodilation through its direct vasoconstriction.

Heusch and Deussen [33] demonstrated that postsynaptic alpha$_2$-adrenoceptor stimulation mediates coronary vasoconstriction produced by sympathetic nerve stimulation during critical reduction of coronary perfusion pressure, and concluded that alpha$_2$-adrenoceptor stimulation is deleterious for myocardial ischemia. Seitelberger et al. [34] also demonstrated that alpha-adrenoceptor blockade attenuates the severity of exercise-induced myocardial ischemia. Both exercise and sympathetic nerve stimulation elevate the systemic norepinephrine level to more than 1000 pg/ml, a concentration two- to three-fold higher than that during regional ischemic conditions. Norepinephrine concentration in the systemic blood is 200–300 pg/ml even when the left anterior descending coronary flow is reduced to one-third of the control, and fractional shortening is reduced to 5% from 25% in the control condition. These observations indicate that if alpha$_2$-adrenoceptor stimulation is potent, enhancement of adenosine-induced vasodilation by alpha$_2$-adrenoceptor stimulation is masked by the direct vasoconstriction.

Alpha$_1$-adrenoceptor stimulation is also reported to be beneficial for myocardial ischemia (Fig. 4) [8]. During coronary hypoperfusion, administration of a low dose of prazosin, which does not cause a direct vasodilation but inhibits the release of adenosine, further decreased coronary blood flow and worsened the severity of ischemia (Fig. 5). When a larger dose of prazosin was employed, direct coronary vasodilation was exerted, thereby attenuating the extent of ischemia [35]. Thus, it is most likely that mild to moderate alpha$_1$-adrenoceptor stimulation exerts beneficial effects on the ischemic myocardium through the augmentation of adenosine release; whereas potent alpha$_1$-adrenoceptor stimulation causes deleterious effects via direct vasoconstriction. Herrmann and Feigl [12] also observed that adrenergic blockade blunts adenosine concentration and coronary vasodilation during hypoxia.

Effects of Alpha-Adrenoceptor Activity and Adenosine on Reperfusion Injury

Contractile dysfunction after a brief period of ischemia is defined as myocardial stunning [36]. Although the pathophysiology of myocardial stunning is extensively discussed, the role of alpha-adrenoceptor activity in this abnormality is hardly known. Our recent observations revealed that administration of methoxamine attenuated myocardial stunning associated with enhanced release of adenosine, and that treatment with theophylline completely abolished this

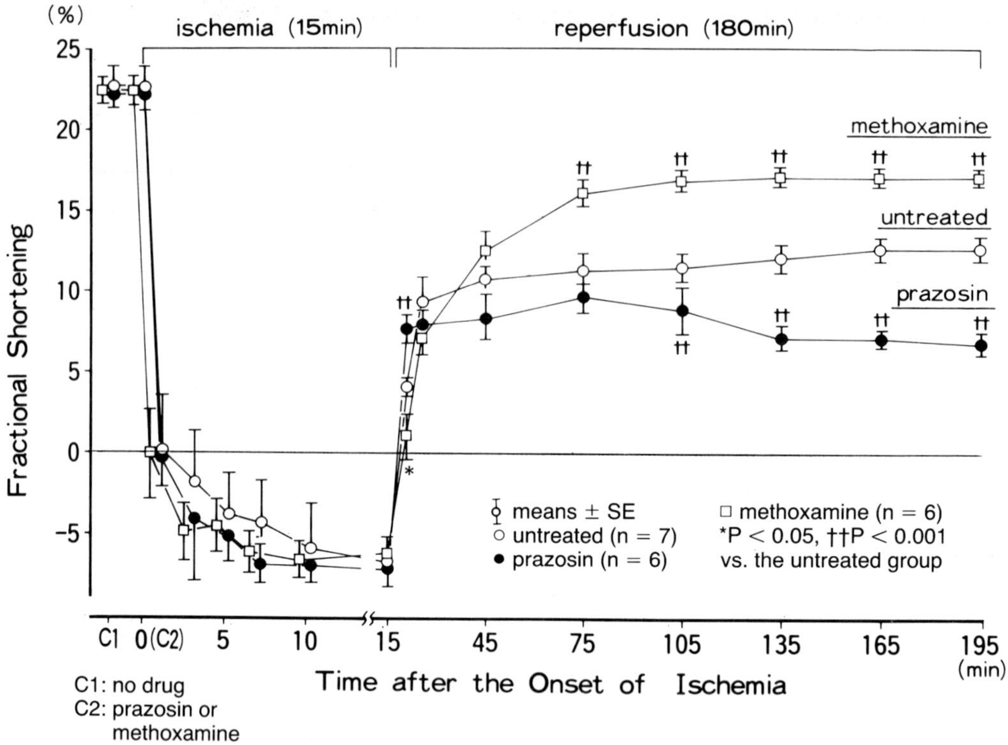

Fig. 4. Serial changes in fractional shortening of the left anterior descending coronary artery area before, during, and after 15 min of myocardial ischemia. Although the pharmacological interventions do not alter the decreases in fractional shortening during myocardial ischemia, in the prazosin (4.0 μg/kg per min, i.c.) and methoxamine-treated conditions, fractional shortening at 3 h of reperfusion is attenuated and augmented compared with the control condition, respectively (From [37], with permission)

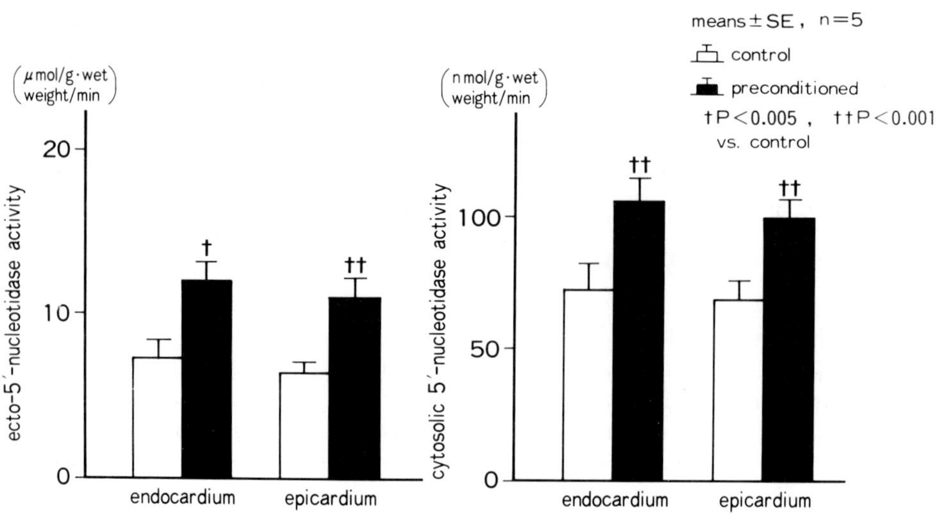

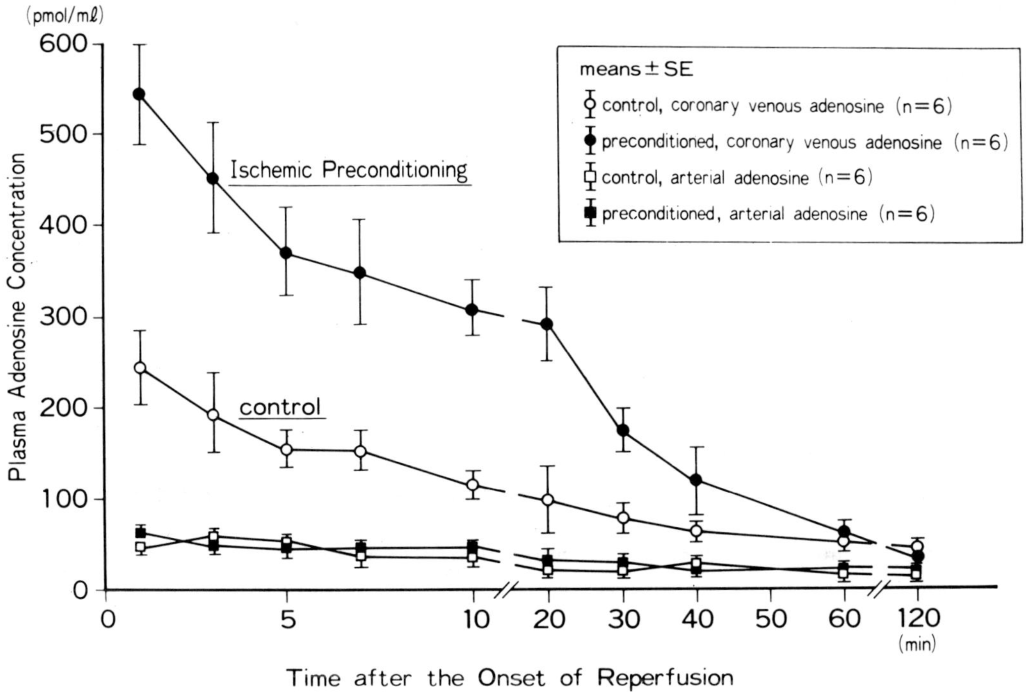

Fig. 6. Graph showing adenosine release during reperfusion after 40 min of coronary occlusion with and without ischemic preconditioning. Adenosine release in the group that underwent ischemic preconditioning is enhanced significantly ($P < 0.01$) for 40 min compared with the untreated control condition (From [60], with permission)

beneficial effect of methoxamine [37]. These results suggest that alpha$_1$-adrenoceptor stimulation can attenuate the severity of myocardial stunning through the enhanced release of adenosine (Fig. 6). This is compatible with other studies supporting the protective effects of adenosine on myocardial stunning [38,39]. However, it should be noted that a high dose of methoxamine blunted the beneficial effects of alpha$_1$-adrenoceptor stimulation. Preservation of ATP may not be a mechanism for the beneficial effects of adenosine since the replenishment of ATP does not necessarily restore the contractile function [40]; however, this hypothesis cannot be completely excluded [41].

Instead, calcium overload may be a primary mechanism of myocardial stunning [42–46]. If this is the case, alpha$_1$-mediated release of adenosine may

←

Fig. 5. Bar graphs showing ectosolic and cytosolic 5′-nucleotidase activities in the control and ischemic preconditioned myocardium before the 40-min coronary occlusion. Both ectosolic and cytosolic 5′-nucelotidase activities were augmented by ischemic preconditioning (From [60], with permission) attenuate myocardial stunning by inhibiting calcium influx through the stimulation of adenosine A_1-receptors [47]. The reason that higher doses of methoxamine blunt the beneficial effects of alpha-adrenoceptor stimulation may be attributed to the fact that the higher dose of methoxamine increases intracellular Ca^{2+} during ischemia and reperfusion [48]. A report that prazosin attenuates Ca^{2+} increases during reperfusion may support this hypothesis [49].

Alpha$_1$-adrenoceptor-mediated release of adenosine also attenuates the activation of neutrophils [50]: free-radical generation is inhibited through adenosine A_2-receptor stimulation, and adherence to endothelial cells is attenuated through adenosine A_1-receptor stimulation. Platelet aggregation may cause reperfusion injury since aggregated platelets impede the microcirculation of the coronary vessels. It is known that adenosine also inhibits platelet aggregation through A_2-receptor stimulation [51], and that endogenous adenosine released from the ischemic myocardium inhibits platelet aggregation in the blood perfused canine heart [52]. Thus, inhibition of platelet aggregation by endogenous adenosine released from ischemic myocardium may attenuate reperfusion injury. Since adenosine is a potent vasodilator, massive release of adenosine during ischemia and reperfusion may attenuate microcirculatory disturbances. Thus, an improvement of the coronary microcirculation by adenosine enhanced by alpha$_1$-adrenoceptor stimulation may largely contribute to the prevention of reperfusion injury.

In contrast, there is no clear consensus whether alpha$_2$-adrenoceptor stimulation is beneficial for stunning. Although alpha$_2$-adrenoceptor stimulation may enhance adenosine-induced coronary vasodilation, there is no close relation between the severity of myocardial stunning and the extent of coronary vasodilation. Alpha$_2$-adrenoceptor stimulation may cause platelet aggregation, which may worsen myocardial stunning. However, this question remains for further investigation.

Role of Alpha$_1$-Adrenoceptor Activity in Salvage of Myocardial Necrosis in Ischemic Preconditioning

It has been clarified that adenosine limits the size of the infarct caused by sustained myocardial ischemia and reperfusion: intracoronary infusion of adenosine reduces myocardial infarct size in dogs by 75% [53]. The attenuation of reduction of ATP during ischemia and reperfusion seems critically important because intracellular ATP concentration is one of the factors which determine the irreversibility of injury to the myocardium. Adenosine may act by preserving ATP [54]. The myocardial ATP concentration and ATP synthesis are increased in the postischemic myocardium when exogenous adenosine is administered to the crystalloid perfused heart [55].

Recently, considerable attention has been paid to ischemic preconditioning not only by basic researchers but also by cardiologists because ischemic preconditioning is believed to limit infarct size to 10%–20% in the reperfused ischemic myocardium [56–58]. The mechanism underlying this phenomenon is being studied actively with an eye towards developing treatments to limit the size of myocardial infarct. Liu et al. [59] have shown that endogenous adenosine mediates ischemic preconditioning, based upon the observation that 8-phenyltheophylline abolishes the necrosis-limiting effects of ischemic preconditioning. They have hypothesized that ischemic preconditioning occurs via adenosine A_1 receptor activation [59]. Increases in blood flow, and inhibitions of neutrophil activation and platelet aggregation, are mediated through adenosine A_2 receptors, eliminating these as mechanisms of action for ischemic preconditioning. In contrast, the inhibition of adrenergic stimulation by adenosine and norepinephrine release may account for the beneficial effects of ischemic preconditioning, since both actions are mediated via adenosine A_1-receptor activation. Indeed, myocardial oxygen consumption during reperfusion was significantly less after ischemic preconditioning [60]. Attenuation of Ca^{2+} overload by activation of adenosine A_1 receptors may also contribute to the beneficial effects of ischemic preconditioning.

Despite this progress in the understanding of the ischemic preconditioning, the mechanism relating adenosine to ischemic preconditioning is unknown. One likely mechanism is that ischemic preconditioning increases adenosine release during sustained ischemia and reperfusion, possibly by augmenting 5′-nucleotidase activity [60]. We have reported that ischemic preconditioning augments the activity of 5′-nucleotidase (Fig. 5), and thereby increases adenosine production (Fig. 6) during ischemia and reperfusion. This augmented adenosine production may contribute to the underlying mechanisms of ischemic preconditioning. Protein kinase C activity increases during ischemia and reperfusion, which also increases adenosine production. Recently, we have observed that alpha$_1$-adrenoceptor activation mediates increases in ectosolic and cytosolic 5′-nucleotidase activities [30] and contributes to reduction of infarct size [61]. Therefore, we postulate the hypothesis that alpha$_1$-adrenoceptor activation during ischemic preconditioning is attributable to the attenuation of the infarct size [55], although we need to continue to study how 5′-nucleotidase activity is enhanced by ischemic preconditioning.

Our study hints that increased adenosine release may be the mechanism by which ischemic preconditioning limits infarct size. It is possible, therefore, that intracoronary administration of adenosine or an adenosine potentiator, e.g., AICA riboside (5-amino-4-imidazole carboxamide-riboside), dilazep, or dipyridamole, may limit infarct size in acute myocardial infarction and reduce contractile dysfunction [62,63]. Additionally, it may be possible to enhance adenosine production during ischemia and reperfusion by activation of 5′-nucleotidase. Alpha$_1$-adrenoceptor stimulation is one approach to increasing 5′-nucleotidase activity. Indeed, alpha$_1$-adrenoceptor stimulation attenuates contractile dysfunction by enhancing the release of adenosine and ultimately limits infarct size [64,65]. Interleukin and tumor necrosis factor also have been reported to increase 5′-nucleotidase activity [66]. Further studies are required to learn how best to stimulate adenosine production and limit infarct size following acute myocardial infarction [67]. Investigation of drugs which increase adenosine production or activate adenosine receptors is a promising approach.

Conclusion

Briefly, we presented and discussed here the beneficial roles of alpha-adrenoceptor activity on the pathogenesis of ischemic heart disease. The major effect of alpha-adrenoceptor stimulation in the coronary arteries is vasoconstriction, which predominantly restricts epicardial coronary vessels and maintains endocardial coronary flow during exercise and ischemia. Recently, our laboratory has revealed the phenomenon that alpha-adrenoceptor activity is tightly related to the metabolism and effect of adenosine: $alpha_1$-adrenoceptor stimulation enhances the release of adenosine through the activation of 5′-nucleotidase, and $alpha_2$-adrenoceptor stimulation increases the sensitivity of the coronary vascular smooth muscle to adenosine. These beneficial effects of alpha-adrenoceptor stimulation attenuate the severity of contractile dysfunction following transient myocardial ischemia and limit the infarct caused by sustained ischemia. Further clinical studies are necessary to clarify the role of alpha-adrenoceptor activity in coronary flow regulation and myocardial function in the human ischemic heart.

References

1. Wollenberger A, Shaab L (1965) Anoxia-induced release of noradrenaline from the isolated perfused heart. Nature 207:88–89
2. Muntz KH, Hapler HK, Boulas JH, Willerson JT, Buja ML (1984) Redistribution of catecholamines in the ischemic zone of the dog heart. Am J Physiol 114:64–78
3. Schömig A, Dart AM, Dietz R, Mayer E, Kubler W (1984) Release of endogenous catecholamines in the ischemic myocardium of the rat. Part A: Locally mediated release. Circ Res 55:689–701
4. Dart AM, Schömig A, Dietz R, Mayer E, Kubler W (1984) Release of endogenous catecholamine in the ischemic myocardium of the rat. Part B: Effects of sympathetic nerve stimulation. Circ Res 55:702–706
5. Zuberbuhler RC, Bohr DF (1965) Responses of coronary smooth muscle to catecholamine. Circ Res 16:431–440
6. Murray PA, Vatner SF (1979) Alpha-adrenoceptor attenuation of the coronary vascular response to severe exercise in the conscious dog. Circ Res 45:654–660
7. Vatner SF (1983) Alpha-adrenergic regulation of the coronary circulation in the conscious dog. Am J Cardiol 52:15A–21A
8. Kitakaze M, Hori M, Tamai J, Iwakura K, Koretsune Y, Kagiya T, Iwai K, Kitabatake A, Inoue M, Kamada T (1987) $Alpha_1$-adrenoceptor activity regulates release of adenosine from the ischemic myocardium in dogs. Circ Res 60:631–639
9. Hori M, Kitakaze M, Tamai J, Koretsune Y, Iwai K, Iwakura K, Kagiya T, Kitabatake A, Inoue M, Kamada T (1988) $Alpha_2$-adrenoceptor activity exerts dual

control of coronary blood flow in canine coronary artery. Am J Physiol 255:H250–H260

10. Hori M, Kitakaze M, Tamai J, Iwakura K, Kitabatake A, Inoue M, Kamada T (1989) Alpha$_2$-adrenoceptor stimulation can augment coronary vasodilation maximally induced by adenosine in dogs. Am J Physiol 257:H132–H140
11. Kitakaze M, Hori M, Gotoh K, Sato H, Iwakura K, Kitabatake A, Inoue M, Kamada T (1989) Beneficial effects of alpha$_2$-activity on ischemic myocardium during coronary hypoperfusion in dogs. Circ Res 65:1632–1645
12 Herrmann SC, Feigl EO (1992) Adrenergic blockade blunts adenosine concentration and coronary vasodilation during hypoxia. Circ Res 70:1203–1216
13. Schömig A, Fischer S, Kurz T, Richardt G, Schömig E (1987) Nonexocytotic release of endogenous noradrenaline in the ischemic and anoxic rat heart: Mechanism and metabolic requirements. Circ Res 60:194–205
14. Corr PB, Gillis RA (1978) Autonomic neural influences on the dysarrhythmia resulting from myocardial infarction. Circ Res 43:1–9
15. Penny WJ (1984) The deleterious effects of myocardial catecholamines on cellular electrophysiology and arrhythmias during ischemia and reperfusion. Eur Heart J 5:960–973
16. Rona G (1985) Catecholamine cardiotoxicity. J Mol Cell Cardiol 17:291–306
17. Gauduel Y, Karagueuzian HS, Leiris JD (1979) Deleterious effects of endogenous catecholamines on hypoxic myocardial cells following reoxygenation. J Mol Cell Cardiol 11:717–731
18. Shaab L, Wollenberger A, Haase M, Schiller U (1969) Noradrenalinabgabe aus dem Hundeherzen nach vorübergehender Okklusion einer Koronararterie. Acta Biol Med Gem 22:135–143
19. Homcy CJ, Graham RM (1985) Molecular characterization of adrenergic receptors. Circ Res 56:635–650
20. Kelley KO, Feigl EO (1978) Segmental alpha-receptor-mediated vasoconstriction in the canine coronary circulation. Circ Res 43:908–917
21. Chillian WM, Layne SM, Eastham CL, Marcus ML (1989) Heterogeneous microvascular coronary alpha-adrenergic vasoconstriction. Circ Res 64:376–388
22. Nathan HJ, Feigl EO (1986) Adrenergic vasoconstriction lessens transmural steal during coronary hypoperfusion. Am J Physiol 250:H645–H653
23. Buffington CW, Feigl EO (1983) Effect of coronary artery pressure on transmural distribution of adrenergic coronary vasoconstriction in the dog. Circ Res 53:613–621
24. Angus JA, Cocks TM, Satoh K (1986) The adrenoceptors on endothelial cells. Fed Proc 45:2355–2359
25. Palmer RMJ, Ferrige AG, Moncada S (1987) Nitric oxide release accounts for the biological activity of endothelium-derived relaxing factor. Nature 327:524–526
26. Horeyseck G, Janig W, Kirchner F, Thamer V (1976) Activation and inhibition of muscle and cutaneous postganglionic neurons to hindlimb during hypothalamically induced vasoconstriction and atropine-sensitive vasodilation. Pflügers Arch 361: 231–240
27. Camazine B, Shannon RP, Guerrero JL, Graham RM, Powell WJ Jr (1988) Neurogenic histaminergic vasodilation in canine skeletal muscle: mediation by alpha$_2$-adrenoceptor stimulation. Circ Res 62:871–883
28. Hori M, Tamai J, Kitakaze M, Iwakura K, Gotoh K, Iwai K, Koretsune Y, Kagiya T, Kitabatake A, Kamada T (1989) Adenosine-induced hyperemia attenuates myo-

cardial ischemia in coronary microembolization in dogs. Am J Physiol 257:H244–H251
29. DeWitt DF, Wangler RD, Thompson CI, Sparks HV Jr (1983) Phasic release of adenosine during steady state metabolic stimulation in the isolated guinea pig heart. Circ Res 53:636–643
30. Kitakaze M, Hori M, Iwakura K, Sato H, Gotoh K, Tada M (1989) Protein kinase C regulates production of adenosine in hypoxic myocytes of rats (abstract). Circulation 80:II-498
31. Berne RM (1980) The role of adenosine in the regulation of coronary blood flow. Circ Res 47:807–813
32. Nayler WG, Price JM, Lowe TE (1967) Inhibition of adenosine-induced coronary vasodilation. Cardiovasc Res 1:63–66
33. Heusch G, Deussen A (1983) The effects of cardiac sympathetic nerve stimulation on perfusion of stenotic coronary arteries in the dog. Circ Res 53:8–15
34. Seitelberger R, Guth BD, Heusch G, Lee JD, Katayama K, Ross J Jr (1988) Intracoronary alpha$_2$-adrenergic receptor blockade attenuates ischemia in conscious dogs during exercise. Circ Res 62:436–442
35. Nayler WG, Gordon M, Stephens DJ, Sturrdock JW (1985) The protective effect of prazosin on the ischemic and reperfused myocardium. J Mol Cell Cardiol 17:685–699
36. Braunwald E, Kloner RA (1982) The stunned myocardium: prolonged, postischemic ventricular dysfunction. Circulation 60:1146–1149
37. Kitakaze M, Hori M, Sato H, Iwakura K, Gotoh K, Inoue M, Kitabatake A, Kamada T (1991) Beneficial effects of alpha$_1$-adrenoceptor activity on myocardial stunning in dogs. Circ Res 68:1322–1339
38. Kitakaze M, Takashima S, Sato H (1990) Stimulation of adenosine A_1 and A_2 receptors prevents myocardial stunning (abstract). Circulation 82[Suppl III]:III-37
39. Brodeur RD, Storey C, Anderson PR, Cabrera BDF, Nunnally RL (1990) Effects of adenosine on functional recovery during reperfusion of the ischemic rabbit myocardium. Circulation [Suppl III]:III–289
40. Taegtmeyer H, Roberts AFC, Raine AEG (1985) Energy metabolism in reperfused heart muscle. Metabolic correlates to return of function. J Am Coll Cardiol 6:864–870
41. Bittl JA, Ingwall JS (1985) Reaction rates of creatine kinase and ATP synthesis in the isolated rat heart: A ^{31}P-NMR magnetization transfer study. J Biol Chem 260:3512–3517
42. Kusuoka H, Porterfield JK, Weisman HF, Weisfeldt ML, Marban E (1987) Pathophysiology and pathogenesis of stunned myocardium. Depressed Ca^{2+} activation of contraction as a consequence of reperfusion-induced cellular calcium overload in ferret hearts. J Clin Invest 79:950–961
43. Steenbergen C, Murphy E, Levy L, London RE (1987) Elevation in cytosolic free calcium concentration early in myocardial ischemia in perfused rat heart. Circ Res 60:700–707
44. Kitakaze M, Weisman HF, Marban E (1988) Contractile dysfunction and ATP depletion after transient calcium overload in perfused ferret hearts. Circulation 77:685–695
45. Kitakaze M, Weisfeldt ML, Marban E (1988) Acidosis during early reperfusion prevents myocardial stunning in perfused ferret hearts. J Clin Invest 82:920–927

46. Marban E, Kitakaze M, Koretsune Y, Yue DT, Chacko VP, Pike MM (1990) Quantification of $[Ca^{2+}]_i$ in perfused hearts. Critical evaluation of the 5F-BAPTA and nuclear magnetic resonance method as applied for the study of ischemia and reperfusion. Circ Res 66:1255–1267
47. Cerbai E, Klockner U, Isenberg G (1988) Ca-antagonistic effects of adenosine in guinea pig atrial cells. Am J Physiol 255:H872–H878
48. Endo M, Blinks JR (1988) Actions of sympathomimetic amines on the Ca^{2+} transients and contractions of rabbit myocardium: Reciprocal changes in myofibrillar responsiveness to Ca^{2+} mediated through alpha- and beta-adrenoceptors. Circ Res 62:247–265
49. Sharma AD, Saffitz JE, Lee BI, Sobel BE, Corr PB (1983) Alpha adrenergic-mediated accumulation of calcium in reperfused myocardium. J Clin Invest 72:802–818
50. Cronstein BN, Levin RI, Belanoff J, Weissmann G, Hirschhorn R (1986) Adenosine: an endogenous inhibitor of neutrophil-mediated injury to endothelial cells. J Clin Invest 78:760–770
51. Agarwal KC, Zielinski BA, Maitra RS (1989) Significance of plasma adenosine in the antiplatelet activity of forskolin: potentiation by dipyridamole and dilazep. Thromb Haemostas 61:106–110
52. Kitakaze M, Hori M, Sato H, Iwakura K, Takashima S, Inoue M, Kitabatake A, Kamada T (1991) Endogenous adenosine inhibits platelet aggregation during myocardial ischemia in dogs. Circ Res 69:1402–1408
53. Olafsson B, Forman MB, Puett DW, Pou A, Cates CU, Friesinger GC, Virmani R (1987) Reduction of reperfusion injury in the canine preparation by intracoronary adenosine: importance of the endothelium and the no-reflow phenomenon. Circulation 76:1135–1145
54. Foker JE, Einzig E, Wang T (1980) Adenosine metabolism and myocardial preservation. J Thorac Cardiovasc Surg 80:506–516
55. Reibel DK, Rovette MJ (1979) Myocardial adenosine salvage rates and restoration of ATP content following ischemia. Am J Physiol 237:H247–H252
56. Murray CE, Jennings RB, Reimer KA (1986) Preconditioning with ischemia: A delay of lethal cell injury in ischemic myocardium. Circulation 74:1124–1136
57. Scott RJ, Rohmann S, Braun ER, Schaper W (1990) Ischemic preconditioning reduces infarct size in swine myocardium. Circ Res 66:1133–1142
58. Li GC, Vasquez JA, Gallagher KP, Lucchesi BR (1990) Myocardial protection with preconditioning. Circulation 82:609–619
59. Liu GS, Thornton J, Van Winkle DM, Stanley AWH, Olsson RA, Downey JM (1991) Protection against infarction afforded by preconditioning is mediated by A_1 adenosine receptors in rabbit heart. Circulation 84:350–356
60. Kitakaze M, Hori M, Takashima S, Sato H, Inoue M, Kamada T (1993) Ischemic preconditioning increases adenosine release and 5′-nucleotidase activity during myocardial ischemia and reperfusion in dogs. Implication for myocardial salvage. Circulation 87:208–215
61. Kitakaze M, Takashima S, Morioka T, Sato H, Hori M (1992) $Alpha_1$-adrenergic activation limits infarct size by augmenting adenosine production and 5′-nucleotidase activity in ischemic preconditioning (abstract). Circulation 86:I-213
62. Gruber HE, Hoffer ME, McAllister DR, Laikand PK, Lane TA, Schmid-Schoenbein GW, Engler RL (1989) Increased adenosine concentration in blood from

ischemic myocardium by AICA riboside. Effects on flow, granulocyte, and injury. Circulation 80:1400–1411
63. Hori M, Kitakaze M, Takashima S (1990) AICA-riboside (5-amino-4-imidazole carboxamide riboside 100), a novel adenosine potentiator, attenuates myocardial stunning (abstract). Circulation 82:III-466
64. Kitakaze M, Hori M, Kamada T (1993) Role of adenosine and its interaction with alpha-adrenoceptor activity in ischemic and reperfusion injury of the myocardium (review). Cardiovasc Res 217:18–27
65. Locke-Winter CR, Winter CB, Nelson DW, Banerjee A (1991) cAMP stimulation facilitates preconditioning against ischemia-reperfusion through norepinephrine and $alpha_1$ mechanisms (abstract). Circulation 84:II-433
66. Savic V, Stefanovic V, Ardaillou N, Ardaioolu R (1990) Induction of ecto-5′-nucleotidase of rat cultured mesangial cells by interleukin 1-beta and tumor necrotic factor-alpha. Immunology 70:321–326
67. Hori M, Kitakaze M (1991) Adenosine, the heart, and coronary circulation. Hypertension 18:565–574

1.11 The Role of Adenosine in Ischemic Preconditioning

JAMES M. DOWNEY[1] and TETSUJI MIURA[2]

Summary. Exposing the heart to only 5 min of regional ischemia followed by reperfusion renders it very resistant to infarction from a subsequent ischemic insult. This change represents a biochemical change in the tissue which we believe is triggered by adenosine A_1 type receptors. The protection lasts for less than an hour and additional periods of ischemia offer no additional protection. Recent studies in rabbit hearts suggest that adenosine receptors are coupled to phospholipase C via a pertussis toxin-sensitive G protein. Phospholipase C activity activates protein kinase C which protects by phosphorylating a protective protein early in the ischemic period. We believe that preconditioning acts to up-regulate protein kinase C, perhaps by translocating it into the sarcolemma. Any receptor in the myocyte coupled to phospholipase C should be capable of putting the heart into the preconditioned state. That has been verified for the alpha-1 and the muscarinic M_2 receptors. Because pharmacologic preconditioning must precede ischemia we have been examining whether adenosine-induced protection can be maintained indefinitely. Unfortunately, after only 3 days of treatment tolerance develops to A_1-selective agonists with a loss of protection as well the ability to protect with ischemic preconditioning.

Key words: Myocardial infarction—Protein kinase C—Phospholipase C—Adenosine—Alpha-1 receptors—A_1 adenosine receptors—G proteins—Pertussis toxin—Muscarinic M2 receptors—Microtubules—Ischemic preconditioning

[1] Department of Physiology, University of South Alabama, Mobile, AL 36688, USA
[2] The Second Department of Internal Medicine, Sapporo Medical University, Sapporo, 060 Japan

Introduction

Myocardial cell death begins 10–20 min after the onset of a coronary artery occlusion and by 3 h involves the entire ischemic zone [1,2]. For several decades there has been a concerted research effort to devise an intervention which could delay the time course of necrosis. While it is now possible with thrombolytic therapy to restore perfusion to ischemic regions of the patient with acute myocardial infarction, reperfusion can seldom be accomplished before a substantial amount of myocardial necrosis has occurred. Despite this effort no such therapy is available. Antioxidants, calcium antagonists, and beta blockers have all been tested but have failed to provide consistent protection in preclinical trials [3–5]. This experience raised questions as to whether it is even possible to render the myocytes more resistant to a transient ischemic insult. That was until Murry and colleagues in 1986 reported that preconditioning the heart with four brief periods of ischemia, each 5 min in duration, caused the heart to tolerate a subsequent 40-min ischemic insult with much less infarction than was seen in nonpreconditioned hearts [6]. If the mechanism of this adaptive response can be understood, it should theoretically be possible to institute this form of protection pharmacologically in the coronary artery disease patient.

Ischemic preconditioning is a potent protector of the reperfused heart and its efficacy has been repeatedly confirmed. We [7,8] and others [9] have shown that as little as a single 5-min period of coronary occlusion could invoke full protection and that the anti-infarct effect lasts for no more than an hour [7,8,10]. In most models of ischemic preconditioning the protection is roughly equivalent to that which would result from shortening the ischemic period by about 20 min. While the exact mechanism of this protection has yet to be disclosed, there is now mounting evidence that adenosine plays an important role in this phenomenon. Adenosine has been the focus of studies in the heart for many years but adenosine has only recently been proposed to have direct cardioprotective effects. This concept was first proposed by Ely and colleagues in the isolated rat heart [11]. It was against that background that we thought to test adenosine as a possible mediator of ischemic preconditioning.

The Rabbit Infarct Model

Most of our studies on preconditioning have been conducted in the rabbit model of myocardial infarction. A prominent branch of the left coronary artery is ligated for 30 min and then reperfused for either several hours or several days. The ischemic zone is marked post mortem with fluorescent particles. Infarct size is determined by staining the heart with triphenyl tetrazolium chloride (TTC) in the 2- to 3-h reperfusion model and with conventional histology using Mallory-Azan stain in the 72-h reperfusion model. TTC reacts with dehydrogenase enzymes and cofactor in the tissue to produce a red pigment. Dead tissue quickly loses these constituents and fails to stain. Because these enzymes and cofactor are vital to the cell, TTC-negative tissue is unambiguously dead. On the other hand, degenerative changes responsible for enzyme loss can be slow to develop and as a result TTC-positive tissue may or may not be dead. The 72-h reperfusion model has the advantage that dead and living tissue are easily delineated and avoids the possibility of false-positive data. Infarct size is generally normalized by expressing it as a percentage of the ischemic zone, often referred to as the region at risk. The normalization procedure allows one to correct for differing heart sizes and variations in vascular anatomy. We consistently find that approximately 35%–45% of the risk region infarcts in a rabbit heart following a 30-min period of regional ischemia using either the TTC or the histology model.

TTC seems to be an accurate indicator of preconditioning-induced salvage in the rabbit heart. We reported infarct size from preconditioned rabbits subjected to a 30-min occlusion and 3 days of reperfusion [12]. Nonpreconditioned hearts had 45% of the risk zone infarcted, which compares favorably to that seen with TTC. Infarct size in preconditioned animals was much smaller and, again, similar to that determined by TTC (13% by histology [12] *vs* 8% by TTC [13]).

We have chosen rabbits for these studies for a number of important reasons. Foremost, rabbits are inexpensive and plentiful and we believe are a better biochemical model of the human heart than the rat. Rabbits also lack preformed coronary collateral vessels, so that it is not necessary to incorporate collateral flow as a covariant in the infarct size analysis, as is the case in dogs [1,14]. Another major advantage of the rabbit heart is the ability to study it in situ or in vitro. We find that 30 min regional ischemia yields the same infarct size whether in situ or in vitro in a Krebs buffer perfused Langendorff mode [15]. The isolated model allows us interventions which either must be confined to the heart or would not be tolerated if given systemically. Finally, rabbits are small which reduces the cost of dosing with expensive compounds such as pertussis toxin. By simplifying the model it has been possible for us to study a large number of rabbits using a wide variety of interventions which have allowed us to learn a great deal about the receptors and intracellular signalling pathways that are involved in the preconditioning phenomenon.

Adenosine A_1 Receptors Mediate Protection

Our original hypothesis was that endogenous adenosine released during the brief ischemia was the initiator of preconditioning. If that were correct then adenosine receptor blockade should prevent protection from ischemic preconditioning. Two broad acting adenosine receptor blockers, 8-*p*-sulfophenyl theophylline (SPT), and *N*-[2-(dimethylamino) ethyl] *N*-methyl-4-(2,3,6,7-tetrahydro-2,6-dioxo-1,3-dipropyl-1*H*-purin-8-yl) benzosulfonamide (PD 115,199), were used. The blockers were given 20 min prior to the 30-min ischemic period. The study design consisted of both ischemically preconditioned (5 min of ischemia followed by 10 min of reperfusion) and nonprecondititioned open-chest anesthetized rabbits. All experienced 30 min of ischemia to induce the infarct.

Thirty eight percent of the ischemic zone infarcted in the unblocked and nonpreconditioned control group. Preconditioning untreated hearts caused significant protection from infarction with only 8.8% ± 2.1% infarction. Pretreatment with SPT had no significant effect on infarct size in nonpreconditioned hearts but completely blocked the protective effect of preconditioning, with 38.9% ± 7.0% of the ischemic zone infarcting (NS *vs* control). Pretreatment with the other adenosine receptor antagonist, PD 115,199, produced an identical result [13] as did the blocker 8-phenyl-theophylline [16]. Thus, adenosine receptor occupation is essential for protection from ischemic preconditioning.

If the adenosine hypothesis is correct, then exposure of the heart to exogenous adenosine should protect the heart as well as exposure to ischemia. To test for a direct myocardial effect we confined the adenosine to the coronary arteries by using an isolated, blood-perfused rabbit heart [13]. Since intracoronary injections are impossible for us to make in the rabbit, a blood-perfused, isolated heart model was used to test the adenosine hypothesis. The hearts were electrically paced to avoid the bradycardia associated with intracoronary adenosine. The hearts underwent 45 min of regional ischemia followed by 2 h of reperfusion to induce an infarct. Infarct sizes in the isolated hearts were similar to those seen in in situ hearts and Fig. 1 reveals that these hearts could still be protected by ischemic preconditioning. In a third group, adenosine was infused directly into the coronary perfusate for 5 min at a total dose of

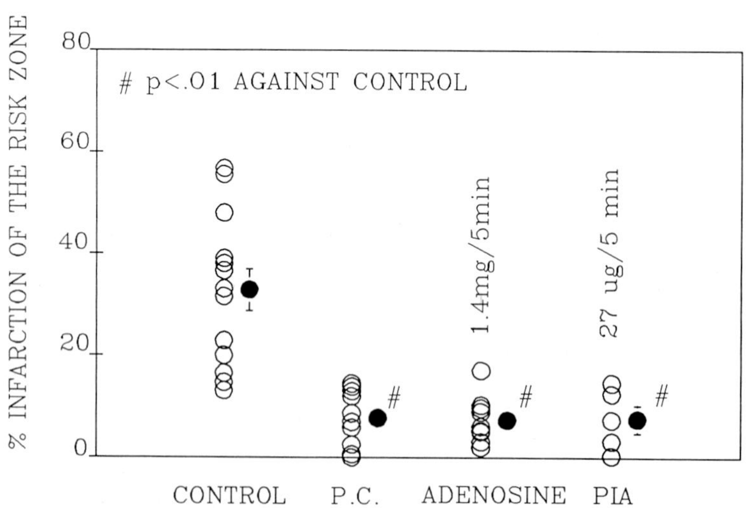

Fig. 1. Intracoronary infusion of adenosine or the A_1-selective agonist, PIA, was equipotent with ischemic preconditioning (*PC*) in protecting the isolated blood perfused rabbit heart from infarction. (From [13], with permission)

1.4 mg. The infusion was then stopped for 10 min to simulate the period of reperfusion which follows a preconditioning ischemia. Intracoronary adenosine protected the isolated heart to the same degree as ischemic preconditioning.

In an attempt to determine which adenosine receptor subtype was initiating the preconditioning protection, we employed the A_1 selective analog N^6-(phenyl-2R-isopropyl)-adenosine, PIA. The right-most panel of Fig. 1 reveals that PIA also protected the isolated heart when infused at a total dose of 26.6 μg over 5 min. That dose of PIA was chosen because it lengthened the P–R interval, an adenosine A_1 effect, but did not lower the coronary resistance, an adenosine A_2 effect. Because the A_1-selective agonist and ischemia were equipotent we concluded that the A_1 adenosine receptor was responsible for ischemic preconditioning's protection. Similar studies have recently been performed in the pig heart by Van Winkle and Davis [17] with identical results.

Others have reported that intravenous adenosine could be given both prior to or after ischemia and salvage myocardium [18,19]. We, however, have had little success in protecting the heart with intravenous adenosine treatment, either prior to ischemia [13] or at reperfusion [20]. We have tried intravenous A_1-selective agonists and have seen some protection [16,21] but the protection has not been equivalent to that seen with ischemic preconditioning, probably due to the hypotensive side effects of A_1 agonists [16]. Finally, we found that dipyridamole, a nucleoside transport inhibitor, lowered the threshold for preconditioning in rabbits to below 2 min of ischemia [22], which is also consistent with the adenosine hypothesis.

How Do Adenosine Receptors Mediate Protection?

In previous studies it had been shown that preconditioning does not involve an increase in coronary collateral blood flow [6]. Furthermore, cyclooxygenase inhibitors failed to block the protective effect of preconditioning against infarction, making it unlikely that activation of prostaglandins mediates protection [23,24].

Preconditioning Is Not the Result of Increased Antioxidants

One possible mechanism is that the antioxidant defence of the preconditioned heart is increased. In a recent experiment we examined the antioxidant status of control and preconditioned rabbit hearts [25]. Tissue was frozen after 5 min of reperfusion following 30 min regional ischemia. Figure 2 reveals that there were no significant differences in catalase, superoxide dismutase (Mn and CuZn), glucose-6-phosphate dehydrogenase, glutathione oxidase, or glutathione reductase between ischemically preconditioned and control hearts. Note that enzyme activities are expressed as a percentage of that in the nonischemic region. None of these antioxidant defenses had been significantly attenuated in the ischemic regions, even though they had experienced an ischemia/reperfusion insult sufficient to kill 40% of the cells.

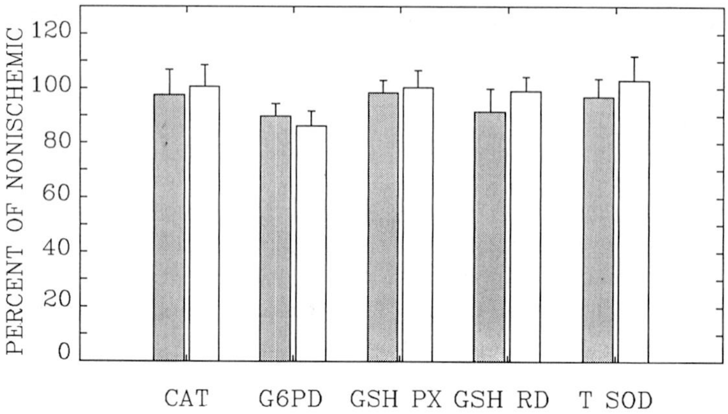

Fig. 2. Enzyme activity in the ischemic zone normalized as a percent of the nonischemic region for nonpreconditioned (*cross-hatched*) and preconditioned (*open*); standard error of the mean is indicated. Hearts had undergone 30 min of ischemia and 5 min of reperfusion. None of the enzymes were different from that in the nonischemic zone. *CAT*, Catalase; *G6PD*, glucose 6 phosphate dehydrogenase; *GSH PX*, glutathione peroxidase; *GSH RD*, glutathione reductase; *T SOD*, total superoxide dismutase. (From [25], with permission)

A similar finding was seen when glutathione levels were measured. Total glutathione was significantly lower in the nonpreconditioned hearts, suggesting that protection might be related to higher glutathione content in preconditioned hearts. On the other hand, glutathione washes out of injured cells quickly and we reasoned that if the cells were protected by some unrelated mechanism we would still see less washout in that tissue after a period of reperfusion. We therefore studied a second series of rabbits in which glutathione was measured just prior to the onset of reperfusion. Those measurements allowed us to determine if there were any differences in glutathione levels at the onset of reperfusion. Glutathione levels were identical in both groups, indicating no increased antioxidant capacity for the preconditioned hearts. There is little evidence that free radicals act as the trigger for preconditioning either [12].

Das et al. [26] recently reported that Mn superoxide dismutase (SOD), glutathione reductase, and glutathione oxidase were all higher in preconditioned as compared to nonpreconditioned swine hearts. It should be pointed out that those measurements were made 6 h after a 1-h period of regional ischemia rather than during the critical peri-reperfusion time when a putative reperfusion injury would have occurred. It is possible that the data of Das et al. again reflected increased washout of antioxidant enzymes from necrotic myocardium in the nonpreconditioned hearts, making the differences an effect of preconditioning rather than a cause. Hoshida et al. [27] also reported increased Mn SOD in preconditioned dog hearts, suggesting that dogs may differ from rabbits in that regard.

Heat Stress Proteins Also Are Not Thought to Be Involved

Heat stress proteins have received special attention [28]. Heat shock [29] and ischemia [30] are known to cause the induction of stress proteins in the heart and they appear in quantity several hours after the insult. In fact, Knowlton et al. [31] found that the message for the 70 KD stress protein, HSP70, was elevated after only 5 min of transient ischemia. Although HSP70 has been correlated with increased heat tolerance, it has also been postulated to offer a similar protection against ischemia. Currie et al. [29] reported that a 15-min heat shock induced both HSP70 and catalase and protected the isolated rat heart against subsequent ischemia. A similar observation was made by Yellon et al. [32] in the rabbit heart. While stress proteins, and HSP70 in particular, may at first seem to be prime candidates as the mediators of preconditioning, there is substantial evidence against this mechanism.

We tested whether synthesis of any protective protein might mediate preconditioning by testing whether blockers of protein synthesis could prevent the protection. Neither cycloheximide (blocks translation) nor actinomycin D (blocks transcription by DNA intercalation) could block the anti-infarct effect of preconditioning in our rabbit model [33]. While the protein synthesis studies argue against the role of a protein, it should be pointed out that it is difficult to block 100% of the stress-protein production with those blockers and thus one of the stress proteins could conceivably still have mediated the protection. Another line of evidence argues against HSP70 as the mediator. Message for HSP70 reaches its peak level in the tissue 2 h after an ischemic event [31] while preconditioning has worn off after 2 h [7,8,34]. Based on these observations we, therefore, think it highly unlikely that expression of a protective protein is involved in this protection.

Adenosine Receptors Couple to Protein Kinase C

Many functions in the cell are regulated by the phosphorylation of key proteins by protein kinases. One such kinase is protein kinase C (PKC). We [35] and others [36] have found that protein kinase C plays an important role in ischemic preconditioning. PKC is under the control of lipid cofactors which are produced primarily by phospholipase C. Phospholipase C, when activated, causes phospholipids in the cell membrane to be degraded producing two second messengers, diacylglycerol (DAG) and inositol triphosphate. While inositol triphosphate is thought to control calcium release at the sarcoplasmic reticulum, DAG is the lipid cofactor for PKC [37–39].

Adenosine A_1-receptors in several tissues including guinea pig myocardium reportedly cause phospholipase C activation [40–44]. Thus, it is possible that the activation of A_1-receptors activates PKC resulting in phosphorylation of a protein which then causes protection. To test that hypothesis, either of two inhibitors of PKC, staurosporine (50 μg/kg) or polymyxin B (24 mg/kg), were administered in vivo as a bolus to rabbits subjected to 30 min regional myocardial ischemia followed by 180 min reperfusion [35]. The drugs were given 5 min prior to the 30-min ischemia in all groups. Half of the rabbits were ischemically preconditioned with 5 min ischemia plus 10 min reperfusion while the other half served as nonpreconditioned controls. Regional ischemia in the latter hearts treated with staurosporine and polymyxin B resulted in 40.5% ± 2.8% and 42.0% ± 7.0% infarction of the risk zone, respectively. Both inhibitors blocked protection in preconditioned hearts with 36.2% ± 2.7% and 40.9% ± 2.5% of the risk zone infarcted, respectively. Only data for the staurosporine studies are shown in Fig. 3.

Staurosporine is a potent inhibitor of PKC and acts by interacting with the ATP-binding site which gives the drug rather poor selectivity against other kinases [45]. On the other hand, polymyxin B acts at the lipid regulatory site of PKC and has no known effect against other kinases such as cAMP-dependent kinase [46]. Taken together, then, these data strongly support a role for PKC in ischemic preconditioning. Staurosporine also reportedly blocks preconditioning in the isolated rat heart as does the PKC regulatory site inhibitor, chelerythrine [36].

Figure 3 also shows the converse experiment (only the PMA data shown). We tested whether activation of PKC with 4β-phorbol 12-myristate 13-acetate

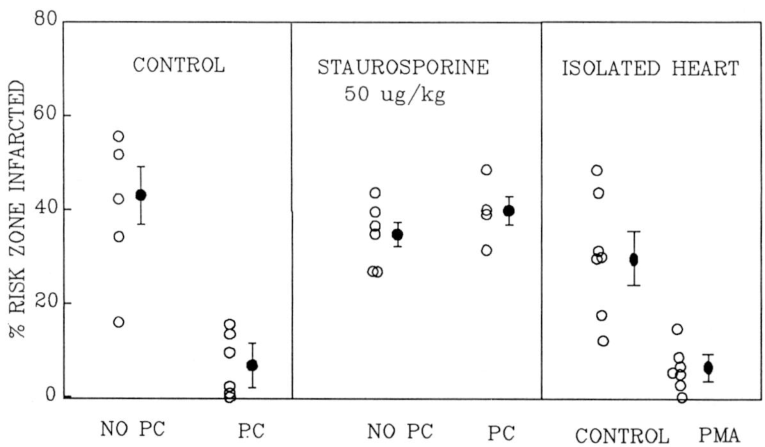

Fig. 3. Infarct size expressed as a percentage of the risk zone. Hearts were studied in situ. *Left panel* depicts untreated hearts and demonstrates protection from ischemic preconditioning (*PC*). *Center panel* shows that preconditioning's protective effect was lost in animals receiving the PKC inhibitor, staurosporine, just prior to the long ischemia. *Right panel* shows infarct size in Krebs-perfused isolated rabbit hearts. Note that 5 min exposure to the PKC activator, PMA, profoundly protected these hearts. *Open symbols*, individual hearts; *solid symbols*, group means. *PMA*, 4β-phorbol 12-myristate 13-acetate

(PMA) or with oleyl acetyl glycerol (OAG) could mimic preconditioning in buffer-perfused hearts. Hearts were exposed to either PMA (0.01 nmol/min) or OAG (10 nmol/min) for 5 min followed by 10 min of normal perfusate. They then experienced 30 min regional ischemia and 120 min reperfusion. Note that infarct size as a percentage of area at risk was significantly reduced in the PMA and OAG groups (6.4% ± 1.4% and 11.7% ± 3.3% *vs* 28.0% ± 4.5% in untreated controls). Because inhibition of PKC eliminates preconditioning's protection and because pretreatment with PKC activators mimic preconditioning's protection, we conclude that activation of PKC is an important step in the mechanism of preconditioning.

Adenosine A_1-Receptors Are Coupled with a Pertussis Toxin-Sensitive G Protein

A_1-receptors invariably have been found to be coupled to pertussis toxin sensitive G-proteins [47,48]. G proteins which couple to the β isoform of phospholipase C are broadly categorized as G_p. This family includes G_o (other) and several of the isoforms of G_i which are pertussis toxin-sensitive, and G_q which is not pertussis toxin-sensitive. If A_1 adenosine receptors effect preconditioning via G_i or G_o, then ribosylation of G proteins with pertussis toxin should block the protective effect of preconditioning. Rabbits received an intravenous bolus of pertussis toxin, 25 μg/kg, 48 hours prior to the surgical procedure and this was found to selectively block the protective effect of ischemic preconditioning [49], thus supporting the PKC theory.

The Translocation Theory of Ischemic Preconditioning

One peculiar feature of the preconditioning phenomenon is that the tissue can somehow remember that it has been preconditioned. For example, exposure of the heart to a single isolated ischemic episode puts the heart into a protected state which lasts for about an hour [7]. Similarly, transient exposure to adenosine protects the heart even when the adenosine is allowed to wash out for 10 min [13]. Any theory that attempts to explain preconditioning must be able to explain this memory.

We propose that the memory reflects translocation of PKC from the cytosol to the membranes. DAG produced by phospholipase C causes both activation of PKC that is already in the cell membranes and a translocation of cytosolic PKC into the membranes where it can become activated. Translocation can be relatively slow and is thought to account for the delayed response often seen with PKC activation since most of the kinase resides in the cytosol of the quiescent cell. Strasser et al. [50] recently reported that translocation of PKC from the cytosolic to the particulate fractions of the rat heart occurs in response to acute myocardial ischemia. Yuan et al. [37] reported that in rat ventricle, translocation induced with phorbol dibutyrate exhibited a 10-min time course which is very compatible with the kinetics of ischemic preconditioning. Seven isoforms of PKC have been identified in heart and the noncalcium dependent forms appear to predominate in rat heart, particularly epsilon [51]. Little is known about the translocation kinetics of individual isoforms during ischemia.

We propose that adenosine receptor activation during ischemic preconditioning initiates translocation of one or more isoforms of PKC into the membranes. Once the enzyme has translocated we propose that it would stay in the membranes for about 1h. If the protein responsible for protection must be phosphorylated in the first few minutes of ischemia in order to realize protection, then the delay imposed by the translocation step would be disastrous in nonpreconditioned myocardium. Such a delay would be absent from preconditioned myocardium since enzyme is already in the membranes and phosphorylation could proceed immediately upon population of A_1 receptors. The translocation theory then states that the only difference between a preconditioned heart and a virgin heart is that the former has PKC translocated into its membranes.

There is circumstantial evidence supporting the translocation theory. For example, blocking adenosine receptors only during the prolonged ischemia should block preconditioning, since reoccupation of adenosine receptors would be required to reactivate the translocated PKC. Indeed we found that to be the case [52]. Blocking adenosine receptors with PD 115,199 did not significantly affect infarction in nonpreconditioned animals when administered either prior to occlusion or at reperfusion (46.3% ± 5.9% and 44.3% ± 6.3% infarction of the risk zone, respectively; NS *vs* control). PD 115,199 completely blocked preconditioning's protection in our rabbit model whether given prior to or after the preconditioning ischemia (38.8% ± 5.4% and 30.1% ± 4.0% infarction, respectively; NS *vs* control). When PD 115,199 was administered just prior to the 180-min reperfusion in preconditioned (PC) rabbits, the protection was unaffected (17.1% ± 4.9% infarction, $P < 0.05$ *vs* control, NS *vs* PC). The alternative hypothesis for the memory is that phosphorylation of some protein constitutes the memory and that protection wears off only when that protein is dephosphorylated. In Fig. 3 the PKC inhibitors were given to the rabbits during the reperfusion phase following the preconditioning ischemia, indicating that phosphorylation must occur during the long ischemia to realize protection. Staurosporine only blocks the kinase activity of PKC and has no effect on its translocation. When we gave staurosporine only during the preconditioning ischemia, protection was retained [35], again showing that phosphorylation of protein is not even necessary during the preconditioning ischemia. Both of these observations argue strongly against the phosphorylation theory.

Translocations in the cell are usually accomplished by microtubules. We recently tested whether disrupting microtubules with colchicine would alter the ability to precondition the rabbit heart (data not yet published). Colchicine (5 mg/kg) was given 30 min prior to study in anesthetized open-chest rabbits. Colchicine pretreatment selectively blocked the protective effect of preconditioning but had no effect on infarct size in the nonpreconditioned group. Infarct size in the preconditioned colchicine group was 34.4% ± 5.8% (in-

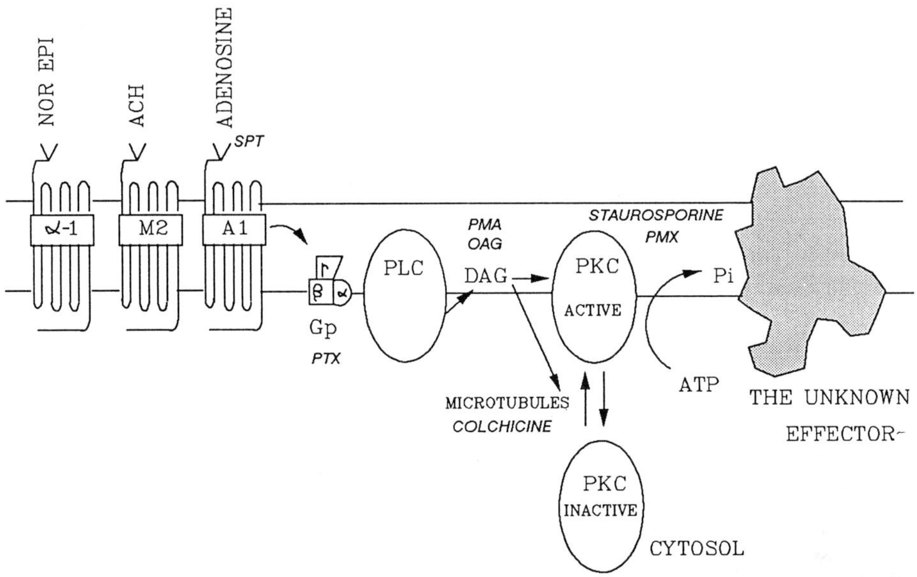

Fig. 4. Diagram of the proposed intracellular signalling system used in preconditioning. In the first ischemic period, adenosine populates A_1 receptors. Adenosine receptors couple to phospholipase C (*PLC*) through a pertussis-toxin-sensitive G protein (*GP*). The diacylglycerol (*DAG*) produced by the lipase causes cytosolic protein kinase C (PKC) to slowly translocate into the membranes where it can be activated. Because of the delay required for translocation, little protein is phosphorylated. PKC remains in the membranes during reperfusion. In the second ischemic period, repopulation of adenosine receptors reactivates the pathway and since translocation has already occurred, an unidentified protein is phosphorylated early in ischemia resulting in protection. Muscarinic (*M2*) or α-1 receptors also couple to phospholipase C and can equally initiate preconditioning. The interventions used to test each leg of the diagram are shown in the figure. *PTX*, pertussis toxin; *PMX*, polymyxin B; *NOR EP1*, norepinephrine; *ACH*, acetylcholine; *SPT*, 8-*p*-sulfophenyl theophylline; *OAG*, oleyl acetyl glycerol; *PMA*, 4β-phorbol 12-myristate 13-acetate; P_i, inorganic phosphate

farction of risk zone) which was not significantly different from that in nonpreconditioned hearts with colchicine (38.3% ± 1.9%) and significantly larger than that in untreated preconditioned hearts. The fact that disrupting microtubules with colchicine selectively blocks the protective effect of preconditioning again strongly supports the translocation hypothesis.

Stimulation of PKC with PMA or OAG also translocates PKC from the cytoplasm to the membranes [37–39]. In experiments not yet published we found that the adenosine receptor blocker, SPT, could block protection from PMA. That would be predicted by the translocation theory because the heart must rely on adenosine to reactivate the PKC pathway during the second occlusion. Figure 4 shows a summary of the intracellular signalling pathways that we think are involved in ischemic preconditioning in the rabbit.

Other Receptors Coupled to Phospholipase C Can Precondition

The translocation theory predicts that any agent which activates phospholipase C would precondition the heart. One such receptor is the α-1 receptor which is well known to couple to phospholipase C. An IV bolus of tyramine displaces cardiac norepinephrine and puts the heart into a preconditioned state [53]. Figure 5 reveals that blockade of α-1 receptors with BE 2254 removes tyramine's protection. Note that the β antagonist, propranolol, has no effect on protection from tyramine. Blocking the adenosine receptors with PD 115,199, however, completely removes the protection. The translocation theory states that the transient occupation of α-1 receptors simply translocated the PKC and that activation of adenosine receptors during the ischemic insult would be needed to reactivate PKC.

Norepinephrine is known to be released with ischemia [54] and, thus, norepinephrine could conceivably be responsible for the protection of ischemic preconditioning. That hypothesis did not prove to be the case, at least in the rabbit. The right-most panel of Fig. 5 reveals that blocking α-1 receptors with BE 2254 did not prevent ischemic preconditioning from protecting the heart. These data suggest that with a 5-min ischemia, adenosine receptors are the

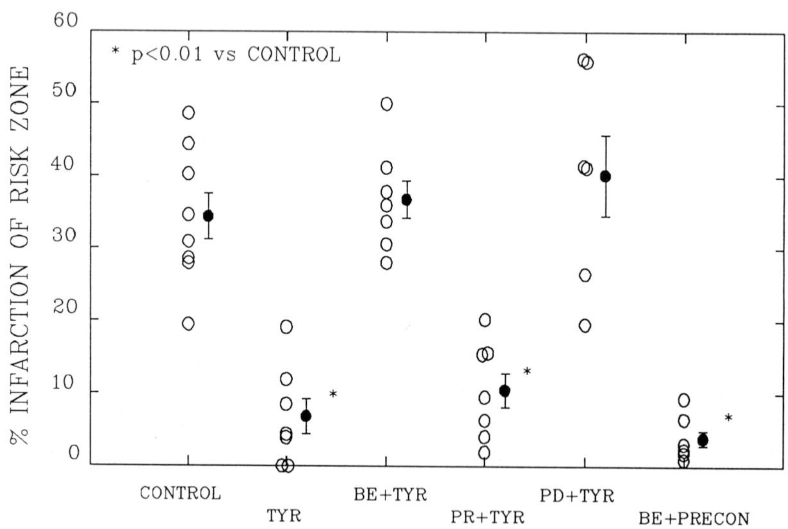

Fig. 5. Infarct size plotted as a percentage of risk zone for rabbits treated with tyramine (*TYR*). Also demonstrated are effects of tyramine on infarct size after pretreatment with BE 2254 (*BE*), propranolol (*PR*), and PD 115,199 (*PD*), and the effect of pretreatment with BE 2254 on ischemic preconditioning (*PRECON*). Both BE 2254 and PD 115,199 successfully blocked the protective effect of tyramine. Propranolol did not affect salvage by tyramine of ischemic tissue. Finally, the ability of ischemic preconditioning to limit infarct size was not diminished by BE 2254

only source of phospholipase C activation in rabbits. Another receptor known to couple to phospholipase C in the heart is the muscarinic M2 and transient exposure to carbachol is known to mimic preconditioning [49].

The Rat May Be Different

While the evidence linking adenosine receptors and PKC to ischemic preconditioning is strong for the rabbit, no such data exist for the rat and that species remains enigmatic. Rats can be protected against infarction with ischemic preconditioning in a manner identical to that seen in the rabbit [55–57]. Yet, neither adenosine receptor blockers [55,56] nor pertussis toxin [58] can block that protection. The explanation for this observation is unclear at this time. We have not examined PKC blockers in the rat model but one group has reported that protection was blocked [36]. Unfortunately, they used recovery of function as their end point rather than necrosis so we cannot be sure that the data can be extrapolated to infarction.

Tolerance to Chronic Adenosine Exposure Could Be a Therapeutic Problem

While receptor-selective adenosine analogs show some promise as cardioprotective agents, administration has to be prior to the onset of ischemia. This could be accomplished by maintaining high-risk groups continuously on a prophylactic dose of an A_1 agonist. To test the feasibility of prophylactic treatment we infused the A_1-selective agonist, N^6-cyclopentyladenosine (CCPA), into rabbits for up to 3 days [59]. To produce myocardial infarction a branch of the left coronary artery of rabbit hearts was occluded for 30 min and reperfused for 3 h. Infarct size was again determined with tetrazolium staining.

Prior to the 30-min ischemia, rabbits were subjected to one of the following six protocols: (1) 6-h IV saline infusion; (2) 6-h IV CCPA (0.043 mg/kg per hr) infusion; (3) 72-h saline infusion; (4) 72-h CCPA infusion; (5) 72-h CCPA infusion followed by preconditioning with 5-min ischemia followed by 10-min reperfusion; (6) 72-h saline infusion followed by ischemic preconditioning. The resulting infarct sizes appear in Fig. 6. Rabbits receiving CCPA for only 6 h had significantly smaller infarct sizes than the 6-h vehicle group, indicating that protection could be maintained continuously for 6 h. After 72 h of CCPA infusion, however, heart rate was seen to return to normal, suggesting that A_1 tolerance had developed. Note that infarct size in the 72-h CCPA infusion group was not different than that in the 72-h vehicle group, indicating that the protective effect of the drug had also been lost. Of particular interest is the observation that ischemic preconditioning could no longer limit infarct size in animals receiving a 72-h infusion of CCPA but did protect animals receiving vehicle for 72 h. These findings indicate that the myocytes become desensitized to the protective effect of an A_1 agonist with prolonged exposure. Furthermore,

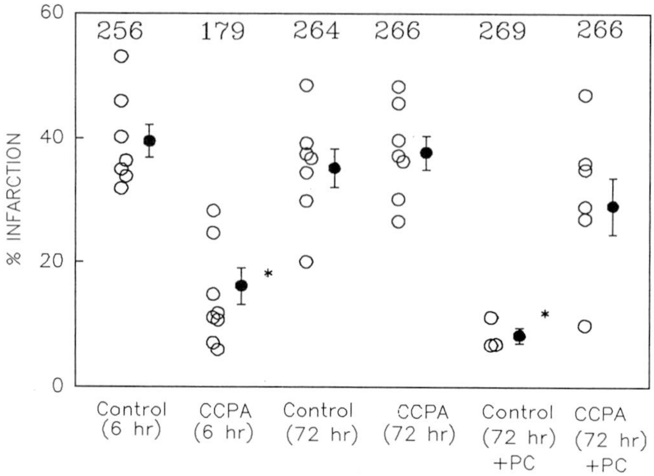

Fig. 6. A plot of the percentage of the risk zone infarcted for the 6 h and 72 h saline and CCPA infusion groups. *Open symbols* depict individual experiments while *solid symbols* show the mean and standard error for each group. Note that after 72 h infusion of CCPA, hearts can no longer be protected with preconditioning (*PC*). Numbers at the *top* of each panel indicate the heart rate at coronary occlusion. Note that the bradycardia induced by CCPA was lost at 72 hours. *CCPA*, N^6-cyclopentyladenosine

when tolerance to adenosine does develop, ischemic preconditioning is no longer protective as would be expected if adenosine mediates preconditioning.

We do not know the mechanism by which desensitization to CCPA occurred. However, previous reports suggest that the desensitization may occur at either the A_1 receptor itself or at the level of the G proteins. Many investigators have reported that A_1-receptor density is reduced after prolonged PIA exposure as revealed by receptor-binding assays in rat adipocyte [60–64], in chick embryo myocytes [65,66], and in Hamster DDT1 MF-2 cells [67]. Longabaugh et al. [61], Liang and Donovan [65], and Ramkumar et al. [67] all reported that the percentage of A_1-receptors in the high-affinity state was also reduced after desensitization with PIA. Because the high-affinity state is thought to occur when the receptor is attached to its G protein, desensitization could be the result of depletion of the G proteins or failure of the G proteins to couple properly to the receptor. Indeed, reduced levels of the inhibitory G protein, Gi, have been reported with desensitization. Green et al. [64,68] and Longabaugh et al. [61] reported reductions of the three alpha subunits of Gi protein (Gia1, Gia2, Gia3) in the A_1-receptors of adipocytes desensitized by PIA. Patients with recurrent angina may also become desensitized: it is thought that patients who have angina prior to a coronary thrombosis may obtain some protection through the preconditioning mechanism. The transient ischemia associated with an attack of angina causes a local release of adenosine, and it has been proposed that the released adenosine may be the actual mediator of the anginal pain [69]. In patients with recurrent angina, however, frequent exposure of those receptors might cause a similar desensitization to adenosine as was seen with CCPA.

To test for this possibility we surgically installed a pneumatic occluder on a branch of the left coronary artery in chronically instrumented rabbits [70]. The rabbits were allowed to recover from surgery for several days before study. This procedure allowed us to occlude and reperfuse the coronary branch at will while the animal was in the conscious state. A 30-min coronary occlusion followed by 3 h reperfusion in the conscious state resulted in 37.7% ± 2.6% infarction of the risk area, and 5 of 8 rabbits developed ventricular arrhythmias. If a cycle of 5 min coronary occlusion/10 min reperfusion preceded the 30-min occlusion, infarction was significantly decreased to 5.6% ± 1.1% ($P < 0.0001$) and ventricular arrhythmias were observed in only 1 of 8 animals ($P < 0.05$). Thus, a single episode of PC diminished infarction and serious arrhythmias even in the absence of anesthesia. After pretreatment with 40–60 5-min occlusions (1 every 30 min) over 3–4 days, a 30-min sustained period of ischemia was instituted 10 min after the last 5-min occlusion. Infarction in those animals was 26.5% ± 2.9% ($P < 0.001$ *vs* single PC), and serious arrhythmias occurred in 50% of animals. Clearly preconditioning's ability to protect was attenuated after multiple episodes of PC, and this suggests that patients with recurrent angina may also become unresponsive to PC or adenosine-based interventions.

Concluding Remarks

These studies make a strong case for adenosine being a potent anti-infarction agent when given prior to ischemia. The heart is apparently able to capitalize on this property of adenosine and employ it in the preconditioning phenomenon. While we have been able to shed some light on the receptor type involved, the coupling G protein, and PKC, the overall mechanism of how PKC activation protects the ischemic heart remains unknown. We do not know what protein gets phosphorylated by PKC in the heart. For example, it could be 5′-nucleotidase, the enzyme responsible for adenosine production [71]. Other candidates might include the ATP-sensitive potassium channel [72], a glycolytic enzyme [73], the β receptor [74], a cytoskeletal element [75], or perhaps even another kinase.

Multiple isoforms of PKC have been identified and it is most likely that protection from preconditioning may reflect the action of a single isoform working on a preferred substrate. It is recognized that the different isoforms have very different translocation patterns in the myocyte [51] and as a result biochemical measurement of total PKC activity may prove to be very misleading. Future work should concentrate of identification of the specific isoform.

Adenosine or A_1-selective analogs do not appear to offer great clinical promise. The requirement for pretreatment is a major problem since most patients with acute myocardial infarction do not seek treatment until after they thrombose. Selection of an agent is also difficult. Adenosine itself can only be infused into the coronary artery to achieve full preconditioning. Parenteral use of A_1-selective agonists still is associated with too many side effects. Furthermore, tolerance soon develops to A_1 agonists, making prophylactic therapy impossible. Finally, because natural tolerance can potentially occur, patients with chronic ischemia may become naturally resistant to any adenosine-based therapy or even ischemic preconditioning itself. Thus, while inroads have been made into the mechanism of ischemic preconditioning, many problems remain to be solved before a practical therapy will result.

References

1. Reimer KA, Jennings RB (1979) The "wavefront phenomenon" of myocardial ischemic cell death. II. Transmural progression of necrosis within the framework of ischemic bed size (myocardium at risk) and collateral flow. Lab Invest 40:633–644
2. Miura T, Downey JM, Ooiwa H, Ogawa S, Adachi T, Noto T, Shizukuda Y, Iimura O (1989) Progression of myocardial infarction in a collateral flow deficient species. Jpn Heart J 30:695–708
3. Kloner RA, Przyklenk K, Whittaker P (1989) Deleterious effects of oxygen radicals in ischemia/reperfusion: resolved and unresolved issues. Circulation 80:1115–1127
4. Reimer KA, Murry CE, Richard VJ (1989) The role of neutrophils and free radicals in the ischemic-reperfused heart: Why the confusion and controversy? J Mol Cell Cardiol 21:1225–1239
5. Hearse DJ, Yellon DM, Downey JM (1986) Can beta blockers limit infarct size? Eur Heart J 7:925–930
6. Murry CE, Jennings RB, Reimer KA (1986) Preconditioning with ischemia: a delay of lethal cell injury in ischemic myocardium. Circulation 74:1124–1136
7. Van Winkle DM, Thornton JD, Downey DM, Downey JM (1991) The natural history of preconditioning: Cardioprotection depends on duration of transient ischemia and time to subsequent ischemia. Coronary Art Dis 2:613–619
8. Miura T, Adachi T, Ogawa T, Iwamoto T, Tsuchida A, Iimura O (1992) Myocardial infarct size limiting effect of ischemic preconditioning: its natural decay and the effect of repetitive preconditioning. Cardiovasc Pathol 1:147–154
9. Li GC, Vasquez JV, Gallagher KP, Lucchesi BR (1990) Myocardial protection with preconditioning. Circulation 82:609–619
10. Li Y, Whittaker P, Kloner RA (1992) The transient nature of the effect of ischemic preconditioning on myocardial infarct size and ventricular arrhythmia. Am Heart J 123:346–353
11. Ely SW, Mentzer RM Jr, Lasley RD, Lee BK, Berne RM (1985) Functional and metabolic evidence of enhanced myocardial tolerance to ischemia and reperfusion with adenosine. J Thorac Cardiovasc Surg 90:549–556
12. Iwamoto T, Miura T, Adachi T, Noto T, Ogawa T, Tsuchida A, Iimura O (1991) Myocardial infarct size-limiting effect of ischemic preconditioning was not attenuated by oxygen free-radical scavengers in the rabbit. Circulation 83:1015–1022

13. Liu GS, Thornton J, Van Winkle DM, Stanley AWH, Olsson RA, Downey JM (1991) Protection against infarction afforded by preconditioning is mediated by A1 adenosine receptors in rabbit heart. Circulation 84:350–356
14. Miura T, Yellon DM, Hearse DJ, Downey JM (1987) Determinants of infarct size during permanent occlusion of a coronary artery in the closed chest dog. J Am Coll Cardiol 9:647–654
15. Ytrehus K, Downey JM (1993) Experimental models assessing the physiology of myocardial ischemia. Curr Opin Cardiol 8:581–588
16. Tsuchida A, Miura T, Miki T, Shimamoto K, Iimura O (1992) Role of adenosine receptor activation in myocardial infarct size limitation by ischemic preconditioning. Cardiovasc Res 26:456–461
17. Van Winkle DM, Davis RF (1991) Ischemic preconditioning of myocardium: effect of the adenosine agonist phenylisopropyl adenosine (PIA) (abstract). Circulation 84[Suppl II]:II-305
18. Toombs CF, McGee DS, Johnston WE, Vinton-Johanson J (1992) Myocardial protective effects of adenosine: infarct size reduction with pretreatment and continued receptor stimulation during ischemia. Circulation 86:986–994
19. Forman M, Virmani R, Puett D (1990) Mechanisms and therapy of myocardial reperfusion injury. Circulation 81[Suppl]:IV69–IV78
20. Goto M, Miura T, Liodoromitis EK, O'Leary EL, Ishimoto R, Yellon DM, Iimura O (1991) Adenosine infusion during early reperfusion failed to limit myocardial infarct size in a collateral deficient species. Cardiovasc Res 25:943–949
21. Thornton JD, Liu GS, Olsson RA, Downey JM (1992) Intravenous pretreatment with A1-selective adenosine analogues protects the heart against infarction. Circulation 85:659–665
22. Miura T, Ogawa T, Iwamoto T, Shimamoto K, Iimura O (1992) Dipyridamole potentiates the myocardial infarct size-limiting effect of ischemic preconditioning. Circulation 86:979–985
23. Li Y, Kloner R (1992) Is ischemic "preconditioning" mediated by cardioprotective prostanoids? Cardiovasc Res 26:226–231
24. Liu GS, Stanley AHS, Downey JM (1992) Cyclooxygenase products are not involved in the protection against myocardial infarction afforded by preconditioning in rabbit. Am J Cardiovasc Path 4:56–63
25. Turrens JF, Thornton J, Barnard ML, Snyder S, Liu G, Downey JM (1992) Protection from reperfusion injury by preconditioning hearts does not involve increased antioxidant defenses. Am J Physiol 262:H585–H589
26. Das DK, Prasad MR, Lu D, Jones RM (1992) Preconditioning of heart by repeated stunning. Adaptive modification of anti oxidative defense system. Cell Mol Biol 38:737–749
27. Hoshida S, Kuzuya T, Fuji H, Oe H, Kimura Y, Sasaki T, Kitabatake A, Tada M (1991) Ischemic preconditioning affects free radical generating and scavenging systems in canine myocardial infarction (abstract). Circulation 84[Suppl]:II-192
28. Yellon DM, Latchman DS (1992) Stress proteins and myocardial protection. J Mol Cell Cardiol 24:113–124
29. Currie WR, Karmazyn M, Kloc M, Mailer K (1988) Heat-shock response is associated with enhanced postischemic ventricular recovery. Circ Res 63:543–549
30. Mestril R, Dillmann WH (1991) Heat shock and adaptive response to ischemia. Trends Cardiovasc Med 1:240–244

31. Knowlton A, Brecher P, Apstein C (1991) Rapid expression of heat shock protein in the rabbit after brief cardiac ischemia. J Clin Invest 87:139–147
32. Yellon DM, Pasini E, Cargnoni A, Marber MS, Latchman DS, Ferrari R (1992) The protective role of heast stress in the ischaemic and reperfused rabbit myocardium. J Mol Cell Cardiol 24:895–907
33. Thornton J, Striplin S, Liu GS, Swafford A, Stanley AWH, Van Winkle DM, Downey JM (1990) Inhibition of protein synthesis does not block myocardial protection afforded by preconditioning. Am J Physiol 259:H1822–H1825
34. Murry CE, Richard VJ, Jennings RB, Reimer KA (1991) Myocardial protection is lost before contractile function recovers from ischemic preconditioning. Am J Physiol 260:H796–H804
35. Ytrehus K, Liu Y, Downey JM (1994) Preconditioning protects ischemic rabbit heart by protein kinase C activation. Am J Physiol 226:H1145–H1152
36. Mitchell MB, Brew EC, Harken AH, Banerjee A (1993) Does protein kinase C mediate functional preconditioning (abstract)? J Mol Cell Cardiol 25:S64
37. Yuan S, Sunahara F, Sen A (1987) Tumor-promoting phorbol esters inhibit cardiac functions and induce redistribution of protein kinase C in perfused beating rat heart. Circ Res 61:372–378
38. Capogrossi M, Kaku T, Filburn C, Pelto D, Hansford R, Spurgeon H, Lakatta E (1990) Phorbol ester and dioctanoylglycerol stimulate membrane association of protein kinase C and have a negative inotropic effect mediated by changes in cytosolic Ca^{2+} in adult rat cardiac myocytes. Circ Res 66:1143–1155
39. Kishimoto A, Takai Y, Mori T (1990) Activation of calcium and phospholipid-dependent protein kinase by diacylglycerol: its possible relation to phosphatidylinositol turnover. J Biol Chem 255:2273–2276
40. Spielman W, Klotz K, Arend L, Olson B, LeVier D, Schwabe U (1992) Characterization of adenosine A_1 receptor in a cell line (28A) derived from rabbit collecting tubule. Am J Physiol 263:C502–C508
41. Schwibert E, Karlson H, Friedman P, Dietl P, Spielman W (1992) Adenosine regulates a chloride channel via protein kinase C and a G protein in a rabbit cortical collecting duct cell line. J Clin Invest 89:834–841
42. Schiemann W, Westfall D, Buxton L (1991) Smooth muscle adenosine A_1 receptors couple to disparate effectors by distinct G proteins in pregnant myometrium. Am J Physiol 261:E141–E150
43. Kohl C, Linck B, Schmitz W, Scholz H, Scholz J, Tóth M (1990) Effects of carbachol and (−)-*N*6-phenylisopropyladenosine on myocardial inositol phosphate content and force of contraction. Br J Pharmacol 101:829–834
44. Stiles G (1992) Adenosine receptors. J Biol Chem 267:6451–6454
45. Tamaoki T (1991) Use and specificity of staurosporine, UCN-01, and calphostin C as protein kinase inhibitors. In: Methods in enzymology, vol 201, pp 340–476
46. Casnellie J (1991) Protein kinase inhibitors: probes for the functions of protein phosphorylation. Adv Pharmacol 22:167–205
47. Brown AM (1990) Regulation of heartbeat by G protein-coupled ion channels. Am J Physiol 259:H1621–H1628
48. Stiles GL (1991) Adenosine receptors: Physiologic regulation and biochemical mechanisms. NIPS 6:161–165
49. Thornton JD, Liu GS, Downey JM (1993) Pretreatment with pertussis toxin blocks the protective effects of preconditioning: evidence for a G-protein mechanism. J Mol Cell Cardiol 25:311–320

50. Strasser RH, Braun-Dullaeus R, Walendzik H, Marquetant R (1992) Alpha 1 receptor-independent activation of protein kinase C in acute myocardial ischemia: mechanism for sensitization of the adenylyl cyclose system. Circ Res 70:1304–1312
51. Bogoyevitch MA, Parker PJ, Sugden PJ (1993) Characterization of protein kinase C isotype expression in adult rat heart. Circ Res 72:757–767
52. Thornton JD, Thornton CS, Downey JM (1993) Effect of adenosine receptor blockade: preventing preconditioning depends on time of initiation. Am J Physiol 265:H504–H508
53. Thornton JD, Daly JF, Cohen MV, Downey JM (1993) Catecholamines induce adenosine receptor-mediated protection of the myocardium but do not participate in ischemic preconditioning in the rabbit. Circ Res 73:649–655
54. Schomig A (1990) Catecholamines in myocardial ischemia: systemic and cardiac release. Circulation 82[Suppl]:II-13–II-22
55. Liu Y, Downey JM (1992) Ischemic preconditioning protects against infarction in rat heart. Am J Physiol 263:H1107–H1112
56. Li Y, Kloner RA (1993) The cardioprotective effects of ischemic "preconditioning" are not mediated by adenosine receptors in rat hearts. Circulation 87:1642–1648
57. Yellon DM, Alkulaifi AM, Browne EE, Pugsley WS (1992) Ischemic preconditioning limits infarct size in the rat heart. Cardiovasc Res 26:983–987
58. Liu Y, Downey JM (1993) Preconditioning against infarction in the rat heart does not involve a pertussis toxin-sensitive G protein. Cardiovasc Res 27:608–611
59. Tsuchida A, Thompson R, Olsson RA, Downey JM (1994) The anti-infarct effect of an adenosine A_1-selective agonist is diminished after prolonged infusion as is the cardioprotective effect of ischemic preconditioning in rabbit heart. J Mol Cell Cardiol 26:303–311
60. Parsons WJ, Stiles GL (1987) Heterologous desensitization of the inhibitory A_1 adenosine receptor-adenylate cyclase system in rat adipocytes. J Biol Chem 262:841–847
61. Longabaugh JP, Didsbury J, Spiegel A, Stiles GL (1989) Modification of the rat adipocyte A_1 adenosine receptor-adenylate cyclase system during chronic exposure to A_1 adenosine receptor agonist. Mol Pharmacol 36:681–688
62. Hoffman BB, Chang H, Dall'aglio E, Reaven GM (1986) Desensitization of adenosine receptor-mediated inhibition of lipolysis: the mechanism involves the development of enhanced cyclic adenosine monophosphate accumulation in tolerant adipocytes. J Clin Invest 78:185–190
63. Green A (1987) Adenosine receptor down-regulation and insulin resistance following prolonged incubation of adipocytes with an A_1 adenosine receptor agonist. J Biol Chem 262:15702–15707
64. Green A, Milligan G, Dobias SB (1990) G_i down-regulation as a mechanism for heterologous desensitization in adipocytes. J Biol Chem 265:5206–5210
65. Liang B, Donovan L (1990) Differential desensitization of A_1 adenosine receptor-mediated inhibition of cardiac myocyte contractility and adenylate cyclase activity. Circ Res 67:406–414
66. Shyrock J, Patel A, Belardinelli L, Linden J (1989) Downregulation and desensitization of A_1 adenosine receptors in embryonic chicken heart. Am J Physiol 256:H321–H327
67. Ramkumar V, Olah ME, Jacobson KA, Stiles GL (1991) Distinct pathway of desensitization of A_1- and A_2-adenosine receptors in DDT1 MF-2 cell. Mol Pharmacol 40:639–647

68. Green A, Johnson JL, Milligan G (1990) Down-regulation of Gi sub-types by prolonged incubation of adipocytes with an A_1 adenosine receptor agonist. J Biol Chem 265:5206–5210
69. Crea F, Pupita G, Galassi AR, El-Tamimi H, Kaski JC, Davies G, Maseri A (1990) Role of adenosine in pathogenesis of anginal pain. Circulation 81:164–172
70. Cohen MV, Yang XM, Downey JM (1994) Conscious rabbits become tolerant to multiple episodes of ischemic preconditioning. Cir Res 74:998–1004
71. Kitakaze M, Hori M, Takashima S, Sato H, Inoue M, Kamada T (1993) Ischemic preconditioning increases adenosine release and 5′ nucleotidase activity during myocardial ischemia and reperfusion in dogs: implications for myocardial salvage. Circulation 87:208–215
72. Gross GJ, Auchampach JA (1992) Blockade of ATP-sensitive potassium channels prevents myocardial preconditioning in dogs. Circ Res 70:223–233
73. Wyatt DA, Edmunds MC, Rubio R, Berne RM, Lasley RD, Mentzer RM Jr (1989) Adenosine stimulates glycolytic flux in isolated perfused rat hearts by A_1-adenosine receptors. Am J Physiol 257:H1952–H1957
74. Vander Heide RS, Reimer KA, Jennings RB (1992) Adenosine mimics ischemic preconditioning and slows ischemic metabolism, possibly by inhibiting the effects of endogenous catecholamines (abstract). FASEB J 6:A-940
75. Armstrong SC, Ganote CE (1992) Flow cytometric analysis of isolated adult cardiomyocytes: vinculin and tubulin fluorescence during metabolic inhibition and ischemia. J Mol Cell Cardiol 24:149–162

1.12 Induction of Myocardial Manganese Superoxide Dismutase and Acquisition of Ischemic Tolerance

T. Kuzuya, S. Hoshida, M. Nishida, N. Yamashita, M. Hori, and M. Tada[1]

Summary. Exposing the myocardium to brief repeated episodes of ischemia and reperfusion has been shown to dramatically limit the size of infarct produced by a subsequent episode of sustained ischemia. We also found that the infarct-limiting effect was observed not only immediately after, but also 24 h after repetitive brief ischemia in dogs. The sublethal ischemia enhanced the myocardial activity of mitochondrial Mn-SOD associated with the increase in its content 24 h after the treatment. Thus, sublethal ischemia-induced protection against myocardial injury could occur biphasically. Induction of Mn-SOD enzyme may contribute to the delayed phase of myocardial adaptation.

Key words: Myocardial reperfusion—Sublethal ischemia—Ischemic preconditioning—Antioxidative enzymes—Manganese superoxide dismutase

If occlusion of a major coronary artery is sustained beyond 15 to 20 min, ischemic cell death begins first in the subendocardial region and then propagates with time toward the subepicardium. Timely reperfusion of the ischemic heart, therefore, can limit the extent of myocardial necrosis and improve the prognosis for survival in patients with acute myocardial infarction. On the other hand, it is also well known that repeated brief episodes of ischemia can render the heart more resistant to ischemic injury [1,2].

In a hypothetical view, salvage of jeopardized myocardial tissue by reperfusion could vary according to the degree of myocardial tolerance against ischemic insult (Fig. 1). In the heart resistant to ischemia, progression of myocardial

[1] Division of Cardiology, First Department of Medicine, and Department of Pathophysiology, Osaka University School of Medicine, 2-2 Yamadaoka, Suita, Osaka, 565 Japan

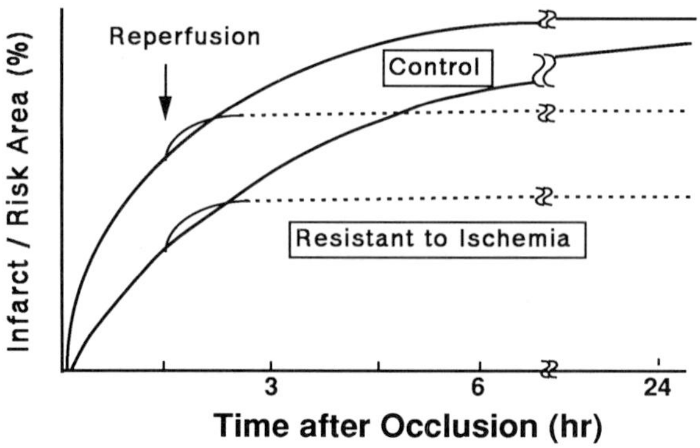

Fig. 1. Progression of myocardial infarction after coronary artery occlusion and reperfusion

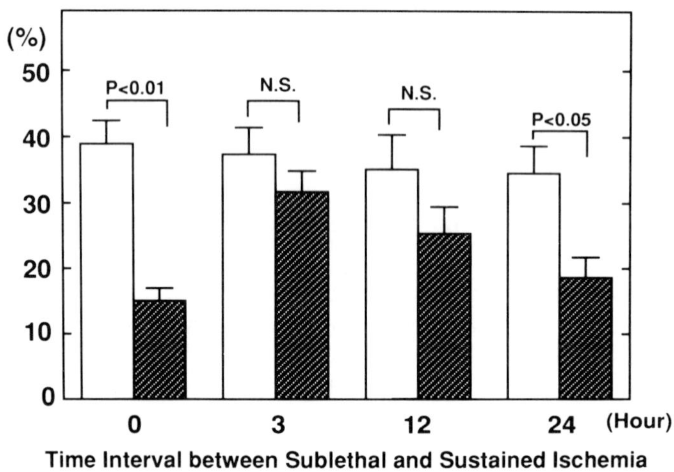

Fig. 2. Bar graph comparing the infarcted area (expressed as a percentage of the area at risk) in preconditioned (*hatched bars*) versus sham-operated (*open bars*) dogs. Values are mean ± SEM (n = 10 each)

necrosis decelerates; as a result, a relatively greater extent of ischemic myocardium can be salvaged even if the reperfusion time after occlusion is identical. So, it is very important to know how the heart is preconditioned before the onset of myocardial infarction.

In the present study, we investigated how the myocardium, preconditioned with sublethal ischemia, acquires resistance to ischemic injury.

Effects of Sublethal Ischemia on the Acquisition of Tolerance to Ischemia

We examined the effect of repeated brief ischemia on limiting infarct size in the open-chest dog [3]. Immediately after, or 3, 12, and 24 h after four cycles of 5 min occlusion–5 min reperfusion of the left anterior descending coronary artery, dogs were subjected to 90 min occlusion followed by 5 h reperfusion. Controls were subjected to the same procedure after sham operation (without repeated brief ischemia). After excision of the heart, the size of the anatomic area at risk and extent of irreversible injury were determined with a dual staining technique, using Evans blue dye and triphenyl tetrazolium chloride (TTC). Arterial blood pressure was monitored and the rate–pressure product was recorded throughout the experiments. We determined regional myocardial blood flow at baseline, during sustained occlusion, and after reperfusion, using colored microspheres.

Figure 2 shows the effect of sublethal ischemia on limiting myocardial infarct size resulting from sustained ischemia. Immediately after sublethal ischemia, the percentage of risk area infarcted was markedly decreased, to 14% compared with 39% in the control. There were no differences in the area at risk between these groups. The dramatic effect of limiting infarct size coincided well with the previous reports [1,2]. The early effect was designated the "preconditioning effect" by Murry and colleagues [1]. When the interval be-

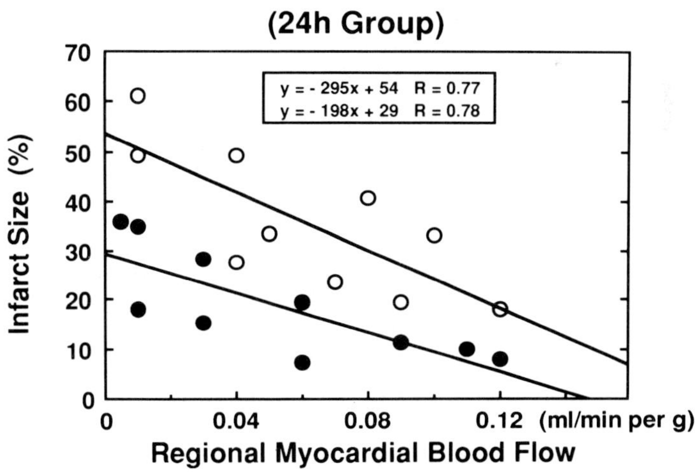

Fig. 3. Linear regression analysis of infarct size expressed as a percentage of the area at risk versus regional myocardial blood flow to the subendocardial left ventricular wall. Dogs in the sham-operated control group (*open circles*, $n = 10$) and the preconditioned group (*closed circles*, $n = 10$) were subjected to 90 min of ischemia followed by reperfusion 24 h after thoracotomy or preconditioning

tween sublethal and sustained ischemia was 3 to 12 h, no statistical differences were seen in the infarct size between pretreated and sham-operated groups. However, it should be noted that the infarct-limiting effect was observed again 24 h after pretreatment with sublethal ischemia: at that time, the percentage of risk area infarcted was about 19% for pretreated and 35% for sham-operated groups, respectively. These results indicate that the so-called "preconditioning effect" occurs not only at early stages but also at a delayed phase after sublethal ischemia.

Figure 3 illustrates the relation between infarct size as a percentage of risk area and collateral blood flow to the inner half of the LAD-dependent myocardium during the sustained ischemic period. Closed circles represent dogs pretreated with sublethal ischemia 24 h before (24-p group) and open circles represent sham-operated controls (24-s group). The regression lines for the control and pretreated groups were significantly different. The regression line in the pretreated group was shifted markedly downward compared with that in the control. Therefore, for a given collateral blood flow, infarct size as a percentage of the risk area was markedly smaller in the pretreated group. No differences were seen in rate–pressure products during sustained coronary occlusion and reperfusion between these two groups. Thus, it is evident that the delayed effect of repeated brief ischemia on limiting infarct size is also based on the acquisition of myocardial tolerance against ischemic insult.

Sublethal Ischemia Alters Myocardial Antioxidant Activity

During ischemia and reperfusion, myocardial tissue undergoes oxidative stress, triggered by reactive oxygen species. In contrast, it is known that superoxide generation can trigger induction of endogenous antioxidant enzymes including mitochondrial manganese-superoxide dismutase (SOD). Recently, hyperthermia [4] and inflammatory mediators that may increase the generation of oxygen-derived free-radicals in vivo, such as endotoxin [5], interleukin-1 (IL-1) [6], and tumor necrosis factor (TNF) [7], have been reported to increase antioxidant activity associated with the acquisition of tolerance against tissue injury. These experiments led us to speculate on the possibility that cellular antioxidant systems may be closely linked to the myocardial adaptation against sublethal ischemia. To elucidate the mechanism for the acquisition of tolerance against myocardial oxidative damage, we further investigated the changes in myocardial antioxidant enzymes after sublethal ischemic insult using a canine coronary occlusion–reperfusion model [8].

After four cycles of 5 min occlusion–5 min reperfusion, hearts were excised, cut into transverse slices, and myocardial samples were taken from the endocardial and epicardial sides of the area at risk and from the nonischemic lesion. As controls, sham-operated hearts were also excised 0–24 h after thoracotomy. After the myocardial tissue samples were homogenized, and centrifuged, the supernatant was sonicated and subjected to biochemical analysis.

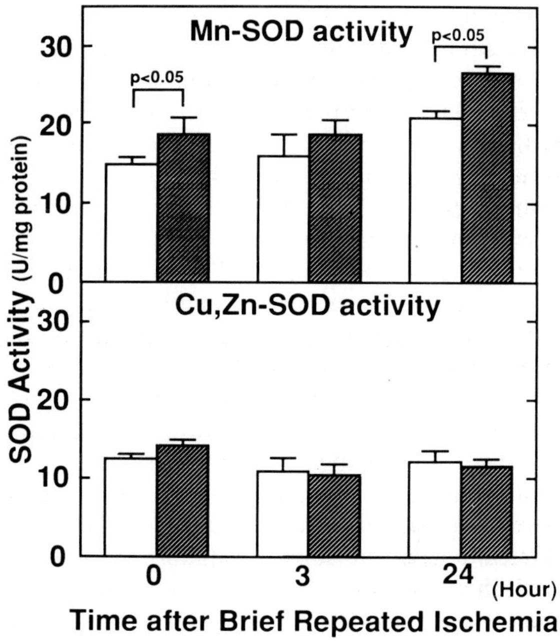

Fig. 4. Superoxide dismutase (*SOD*) activity in the ischemic (*hatched bars*) and nonischemic (*open bars*) myocardium at 0, 3, and 24 h after brief repeated ischemia. Values are mean ± SEM

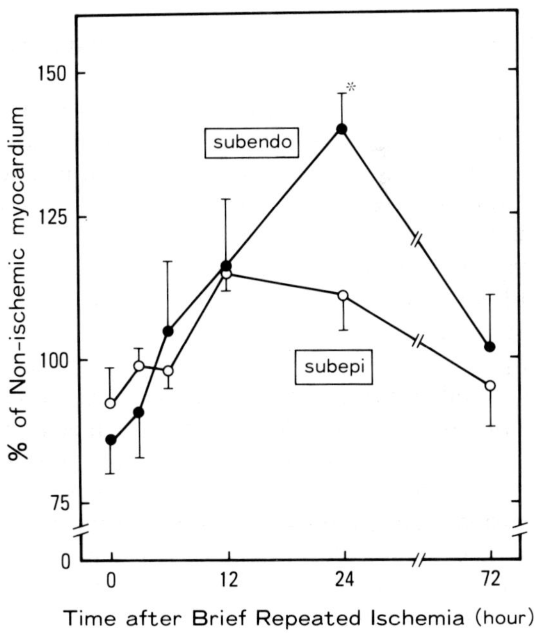

Fig. 5. Serial changes of manganese SOD protein in subepicardial (*subepi*) and subendocardial (*subendo*) sides of ischemic myocardium. Each point shows percent change in manganese-SOD level over that in each side of non-ischemic myocardium at respective time. Values are mean ± SEM ($n = 5$ each)

We determined SOD activity in the myocardial samples by the nitroblue tetrazolium method. Manganese-SOD activity, shown in the Fig. 4a, was measured by adding potassium cyanide (KCN) to inhibit copper-zinc-SOD activity. Copper-zinc SOD activity (Fig. 4b) was obtained by subtracting manganese-SOD from total SOD activity. Manganese-SOD activity was significantly higher both immediately after and 24 h after pretreatment with sublethal ischemia, than in the sham-operated controls. It should also be noted that, 24 h after pretreatment, manganese-SOD activity was increased by about 80% over the normal control. There was no difference in copper-zinc-SOD activity between pretreated and sham-operated groups. In the preliminary study, we could not also see any difference in the activities of glutathione-related enzymes and catalase (data not shown). It is, therefore, important to define the mechanism of augmentation in mitochondrial manganese-SOD activity, in terms of myocardial adaptation to ischemic insult.

Myocardial manganese-SOD contents were measured by enzyme-linked immunosorbent assay using anti-canine manganese-SOD antibody. Figure 5 shows serial changes in manganese-SOD content in the subendocardium (closed circles) and in the subepicardium (open circles) after sublethal ischemia. Each plot shows the percent change in manganese-SOD levels over those in non-ischemic myocardium. In the subendocardial side of the ischemic myocardium, manganese-SOD slightly decreased immediatedly after ischemia, and then gradually increased to a peak at 24 h after. However, 72 h after ischemia there was no difference in the level of manganese-SOD. These results indicate that manganese-SOD protein could be initially denatured by ischemic insult but thereafter be markedly induced over the baseline level.

In summary, the infarct-limiting effect was observed not only immediately after, but also 24 h after repetitive brief ischemia in dogs. The sublethal ischemia enhanced the myocardial activity of mitochondrial manganese-SOD associated with the increase in its content 24 h after the treatment. Thus, sublethal ischemia-induced protection against myocardial injury could occur biphasically. Induction of manganese-SOD enzyme may contribute to the delayed phase of adaptation.

References

1. Murry CE, Jennings RB, Reimer KA (1986) Preconditioning with ischemia: a delay of lethal cell injury in ischemic myocardium. Circulation 74:1124–1136
2. Schott RJ, Rohmann S, Braun ER, Schaper W (1990) Ischemic preconditioning reduces infarct size in swine myocardium. Circ Res 66:1133–1142
3. Kuzuya T, Hoshida S, Yamashita N, Fuji H, Oe H, Hori M, Kamada T, Tada M (1993) Delayed effects of sublethal ischemia on the acquisition of tolerance to ischemia. Circ Res 72:1293–1299
4. Karmazyn M, Mailer K, Currie W (1990) Acquisition and decay of heat-shock-enhanced postischemic ventricular recovery. Am J Physiol 259:H424–H431

5. Brown JM, Grosso MA, Terada LS, Whitman GJR, Banerjee A, White CW, Harken AH, Repine JE (1989) Endotoxin pretreatment increases endogenous myocardial catalase activity and decreases ischemia-reperfusion injury of isolated rat hearts. Proc Natl Acad Sci USA 86:2516–2520
6. Brown JM, White CW, Terada LS, Grosso MA, Shanley PF, Mulvin DW, Banerjee A, Whitman GJ, Harken AH, Repine JE (1990) Interleukin-1 pretreatment decreases ischemia/reperfusion injury. Proc Natl Acad Sci USA 87:5026–5030
7. Tsan MF, White JE, Treanor C, Schaffer JB (1990) Molecular basis for tumor necrosis factor-induced increase in pulmonary superoxide dismutase activities. Am J Physiol 259:L506–L512
8. Hoshida S, Kuzuya T, Fuji H, Yamashita N, Oe H, Hori M, Suzuki K, Taniguchi N, Tada M (1993) Sublethal ischemia alters myocardial antioxidant activity in the canine heart. Am J Physiol 264:H33–H39

Part 2

Cardiac Adaptation to Mechanical Workload

Molecular Aspects

2.1 Adaptation of the Left Ventricular Wall Under Pathological Circumstances

Molecular and Mechanical Aspects

ROBERT S. RENEMAN[1], THEO ARTS[2], MARC VAN BILSEN[1], LUC H.E.H. SNOECKX[1], and GER J. VAN DER VUSSE[1]

Summary. As a reaction to hormonal and mechanical stimuli, the ventricular wall adapts to enhanced workload through hypertrophy of individual myocytes. In the hypertrophic process, the growth of cardiac cells results from an increase in protein content per myocardial cell. The most important cellular features of the myocardial hypertrophic response are an increase in the content of contractile proteins, such as myosin heavy chain, myosin light chain-2, β-tropomyosin, and α-skeletal and α-cardiac actin, the induction of contractile protein isoforms—at least in some species—and the expression of embryonic markers. The expression of proto-oncogenes, genes related to growth, is an early phenomenon in the hypertrophic response. In pressure-overload hypertrophy, the sarcoplasmic reticular (SR)-Ca^{2+} ATPase content, and hence activity, is decreased. In cardiac hypertrophy, the extracellular content (mg) of both collagen and fibronectin increases, mainly in the interstitial space. The collagen concentration (mg/g), however, does not necessarily change and there is increasing evidence that the functional consequences of the changes in extracellular matrix collagen have to be ascribed to the type of collagen expressed and/or cross-linking of collagen. These changes combined with the decrease in SR-Ca^{2+} ATPase activity, enhancing cytoplasmic Ca^{2+} content, probably explain the increased diastolic stiffness of the left ventricle observed during pressure- and volume-overload hypertrophy. Although the molecular changes occurring during a hypertrophic response have been well documented, the way in which myocardial cells sense the change in loading, and the mechanisms through which forces are converted to biomechanical signals regulating cardiac genes during growth, are still incompletely understood. Both stretching of cardiomyocytes and contraction of myofibrils induce the expression of proto-

[1] Department of Physiology and [2] Department of Biophysics, Cardiovascular Research Institute Maastricht (CARIM), University of Limburg, P.O. Box 616, 6200 MD, Maastricht, The Netherlands

oncogenes followed by protein translation. Although the signal responsible for the induction of the hypertrophic response is not precisely known, there is increasing evidence that protein kinases, especially protein kinase C, play an important role. Most of the data obtained on the hypertrophic response are derived from studies using pressure- or volume-overload as a stimulus. One should realize, however, that the molecular changes observed under these circumstances do not necessarily hold for other forms of hypertrophy. For example, differences between pressure-overload hypertrophy and hypertrophy induced by thyroid hormone have been described. Even so, species differences have to be appreciated. Most of the information about the molecular changes in the hypertrophic response of the heart has been obtained in studies performed on cardiomyocytes in culture. Although the set-ups used seem to mimic the pathophysiological situation rather well, it remains to be seen whether the results obtained in these models can be extrapolated to the in vivo situation.

Keywords: Cellular growth—Signal transduction—Gene products—Cytoskeleton—Extracellular matrix—Pressure load—Stretch—Fiber stress/strain—Fiber direction

Introduction

As a reaction to hormonal stimuli and mechanical stimuli such as pressure- and volume-overload, the ventricular wall adapts through hypertrophy of individual myocytes, practically without change in myocyte number: adult myocytes have lost their ability to proliferate. In the hypertrophic process, the growth of cardiac cells results from an increase in protein content per myocardial cell. The most important features of the myocardial hypertrophic response are an increase in contractile protein content, the induction of contractile protein isoforms, and the expression of embryonic markers such as atrial natriuretic factor (ANF [1–3]). Insights into the regulation of the expression of these markers allows identification of the molecular mechanisms involved in the adaptational processes. In these processes, not only intracellular components are expressed, but also constituents of the extracellular matrix, such as fibronectin [4,5] and collagen [6–8]. The different types of collagen are expressed, but not in a coordinated way [7,9]. It is interesting to note that in the early phase of adaptation the expression of both contractile proteins and extracellular matrix components tends to shift towards embryonic forms of these constituents.

Although a large body of information about gene expression during myocardial hypertrophy has been obtained previously, the signaling mechanism regulating cardiac genes during growth and hypertrophy is still incompletely understood. There is increasing evidence that protein kinase C (PKC) plays a central role in the signaling mechanism [10]. An even more fundamental question concerns the way in which cells are able to sense changes in physical forces and to convert these forces to biochemical signals ultimately leading to alterations in gene expression. Recently, interesting results have been obtained in studies looking into the mechanoreceptor and mechanotransduction function of cells (see [11] for review).

It should be realized that quite a bit of the information about the molecular changes in the hypertrophic response of the heart has been obtained in studies performed on cardiomyocytes in culture. Although the set-ups used seem to mimic the pathophysiological situation rather well [12], it remains to be seen whether the results obtained in these models can be extrapolated to the in vivo situation. Even so, species differences have to be appreciated. For example, the shift from α-myosin heavy chain (MHC) to β-MHC during the hypertrophic response, a phenomenon well documented in the rat [13–15], does not occur in the guinea pig [16] or in humans [17,18]. In cardiomyocytes of the latter species, β-MHC is constitutively expressed, while the content of α-MHC is very limited. It is interesting to note that different stimuli, causing hypertrophy, may induce different phenotypes of the cardiomyocyte. For example, sarcoplasmic reticular (SR)-Ca^{2+} ATPase content, and hence its overall activity, is reduced in pressure-overload hypertrophy [19–21], but increased in thyroid hormone-induced hypertrophy [22].

It is well-known that there are limits to the adaptational process in cardiac hypertrophy and that long-existing hypertrophy often leads to heart failure. It is unknown, however, whether the onset of heart failure results from a loss of capacity to adapt to increased workload, for instance due to aging, or whether the adaptation is not optimal right from the beginning.

Not only cellular growth, but also adaptation of fiber orientation occurs in response to increases in workload [23]. Through this adaptation, fiber stress across the ventricular wall will be kept homogeneously distributed [24–26].

Adaptation of the myocardium can also be observed in chronic asynchronous electrical activation of the heart, as during ventricular pacing, and in patients with bundle branch block. During asynchronous electrical activation, fiber shortening [27], total mechanical power [28], and myocardial blood flow [27,28] are significantly reduced in early-activated areas and increased in late-activated areas. In the early-activated regions, a decrease in workload reduces wall mass. Despite the increase in workload, in late-activated regions wall mass increases only slightly and not significantly [29,30]. Similar changes are observed in patients with left bundle branch block [29]. These observations indicate that asynchronous electrical activation results in an asymmetric geometry of the left ventricular wall and that reduced workload leads to wall thinning.

In this chapter, we will discuss various aspects of the basic mechanisms involved in cardiac adaptation under pathological circumstances. Because most of the studies have been performed in relation to pressure- and volume-overload, in general, we will limit ourselves to these pathological conditions.

Changes at the Molecular Level in Myocardial Adaptation to Pressure- and Volume-Overload

Cellular Changes

Introduction

The changes in expression of contractile proteins and other cardiac genes during ventricular hypertrophy have been documented and characterized in a variety of experimental models. The signaling mechanism leading to transcrip-

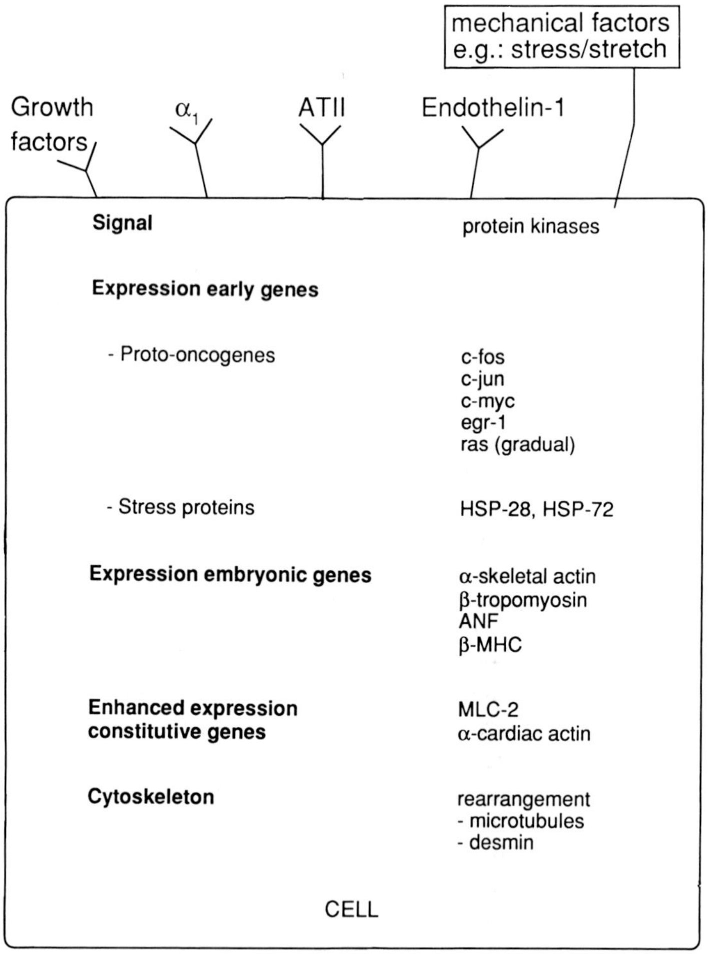

Fig. 1. Candidates for involvement in hypertrophic response. α_1, α_1-adrenoceptor agonists; *ATII*, angiotensin II; *HSP*, heat shock protein; *ANF*, atrial natriuretic factor; *MHC*, myosin heavy chain; *MLC*, myosin light chain

tional activation of these proteins and other target genes, however, is still incompletely understood. The signals generated by the hypertrophic stimuli will ultimately reach the nucleus and activate the cardiac genes involved. A comparable hypertrophic response can be induced by different stimuli (Fig. 1), but differences between the stimuli have to be appreciated (see later section). The candidates possibly involved in this response are depicted in Fig. 1.

Signal Transduction

Several signaling molecules have been proposed as a candidate for inducing the hypertrophic response. There is, however, increasing evidence that the activation of protein kinases (PK), especially PKC, plays an important role in the induction of this response. Hypertrophic stimuli, like norepinephrine, endothelin, and angiotensin, have the ability to activate PKC (see [12] for survey). The activation of PKC may be induced by diacylglycerol [31], that is formed together with inositol phosphates by phospholipase C-induced hydrolysis of phosphatidylinositol, a constituent of cellular membranes, upon stimulation with, for instance, endothelin-1 [32]. The involvement of PKC in inducing the hypertrophic response is supported by the observations that stimulation of PKC with phorbol esters leads to phenomena related to cardiac hypertrophy [33] and that nuclear PKC activity is increased in cardiomyocytes during growth-stimulation [10].

Early Gene Products

Proto-oncogenes. In most cell types, the transient induction of proto-oncogenes, growth-related genes, is one of the earliest detectable genetic effects (within hours after induction of the load to the heart) involved in the hypertrophic response ([34–36]; for reviews see [37,38]). Several of these proto-oncogenes have been identified in the heart [37] and have been well characterized in relation to the proteins they encode (Table 1). An important class of proto-oncogenes are the nuclear proteins, which encode for transcription factor AP-1 and DNA-binding protein. During pressure loading, the expression of the proto-oncogenes c-*fos* and c-*myc* is indeed followed by protein translation [36], indicating that the expression of these genes is functional. In a study with neutralizing antibodies against c-*fos* in fibroblasts, it was confirmed that c-*fos* induction is required for the activation of cell proliferation following stimulation with growth factors [39]. One should realize, however, that differences between proto-oncogenes have to be appreciated. For example, c-*fos*, which is constitutively present only in the media of coronary arteries, is expressed in cardiomyocytes during pressure-overload, while c-*myc*, which is constitutively present in coronary artery endothelium and other nonmuscle cells, is expressed only slightly in cardiomyocytes during pressure-overload [36].

Table 1. Examples of well-characterized proto-oncogenes and the proteins they encode, as well as their presence in the heart.

Classification/oncogenes	Location	Encodes	In heart
Class 1: growth factors			
sis	Secreted	PDGF	+/−
Class 2: growth factor receptors			
erb B	Membrane	Receptor for EGF	+/−
trk	Membrane	Receptor for NGF	?
Class 3: intracellular transducers			
src	Cytoplasm	Protein-tyrosine kinase	+
raf	Cytoplasm	Protein-serine kinase	+
gsp	Cytoplasm	G protein subunit	?
ras	Cytoplasm	GTP/GDP-binding protein	+
Class 4: nuclear proteins			
c-*jun*	Nucleus	Transcription factor (AP-1)	+
c-*fos*	Nucleus	Transcription factor (AP-1)	+
c-*myc*	Nucleus	DNA binding protein	+

PDGF, platelet derived growth factor; *EGF*, epidermal growth factor; *NGF*, nerve growth factor. +, identified; +/−, contradictory results in literature; ?, unknown. Modified after Watson et al. [78], with permission. Most of the data on the heart are derived from Simpson [37]

Stress Proteins. Heat shock proteins (HSP's) were found to be expressed following pressure- and volume-overload [40], but one should bear in mind that the degree of expression of these stress proteins may be the same in sham-operated and pressure-overloaded animals [36,40], reflecting a general response to the surgical procedure rather than a specific reaction to loading. The HSP's commonly found in relation to cellular growth are HSP-28 and HSP-72 [41]. The function of these stress proteins in the hypertrophic response is not precisely known. HSP's bind to actin in nonmuscle cells and recently were found to protect the normal [42,43] and hypertrophic heart [44] (the latter is known to be very susceptible to ischemia [45,46]) against the ischemic insult. There are indications that HSP's cover essential proteins, preventing them from degradation [47].

Secondary Gene Products

A variety of embryonic genes are expressed during the hypertrophic response (Fig. 1). The embryonic genes indicated are given as examples, and represent an overall picture. One should realize, after all, that species differences have to be appreciated.

Two sarcomeric actins can be distinguished: the α-cardiac and the α-skeletal isoform. In the adult heart of small mammals, α-cardiac actin is the predominant isoform [48–50], whereas α-skeletal actin is also present in larger mammals [50,51]. In rat hearts, α-skeletal actin significantly accumulates following pressure-overload [52–54]. The accumulation of α-skeletal actin is seen throughout the left ventricle as early as 4 h after induction of the pressure-overload, and in the left atrium after 12 h. Despite the fact that hypertrophy progresses, as far as the increase in muscle mass is concerned, the expression of this actin isoform reaches a maximum about 4 days after the onset of the pressure load and declines thereafter [52,53]. In contrast, β-MHC is hardly detectable before day 1 and after 2–3 days accumulates mainly in the subendocardial layers of the left ventricle and around coronary arteries [54]. This inhomogeneity in β-MHC accumulation was also found by Bugaisky and colleagues [55]. These investigators not only showed that β-MHC increased most significantly in the subendocardial layers, as compared to the subepicardial ones, but also observed a relatively high degree of inhomogeneity in β-MHC expression throughout a given layer. The accumulation of β-MHC during myocardial hypertrophy, which actually only occurs in the rat and other rodents where a shift from α-MHC to β-MHC can be observed during the hypertrophic response [13–15], is a relatively slow phenomenon. It is of interest to note that also in species which do not show a shift from α-MHC to β-MHC upon pressure-overload (see Introduction), the myosin ATPase activity is significantly reduced under these circumstances, in both the left and the right ventricle [16]. The expression of myosin light chain (MLC)-2, a cardiac myofibrillar gene, has been shown to increase following hypertrophic stimulation [56]. In adult cardiac muscle of small mammals, no expression of β-tropomyosin can be found [57], but following pressure-overload a rapid induction of β-tropomyosin in striated muscle, smooth muscle, and nonmuscle tissue can be observed [53].

In relation to the expression of contractile proteins, it is important to briefly consider Ca^{2+}-homeostasis in the adaptational process. In cardiac hypertrophy induced by pressure-overload, sarcoplasmic reticular (SR) function and SR-Ca^{2+} ATPase activity are reduced [19,21]. The data obtained in these studies strongly suggest that the decrease in SR-Ca^{2+} ATPase activity results from a relative reduction in the total content of the biologically active protein rather than a decrease in activity per mole of Ca^{2+} ATPase. The results obtained in the study performed by Levitsky and colleagues [21] indicate that the velocity of Ca^{2+} transport in SR is diminished in hypertrophied hearts. Also, in the ventricles of humans with end-stage heart failure, the SR-Ca^{2+} ATPase mRNA was found to be decreased [20].

During embryonic development, ANF is expressed in both atrial and ventricular myocardium [58]. In the adult myocardium the expression of ANF is down-regulated in the ventricle and the primary site of ANF synthesis is in the atrium. ANF is reexpressed in the ventricle following the induction of ventricular hypertrophy [1–3]. The role of ANF reexpression in the hypertrophic response is not known. It has been suggested that ventricular ANF plays a role in regulating circulatory ANF levels and, hence, in controlling blood pressure and natriuresis in pathological hypertrophy [12].

Cytoskeleton

Changes in the cytoskeletal proteins can also be observed during the process of hypertrophy. In cardiomyocytes changes have been observed in tubulin and desmin, the constituent proteins of microtubules and intermediate filaments, respectively. In hypertrophied hearts, considerable increases in tubulin are observed near the nuclei and along myofibrils, whereas desmin is distributed transversely, as in the control situation, linking Z-disks which are out of register [59]. It has been indicated that desmin filaments are primarily involved in maintaining the myofibrils in register and that the assembly of microtubules is related to protein synthesis and myofibrillogenesis [59].

Differences Between Different Hypertrophic Stimuli

As mentioned before, the molecular changes following pressure- and occasionally volume-overload are not necessarily similar in other forms of hypertrophy. For example, pressure-overload in rats leads to hypertrophy characterized by a reduction in SR-Ca^{2+} ATPase content, and, hence, in activity [19,21] and a shift from α-MHC to β-MHC isoform expression [13–15]. In contrast, in the same species hypertrophy induced by thyroid hormone is associated with increased SR-Ca^{2+} ATPase activity [22], while α-MHC isoform expression is enhanced in exercise-induced hypertrophy [60]. Even so, differences in the expression of proto-oncogenes have to be appreciated. It was, for instance, shown that pressure-overload-induced hypertrophy leads to increased levels of c-H-*ras* mRNA [61]; and thyroid hormone induced hypertrophy, to a reduction of the c-H-*ras* mRNA level [62]. Differences in proto-oncogene expression have also been observed between α- and β-adrenoceptor stimulation. There is increasing evidence that stimulation of these adrenoceptors leads to a different type of response and that the results obtained with this kind of hypertrophic stimulation are different in vitro and in vivo (see [63] for review).

Extracellular Matrix Changes

Myocytes are surrounded by a matrix of connective tissue, consisting of collagen and elastin. In the rat [64,65] and in nonhuman primates [9] the collagen in the extracellular matrix of the myocardium consists mainly of type I collagen and, to a lesser extent, type III collagen. The collagen runs between and connects neighbouring myocytes and surrounds them, grouping myocytes together [9]. Type IV collagen is found in the basement membrane of cardiomyocytes and in the extracellular matrix [65]. Another important extracellular matrix component in the myocardium is fibronectin [66].

In pressure-overload cardiac hypertrophy, the content of both collagen [5,6,8] and fibronectin [4,5] increases, the expression of fibronectin occurring earlier than that of collagen [5]. Expression of fibronectin can already be observed one day after onset of the pressure-overload [4], while the expression of collagen generally occurs 2–4 days after induction of the stimulus. In pressure-overload, not only are the adult forms of fibronectin expressed but reexpression of the fetal forms also occurs [4]. Fibronectins were found to be localized in the interstitial space and in the media of the coronary arteries. Collagen was observed throughout the interstitial space.

Although the content (mg) of collagen generally increases, the collagen concentration (mg/g) may stay the same [7] or may even decrease. In this study, performed on spontaneously hypertensive rats (SHR's), it was also shown that the various types of collagen are not coordinately expressed in the myocardium during the hypertrophic process. In 10-week-old rats the collagen type I:III ratio was significantly lower in SHR's than in control rats. In 34-week-old rats the opposite was observed: a higher ratio in SHR's. At an age of 86 weeks, the collagen type I:III ratio significantly decreased again, reaching an average value similar to the one observed after 10 weeks. This finding indicates that in the early phase of cardiac hypertrophy and when the rat hearts begin to fail (86 weeks) the expression of the immature type III collagen is more pronounced than the expression of the adult type I. A similar pattern of expression of the various types of collagen was seen in hypertrophic hearts of nonhuman primates [9]. In this study, in the early phase of hypertrophy the content of type I collagen was found to be decreased and that of type III collagen increased, whereas during the stable phase of hypertrophy the content of type I increased and that of type III normalized. A noncoordinated expression of type I and type IV collagen was also observed in a rat model of volume-overload hypertrophy [67]. These observations impose the question as to whether the functional consequences of the changes in extracellular matrix collagen have to be ascribed to an increase in collagen content or to differences in function between the various types of collagen. The possibility that functionally the total collagen content is of less importance is emphasized by the finding of Iimoto and colleagues [68] in a canine model of volume-overload hypertrophy. In this form of hypertrophy the collagen concentration did not significantly change, but the extractible amount of type I and type III collagen was significantly reduced. The latter suggests that the cross-linking of these types of collagen increases in volume-overload hypertrophy [68]. The reduced extractibility of collagen was associated with an increased diastolic stiffness of the left ventricle.

Possible Consequences for Cardiac Function

The increase in ventricular wall thickness in the adaptational process, resulting from the increase in cellular proteins and in fibronectin and collagen in the extracellular matrix, will reduce wall stress. The increased fibronectin and collagen content may reduce ventricular dilatation during left ventricular failure, improving mechanical efficiency [69]. The increased diastolic stiffness observed during pressure- and volume-overload-induced left ventricular hypertrophy may result from the expression of immature forms of collagen and/or cross-linking of collagen, and an increased cytoplasmic Ca^{2+} content due to reduced SR-Ca^{2+} ATPase activity. The increased cytoplasmic Ca^{2+} content, however, will enhance systolic left ventricular function.

The enhanced expression of contractile proteins leads to an increase in the number of contractile units, probably kept in register by the cytoskeletal protein desmin. One may wonder whether new sarcomeres formed with the use of α-skeletal actin are adequately equipped for their function in the left ventricle. The decrease in myosin ATPase activity, whether or not associated with a shift from α-MHC to β-MHC, will decrease the velocity of shortening of cardiac muscle [14] and possibly enhance the economy of isometric force development [70].

Mechanoreception and Mechanotransduction

Although in vivo humoral factors may play a role in the induction of the hypertrophic response, studies on isolated cells have shown that direct pathways are involved in this induction. However, the way in which myocardial cells sense the change in loading and the mechanisms through which physical forces are converted to biochemical signals (mechanotransduction) are still incompletely understood. In this section we will briefly discuss the conversion of mechanical stimuli to cell growth.

(Cyclic) stretching of cardiomyocytes, simulating cellular loading, leads to the immediate (within 15 min) expression of the proto-oncogene c-*fos* followed by an increase in amino acid incorporation into proteins, the increases being dependent on the duration of stretching [71]. c-*Fos* was found to increase in a stretch length-dependent way. That this expression of proto-oncogenes may indeed lead to cell growth is indicated by the finding that myocyte stretching results in pronounced increases in nuclear RNA labeling and in cytoplasmic protein translation [72]. These observations indicate that an increase in load may be a direct regulator of cardiac growth in vivo. However, contractile activity of cardiomyocytes also accelerates growth of these cells [73], indicating that fiber shortening may also be considered as a direct cardiac growth regulator. Cellular deformation due to external forces, like stress, may also be considered as a regulator of cellular growth.

In an excellent review, Watson [11] recently discussed the possible mechanisms involved in mechanotransduction. Based upon studies on, for example, endothelial cells and fibroblasts, he comes to the conclusion that in addition to stretch-activated and stretch-inactivated channels, and the cytoskeleton, the Na^+-H^+ exchanger may play a role in converting cellular deformation to growth signals. Under a variety of circumstances, cellular deformation and growth is associated with activation of the Na^+-H^+ exchanger, leading to cytoplasmic alkalinization. There are indications that the cytoskeleton acts as an intermediate in the transduction of mechanical information to the Na^+-H^+ exchanger [11].

It is not necessarily the case that the stimulus for growth, as induced by physical forces, is generated by the myocytes themselves, because paracrine mechanisms of growth stimulation have to be considered. Recently, it has been shown that in cyclically strained endothelium the production of endothelin-1, a known mitogen, is enhanced [74]. It is interesting to see that endothelial cells have the ability to distinguish between cyclic strain and shear stress as far as the production of this autocoid is concerned. Unlike cyclic strain, shear stress suppresses the production of endothelin-1 [75].

Myocardial Fiber Direction and Hypertrophy

In previous studies it has been shown that fiber direction is an important determinant of fiber stress distribution across the left ventricular wall [24–26]. Despite the increase in left ventricular mass during cardiac hypertrophy, the fiber orientation within the wall seems to be maintained. This raises the question as to how the heart controls this adaptational process and which of the mechanical stimuli are sensed by the myocardial cells in this control mechanism. Fiber stress is one of the best candidates to control fiber direction during myocardial growth, because of the practically linear relation between the ratio of myocardial fiber stress (σ_{mf}) to left ventricular pressure (P_{lv}) and the ratio of ventricular cavity volume (V_{lv}) to wall volume V_{wall} according to [76]:

$$\frac{\sigma_{mf}}{P_{lv}} = \frac{1 + 3V_{lv}}{V_{wall}}$$

To further investigate the stress feedback hypothesis, a section of the left ventricular wall was simulated using the model as previously described in detail [24,25]. In this approach, it was assumed that in hypertrophy, fiber direction is controlled by fiber stress and end-diastolic sarcomere length (stretch), the latter being set homogeneously across the wall. Stretch was included because of its growth stimulating effect. When, as a first approximation, the transmural course of fiber orientation was taken to be linear, calculated fiber stress appeared to be minimum in the subepicardial layers and maximum in the subendocardial ones [23]. In the stress feedback hypothesis, the layers with low stress will decrease in mass whereas the ones with high stress will hypertrophy. As a result, the transmural course of fiber orientation modifies. The transmural distribution of fiber stress associated with this new fiber orientation is much more homogeneous [23]. This sequence is schematically depicted in Fig. 2. This control mechanism, however, does not provide a stable solution as far as fiber orientation is concerned: after more than 100 iterations irregularities in the transmural course of fiber orientation tend to grow. This finding indicates that in the hypertrophying heart, fiber direction cannot be controlled by fiber stress and end-diastolic stretch alone.

First approximation: linear transmural course of fiber orientation

→ accessory calculated transmural course of fiber stress

↙ endocardium maximum ↓ increased wall mass

↘ epicardium minimum ↓ decreased wall mass

↘ transmural course of fiber orientation modifies ↙

↓

more homogeneous transmural distribution of fiber stress

Fig. 2. Model for evaluation of the possible mechanism for the control of fiber orientation in the hypertrophic process, using fiber stress and end-diastolic sarcomere length as feedback

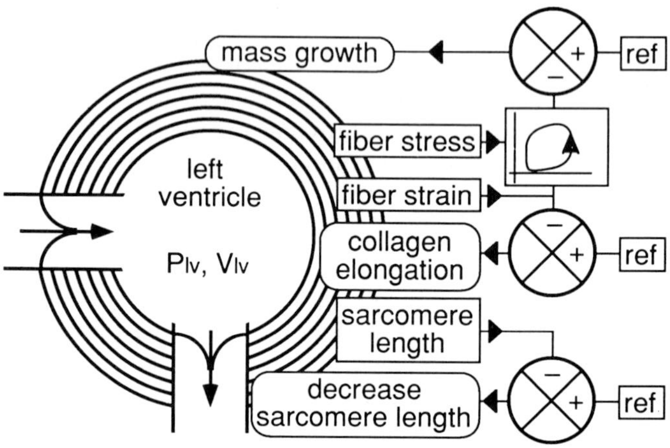

Fig. 3. Schematic representation of the mechanical factors possibly responsible for the control of fiber orientation and myocardial growth. In this model, the systolic fiber stress–strain relation induces adaptive changes in muscle mass, fiber strain during ejection modifies collagen stiffness or length, and sarcomere length (end-diastolic stretch) is controlled directly. P_{lv}, V_{lv}; pressure, volume of left ventricle

In the myocardium the fibers are not as perfectly arranged in parallel as in skeletal muscle and dispersion around the average fiber orientation of about ±10° has to be taken into account. Since in the myocardial layers, shortening during the ejection phase depends on the actual fiber orientation with respect to the local deformation field, in a particular region fibers might sense the direction where fiber shortening is optimal. Assuming that fibers orientate in this direction by a hypothetical local feedback mechanism, fiber shortening was included in the model. In this approach, a linear transmural course of fiber orientation develops to a new stable distribution (for several thousand iterations), close to the distributions found experimentally in a variety of species [23]. These model studies indicate that fiber orientation cannot be controlled by fiber stress alone and that additional feedback through end-diastolic stretch and strain is required to obtain a stable fiber direction. It is proposed that the unique fiber orientation, maintaining an even distribution of the mechanical load in the heart, is a remodelling mechanism based upon control of fiber stress, fiber shortening, and end-diastolic sarcomere length [77]. This remodelling mechanism is schematically depicted in Fig. 3.

Acknowledgments. The authors are indebted to Jos Heemskerk, Karin Van Brussel, Claire Bollen, and Emmy Van Roosmalen for their help in preparing the manuscript.

References

1. Gutkowska J, Horky K, Lachance C, Racz K, Garcia R, Thibault G, Kuchel O, Genest J, Cantin M (1986) Atrial natriuretic factor in spontaneously hypertensive rats. Hypertension 8[Suppl 1]:137–140
2. Lee TR, Bloch KD, Pfeffer JM, Pfeffer MA, Neer EJ, Seidman CE (1988) Atrial natriuretic factor gene expression in ventricles of rats with spontaneous ventricular hypertrophy. J Clin Invest 81:431–434
3. Arai H, Nakao K, Saito Y, Morii N, Sugawara A, Yamada T, Itoh H, Shiono S, Mykoyama M, Ohkubo H, Nakanishi S, Imura H (1988) Augmented expression of atrial natriuretic polypeptide gene in ventricles of spontaneously hypertensive rats (SHR)-stroke prone. Circ Res 62:926–930
4. Samuel JL, Barrieux A, Dufour S, Dubus I, Contard F, Koteliansky V, Farhadian F, Marotte F, Thiéry J-P, Rappaport L (1991) Accumulation of fetal fibronectin mRNA's during the development of rat cardiac hypertrophy induced by pressure overload. J Clin Invest 88:1737–1746
5. Contard F, Koteliansky V, Marotte F, Dubus I, Rappaport L, Samuel J-L (1991) Specific alterations in the distribution of extracellular matrix components within rat myocardium during the development of pressure overload. Lab Invest 64:65–75
6. Weber KT, Janicki JS, Shroff SG, Pick R, Chen RM, Bashey RI (1988) Collagen remodeling of the pressure-overloaded, hypertrophied nonhuman primate myocardium. Circ Res 62:757–765
7. Mukherjee D, Sen S (1990) Collagen phenotypes during development and regression of myocardial hypertrophy in spontaneously hypertensive rats. Circ Res 67: 1474–1480
8. Chapman D, Weber KT, Eghbali M (1990) Regulation of fibrillar collagen types I and III and basement membrane type IV collagen gene expression in pressure overloaded rat myocardium. Circ Res 67:787–794

9. Weber KT, Clark WA, Janicki JS, Shroff SG (1987) Physiologic versus pathologic hypertrophy and the pressure-overloaded myocardium. J Cardiovasc Pharmacol 10[Suppl 6]:S37–S49
10. Allo SN, Carl LL, Morgan HE (1992) Acceleration of growth of cultured cardiomyocytes and translocation of protein kinase C. Am J Physiol 263:C319–C325
11. Watson PA (1991) Function follows form: generation of intracellular signals by cell deformation. FASEB J 5:2013–2019
12. Chien KR, Knowlton KU, Zhu H, Chien S (1991) Regulation of cardiac gene expression during myocardial growth and hypertrophy: molecular studies of an adaptative physiologic response. FASEB J 5:3037–3046
13. Mercadier J-J, Lompré A-M, Wisnewsky C, Samuel J-L, Bercovici J, Swynghedauw B, Schwartz K (1981) Myosin isoenzymic changes in several models of rat cardiac hypertrophy. Circ Res 49:525–532
14. Schwartz K, Lecarpentier Y, Martin JL, Lompré AM, Mercadier J-J, Swynghedauw B (1981) Myosin isoenzymic distribution correlates with speed of myocardial contraction. J Mol Cell Cardiol 13:1071–1075
15. Izumo S, Lompré A-M, Matsuoka R, Koren G, Schwartz K, Nadal-Ginard B, Mahdavi V (1987) Myosin heavy chain messenger RNA and protein isoform transition during cardiac hypertrophy. J Clin Invest 79:970–977
16. Malhotra A, Siri FM, Aronson R (1992) Cardiac contractile proteins in hypertrophied and failing guinea pig heart. Cardiovasc Res 26:153–161
17. Mercadier J-J, Bouveret P, Gorza L, Schiaffino S, Clark WA, Zak R, Swynghedauw B, Schwartz K (1983) Myosin isoenzymes in normal and hypertrophied human ventricular myocardium. Circ Res 53:52–62
18. Clark WA, Everett AW, Chizzonite RA, Eisenberg BR, Zak R (1984) Classification and characterization of cardiac isomyosins. Eur Heart J 5:69–75
19. De la Bastie D, Levitsky S, Rappaport L, Mercadier J-J, Marotte F, Wisnewsky C, Brovkovich V, Schwartz K, Lompré A-M (1990) Function of the sarcoplasmic reticulum and expression of its Ca^{2+}-ATPase gene in pressure overload-induced cardiac hypertrophy in the rat. Circ Res 66:554–564
20. Mercadier J-J, Lompré A-M, Duc P, Boheler KR, Fraysse J-B, Wisnewsky C, Allen PD, Komajda M, Schwartz K (1990) Altered sarcoplasmic reticulum Ca^{2+}-ATPase gene expression in the human ventricle during end-stage heart failure. J Clin Invest 85:305–309
21. Levitsky D, de la Bastie D, Schwartz K, Lompré A-M (1991) Ca^{2+} ATPase and function of sarcoplasmic reticulum during cardiac hypertrophy. Am J Physiol 261: 23–26
22. Sayen MR, Rohrer DK, Dillmann WH (1992) Thyroid hormone response of slow and fast sarcoplasmic reticulum Ca^{2+} ATPase mRNA in striated muscle. Mol Cell Endocrinol 87:87–93
23. Arts T, Bovendeerd PHM, Prinzen FW, Reneman RS (1989) Integrity of myocardial fiber structure maintained by fiber load induced local growth. In: Hori M, Suga H, Baan J, Yellin EL (eds) Cardiac mechanics and function in the normal and diseased heart. Springer, Berlin Heidelberg New York Tokyo, pp 75–80
24. Arts T, Veenstra PC, Reneman RS (1982) Epicardial deformation and left ventricular wall mechanics during ejection in the dog. Am J Physiol 243:H379–H390
25. Arts T, Reneman RS (1989) Dynamics of left ventricular wall and mitral valve mechanics, a model study. J Biomech 22:261–271

26. Bovendeerd PHM, Arts T, Huyghe JM, Van Campen DH, Reneman RS (1992) Dependence of local left ventricular wall mechanics on myocardial fiber orientation: a model study. J Biomech 25:1129–1140
27. Prinzen FW, Augustijn CH, Arts T, Allessie MA, Reneman RS (1990) Redistribution of myocardial fiber strain and blood flow by asynchronous activation. Am J Physiol 259:H300–H308
28. Delhaas T, Arts T, Prinzen FW, Reneman RS (In press) Regional fibre stress-fibre strain area as estimate of regional blood flow and oxygen demand in the canine heart. J Physical (Lond)
29. Reneman RS, Prinzen FW, Cheriex ER, Arts T, Delhaas T (1993) Asymmetrical changes in left ventricular diastolic wall thickness induced by chronic asynchronous electrical activation in man and dogs (abstract). FASEB J 7(4):4341
30. Prinzen FW, Delhaas T, Arts T, Reneman RS (1993) Asymmetrical changes in ventricular wall mass by asynchronous electrical activation of the heart. In: Sideman S, Beyer R (eds) Interactive phenomena in the cardiac system. Plenum Publ., pp 257–264
31. Mochly-Rosen D, Henrich CJ, Cheever L, Khaner H, Simpson PC (1990) A protein kinase C isozyme is translocated in cytoskeletal elements on activation. Cell Regul 1:693–706
32. Shubeita HE, McDonough PM, Harris A, Knowlton KU, Glembotski C, Brown JH, Chien KR (1990) Endothelin induction of sarcomere assembly and cardiac gene expression in ventricular myocytes: a paracrine mechanism for myocardial cell hypertrophy. J Biol Chem 265:20555–20562
33. Dunnmon P, Iwaki K, Henderson S, Sen A, Chien KR (1990) Phorbol esters induce immediate-early genes and stimulate cardiac gene transcription in neonatal rat myocardial cells. J Mol Cell Cardiol 22:901–910
34. Starksen NF, Simpson PC, Bishopric N, Coughlin SR, Lee WMF, Escobedo JA, Williams LT (1986) Cardiac myocyte hypertrophy is associated with c-*myc* protooncogene expression. Proc Nat Acad Sci USA 83:8348–8350
35. Komuro I, Kurabayashi M, Takaku F, Yazaki Y (1988) Expression of cellular oncogenes in the myocardium during the developmental stage and pressure-overloaded hypertrophy of the rat heart. Circ Res 62:1075–1079
36. Snoeckx LHEH, Contard F, Samuel JL, Marotte F, Rappaport L (1991) Expression and cellular distribution of heat-shock and nuclear oncogene proteins in rat hearts. Am J Physiol 261:H1443–H1451
37. Simpson PC (1988) Proto-oncogenes and cardiac hypertrophy. Annu Rev Physiol 51:189–202
38. Parker TG, Schneider MD (1991) Growth factors, proto-oncogenes, and plasticity of the cardiac phenotype. Annu Rev Physiol 53:179–200
39. Riabowol KT, Vosatka RJ, Ziff EB, Lamb NJ, Feramisco JR (1988) Microinjection of *fos*-specific antibodies blocks DNA synthesis in fibroblast cells. Mol Cell Biol 8:1670–1676
40. Delcayre C, Samuel J-L, Marotte F, Best-Belpomme M, Mercadier JJ, Rappaport L (1988) Synthesis of stress proteins in rat cardiac myocytes 2–4 days after imposition of hemodynamic overload. J Clin Invest 82:460–468
41. Welch WJ (1992) Mammalian stress response: cell physiology, structure/function of stress proteins, and implications for medicine and disease. Physiol Rev 72: 1063–1081

42. Currie R, Karmazyn M, Kloc M, Mailer K (1988) Heat-shock response is associated with enhanced post-ischemic ventricular recovery. Circ Res 63:543–549
43. Yellon DM, Pasini E, Cargnoni A, Marber MS, Latchman DS, Ferrari R (1992) The protective role of heat stress in the ischaemic and reperfused rabbit myocardium. J Mol Cell Cardiol 24:895–907
44. Cornelussen R, Snoeckx LHEH, de Bruin LG, Van der Vusse GJ, Reneman RS (1993) Hyperthermic preconditioning improves ischemia tolerance in the hypertrophied and non-hypertrophied rat heart (abstract). J Mol Cell Cardiol 25[Suppl I]:S56
45. Snoeckx LHEH, Van der Vusse GJ, Coumans WA, Willemsen PHM, Van der Nagel T, Reneman RS (1986) Myocardial function in normal and spontaneously hypertensive rats during reperfusion following a period of global ischaemia. Cardiovasc Res 20:67–75
46. Snoeckx LHEH, Van der Vusse GJ, Coumans WA, Willemsen PHM, Reneman RS (1993) Differences in tolerance to ischemia between hypertrophied hearts of adult and aged spontaneously hypertensive rats. Cardiovasc Res 27:874–881
47. Dubois M, Movanessian A, Beusaude O (1991) Heat-shock induced denaturation of proteins. J Biol Chem 266:9707–9711
48. Minty AJ, Alonso S, Caravatti M, Buckingham ME (1992) A fetal skeletal muscle actin mRNA in the mouse and its identity with cardiac actin mRNA. Cell 30: 185–192
49. Mayer Y, Czosnek H, Zeelon PE, Yaffe D, Nudel U (1984) Expression of the genes coding for the skeletal muscle and cardiac actins in the heart. Nucleic Acids Res 12:1087–2000
50. Vandekerckhove J, Bugaisky G, Buckingham M (1986) Simultaneous expression of skeletal muscle and heart actin proteins in various striated muscle tissues and cells: A quantitative determination of the two actin isoforms. J Biol Chem 241: 1836–1843
51. Gunning P, Ponte P, Blau H, Kedes L (1983) α-Skeletal and α-cardiac actin genes are coexpressed in adult human skeletal muscle and heart. Mol Cell Biol 8: 1985–1995
52. Schwartz K, De la Bastie D, Bouveret P, Oliviéro P, Alonso S, Buckingham M (1986) α-Skeletal muscle actin mRNA's accumulate in hypertrophied adult rat hearts. Circ Res 59:551–555
53. Izumo S, Nadal-Ginard B, Mahdavi V (1988) Protooncogene induction and reprogramming of cardiac gene expression produced by pressure overload. Proc Nat Acad Sci USA 85:339–343
54. Schiaffino JL, Samuel JL, Sassoon D, Lompré AM, Garner I, Marotte F, Buckingham M, Rappaport L, Schwartz K (1989) Nonsynchronous accumulation of α-skeletal actin and β-myosin heavy chain mRNAs during early stages of pressure-overload-induced cardiac hypertrophy demonstrated by in situ hybridization. Circ Res 64:937–948
55. Bugaisky LB, Anderson PG, Hall RS, Bishop SP (1990) Differences in myosin isoform expression in the subepicardial and subendocardial myocardium during cardiac hypertrophy in the rat. Circ Res 66:1127–1132
56. Lee HR, Henderson SA, Reynolds R, Dunnmon P, Yuan D, Chien KR (1988) α_1-Adrenergic stimulation of cardiac gene transcription in neonatal rat myocardial cells. J Biol Chem 263:7352–7358
57. Swijnghedauw B (1986) Developmental and functional adaptation of contractile proteins in cardiac and skeletal muscle. Physiol Rev 66:710–771

58. Bloch KD, Seidman JG, Naftilan JD, Fallon JT, Seidman CE (1986) Neonatal atria and ventricles secrete atrial natriuretic factor via tissue-specific secretory pathways. Cell 47:695–702
59. Watkins SC, Samuel JL, Marotte F, Bertier-Savalle B, Rappaport L (1987) Microtubules and desmin filaments during onset of heart hypertrophy in rat: a double immunoelectron microscope study. Circ Res 60:327–336
60. Scheuer J, Buttrick P (1987) The cardiac hypertrophic responses to pathologic and physiologic loads. Circulation [Suppl 1] 75:63–68
61. Komuro I, Kurabayashi M, Takaku F, Yazaki Y (1988) Expression of cellular oncogenes in the myocardium during the developmental stage and pressure-overloaded hypertrophy of the rat heart. Circ Res 62:1075–1079
62. Green NK, Gammaga MD, Franklyn JA, Sheppard MC (1991) Regulation by thyroid status of c-*myc*, c-*fos* and H-*ras* mRNAs in the rat myocardium. J Endocrin 130:239–244
63. Van Bilsen M, Chien KR (1993) Growth and hypertrophy of the heart: towards an understanding of cardiac specific and inducible gene expression. Cardiovasc Res 27:1140–1149
64. Medugorac I, Jacob R (1983) Characterization of left ventricular collagen in the rat. Cardiovasc Res 17:15–21
65. Eghbali M, Blumenfeld OO, Seifter S, Buttrick PM, Leinwand LA, Robinson TF, Zern MA, Giambrone MA (1989) Localization of types I, III and IV collagen mRNAs in rat heart cells by in situ hybridization. J Mol Cell Cardiol 21:103–113
66. Ahumada GG, Saffitz JE (1984) Fibronectin in rat heart. A link between cardiac myocytes and collagen. J Histochem Cytochem 32:383–388
67. Penney DG, Bugaisky LB (1992) Non-coordinate expression of collagen mRNAs during carbon monoxide-induced cardiac hypertrophy. Mol Cell Biochem 109: 37–41
68. Iimoto DS, Covell JW, Harper E (1988) Increase in cross-linking of type I and type III collagens associated with volume-overload hypertrophy. Circ Res 63:399–408
69. Katz AM (1990) Cardiomyopathy of overload. N Eng J Med 322:100–110
70. Alpert NR, Mulieri LA (1982) Increased myothermal economy of isometric force generation in compensated cardiac hypertrophy induced by pulmonary artery constriction in the rabbit. Circ Res 50:491–500
71. Komuro I, Kaida T, Shibazaki Y, Kurabayashi M, Katoh Y, Hoh E, Takaku F, Yazaki Y (1990) Stretching cardiac myocytes stimulates protooncogene expression. J Biol Chem 265:3595–3598
72. Mann DL, Kent RL, Cooper IVG (1989) Load regulation of the properties of adult feline cardiocytes: growth induction by cellular deformation. Circ Res 64: 1079–1090
73. McDermott PJ, Rothblum LI, Smith SD, Morgan HE (1989) Accelerated rates of ribosomal RNA synthesis during growth of contracting heart cells in culture. J Biol Chem 264:18220–18227
74. Carosi JA, Eskin SG, Mclntire LV (1992) Cyclical strain effects on production of vasoactive materials in cultured endothelial cells. J Cell Physiol 151:29–36
75. Sharefkin JB, Diamond SL, Eskin SG, McIntire LV, Dieffenbach CW (1991) Fluid flow decreases preproendothelin mRNA levels and suppresses endothelin-1 peptide release in cultured human endothelial cells. J Vasc Surg 14:1–9
76. Arts T, Bovendeerd PHM, Prinzen FW, Reneman RS (1991) The relation between left ventricular cavity pressure and volume and systolic fiber stress and strain in the wall. Biophys J 59:93–102

77. Arts T, Prinzen FW, Reneman RS (1993) Mechanics of the wall of the left ventricle. In: Strackee J, Westerhof N (eds) Physics of heart and circulation. Institute of Physics Publishing, Bristol and Philadelphia, pp 153–173
78. Watson JD, Gilman M, Witkowski J, Zoller M (1992) Recombinant DNA. Scientific American Books, WH Freeman, p 339

2.2 Abnormalities in β-Adrenergic Signal Transduction with Myocardial Decompensation and Failure

Dorothy E. Vatner[1]

Summary. The progression of changes in β-adrenergic receptor signalling was studied over several time points during the development of pacing-induced heart failure in long-term instrumented, conscious dogs. Animals were paced at 240 beats per minute for one month and data were averaged at 1 day, 1 week, and 3–4 weeks after pacing. The rate of change in left ventricular pressure (LV dP/dt) was decreased at 1 day, LV end-diastolic pressure and heart rate were increased at 1 week, but heart failure occurred only after 3–4 weeks of pacing. Circulating levels of norepinephrine were elevated after 1 day of pacing, and tissue levels of norepinephrine were reduced only after 3–4 weeks of pacing. High-affinity β-adrenergic receptors and adenylyl cyclase activity decreased after one day of pacing. β_1-adrenergic receptor density decreased after one week of pacing. G_s functional activity was not reduced, but $G_{i\alpha 2}$ rose after 3–4 weeks of pacing. Thus, β-adrenergic receptor signal transduction is significantly altered early, i.e., 1 day after the initiation of rapid ventricular pacing, prior to the development of heart failure. Changes occurring at 1 day after rapid ventricular pacing include increases in plasma catecholamines, uncoupling of the β-adrenergic receptor from adenylyl cyclase, and a decrease in adenylyl cyclase activity. After more prolonged pacing there is a decrease in β_1-adrenergic receptors, decreases in myocardial tissue catecholamines, and increases in $G_{i\alpha 2}$. Therefore, physiological changes in β-adrenergic receptor function during the initial development of heart failure appear to be mediated by different mechanisms than those changes that occur later as heart failure becomes manifest.

[1] Departments of Medicine, Harvard Medical School; the New England Regional Primate Research Center, Southborough, MA 01772; and the Children's Service, Massachusetts General Hospital, Boston MA 02114, USA

Introduction

Heart failure is characterized by abnormalities in the autonomic nervous system including sympathetic, parasympathetic, and baroreceptor responses [1]. Plasma catecholamines are elevated [2–5], myocardial catecholamine levels are depleted [6,7], and these measurements correlate positively with the degree of left ventricular (LV) dysfunction [2–4]. The mechanism of altered autonomic cardiovascular responsiveness and reduced catecholamine responsiveness in the failing heart involves changes in end-organ sensitivity to β-adrenergic receptor stimulation. Several animal models of heart failure as well as in vitro studies of failing human ventricle have been studied for changes in the β-adrenergic receptor–adenylyl cyclase signal transduction system. In experimental animals with heart failure, cardiac β-adrenergic receptor density has been demonstrated to be increased [8,9], unchanged [10], or decreased [11–14]. Human studies of heart failure have shown a reduction in β-adrenergic receptors, particularly β_1-receptors [14–16]. These studies examined end-stage heart failure, or a single component of the β-adrenergic receptor–G_s–adenylyl cyclase pathway, resulting in an incomplete picture of the development of abnormalities in β-adrenergic signal transduction. Understanding the inciting events may be more important than understanding the terminal events in the development of heart failure, in that therapeutic treatments designed to prevent these derangements may be more effective than strategies designed to reverse the derangements at end-stage heart failure where other complications have also developed.

To examine the differences in altered β-adrenergic receptor signal transduction mechanisms during the development of heart failure, the pacing-induced heart failure model was utilized. Rapid ventricular pacing was initiated for 1 day, 1 week, and 3–4 weeks. During this time, progressive severe congestive cardiomyopathy developed [17–19]. Cardiac sarcolemma were prepared at these different time points and β-adrenergic receptor density, affinity, β_1- and β_2-adrenergic receptor subpopulations, and adenylyl cyclase activity were determined. In addition, agonist competition curves were used to quantitate those G_s-coupled receptors binding agonist with high affinity. Finally, the guanine nucleotide-binding regulatory proteins that stimulate or inhibit adenylyl cyclase activity were quantitated. This article represents a review of work from our laboratory, which has been published previously [19].

Methods

The methods used have been described previously [19]. Briefly, surgical instrumentation was performed under general anesthesia using sterile technique. Catheters were placed in the descending thoracic aorta and left atrium. A solid-state miniature pressure transducer was implanted in the apex of the left ventricle and pacing wires were placed on the right ventricle. Rapid ventricular pacing at a rate of 240 beats/min was started 2 weeks after surgery.

Hemodynamic measurements were made 2–3 weeks after surgery in the awake state, and again at 1 day, 1 week, and 3–4 weeks after rapid, continuous ventricular pacing. The data were collected in spontaneous rhythm 30 min after the pacemaker was turned off.

Biochemical measurements were performed on left ventricular (LV) crude sarcolemmal membranes [19]. β-adrenergic receptor antagonist and agonist binding studies were performed with ^{125}I-cyanopindolol (^{125}I-cyp). $G_{s\alpha}$ activity was determined with cyc- membrane reconstitution techniques [20]. $G_{i\alpha2}$ was quantitated with immunoblotting [21]. Adenylyl cyclase activity was measured by the method of Salomon et al. [22]. Tissue and plasma catecholamine levels were determined by a radioenzymatic assay [23].

Results

Hemodynamics

There were no significant baseline hemodynamic differences before pacing among the four groups. As shown in Fig. 1, LV systolic pressure and mean arterial pressure declined after one day of pacing, but they did not decrease significantly until one week after pacing [19]. Similarly, LV end-diastolic pressure and heart rate began to increase at one day of pacing. However, the rate of change of LV pressure (dP/dt) was significantly depressed, by 41% ± 3.4%, at one day and was further decreased at one and 3–4 weeks of pacing. Only after 3–4 weeks of rapid ventricular pacing were signs and symptoms of congestive heart failure manifest, e.g., exertional dyspnea, ascites, and pulmonary and peripheral edema.

Biochemistry

Plasma norepinephrine levels increased after one day of pacing (552 ± 62 pg/ml) from a control level of 197 ± 14 pg/ml and remained elevated after 3–4 weeks of pacing (611 ± 95 pg/ml). However, LV tissue norepinephrine levels were similar to control levels at one day (542 ± 80 pg/ml) and one week (624 ± 122 pg/ml) of pacing. After 3–4 weeks of pacing, LV tissue norepinephrine (591 ± 34 pg/ml) decreased significantly (146 ± 28 pg/ml) (Fig. 2).

Receptor binding studies of β-adrenergic receptor antagonist binding showed no significant differences in total β-adrenergic receptor density or affinity among the four groups (sham-operated: 71 ± 2; 1 day: 70 ± 3; 1 week: 73 ± 3; 3–4 weeks: 71 ± 5 fmol/mg). Computer modeling of the data from competition binding curves using ^{125}I-cyp and with the subtype selective β_1-antagonist betaxolol, and with the selective β_2 antagonist ICI-118,551, indicated that a two-site model was preferred for these competition curves. Despite the fact that plasma catecholamine levels had already increased at 1 day of pacing,

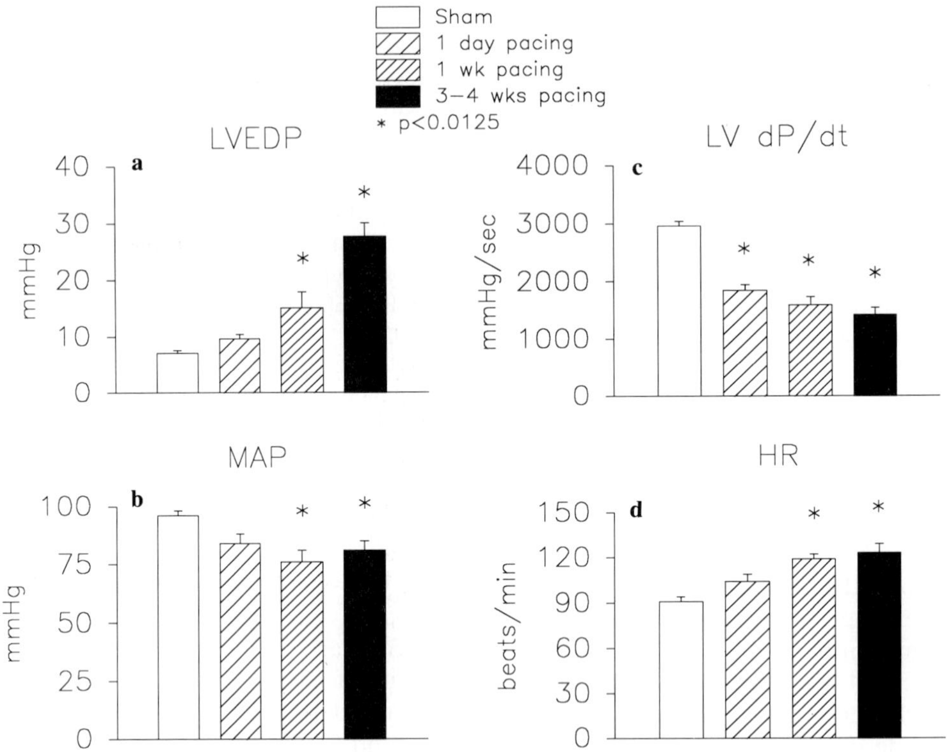
Sham
1 day pacing
1 wk pacing
3–4 wks pacing
* p<0.0125
LVEDP
a
mmHg
LV dP/dt
c
mmHg/sec
MAP
b
mmHg
HR
d
beats/min

1

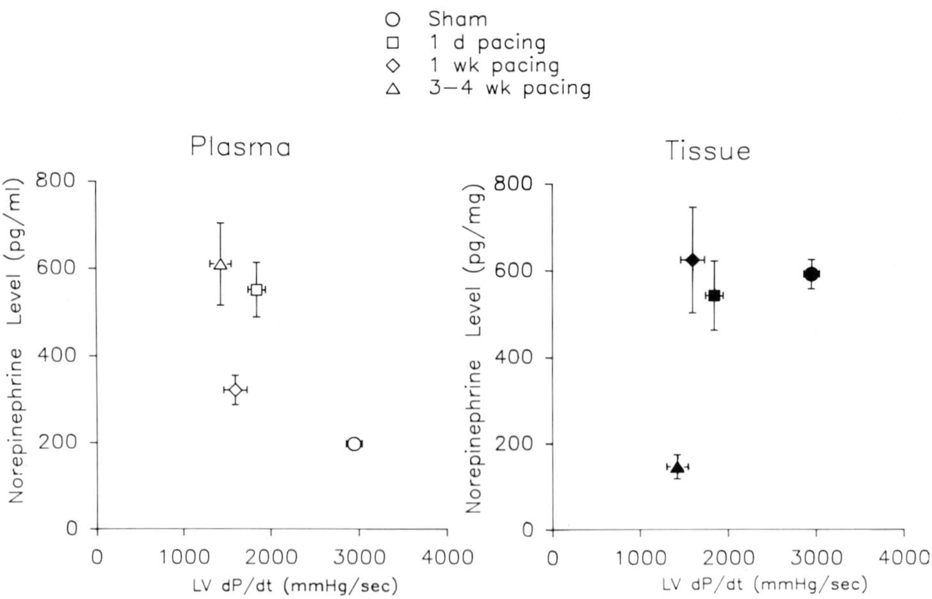
Sham
1 d pacing
1 wk pacing
3–4 wk pacing
Plasma
Norepinephrine Level (pg/ml)
Tissue
Norepinephrine Level (pg/mg)
LV dP/dt (mmHg/sec)

2

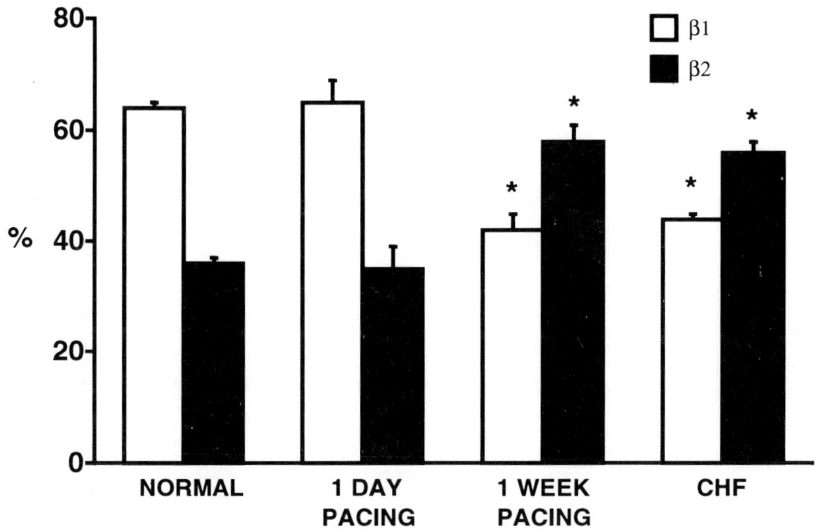

3

Fig. 3. Using betaxolol, a β_1-specific antagonist in competitive binding experiments, the proportion of β_1- to β_2-adrenergic receptor subpopulations was determined in hearts from animals with 1 day, 1 week, and 3–4 weeks of rapid pacing-induced heart failure (*CHF*). There were no significant differences in the proportion of β_1- and β_2-adrenergic receptors after 1 day of pacing. After 1 week and 3–4 weeks of pacing, there was a significant loss of β_1-adrenergic receptors, and increase in β_2-adrenergic receptors, as reflected by the *asterisks*. (Redrawn from data contained in [19] with permission of The American Society for Clinical Investigation)

←

Fig. 1a–d. The absolute levels of **a** left ventricular end-diastolic pressure (*LVEDP*), **b** mean arterial pressure (*MAP*), **c** rate of change of LV pressure (*LV dP/dt*), and **d** heart rate (*HR*) are compared at different stages of pacing-induced heart failure. Heart rate and LV end-diastolic pressure began to increase at 1 day after pacing, but were not significantly increased until 1 week (*wk*) of pacing. Similarly, mean arterial pressure began to decrease at 1 day of pacing, but was not significantly decreased until 1 week of pacing. In contrast, LV dP/dt was significantly decreased at 1 day and was further depressed at 1 week and 3–4 weeks of pacing. (Redrawn from data contained in [19] with permission of The American Society for Clinical Investigation)

Fig. 2. Relationship between LV function and plasma or myocardial norepinephrine content is shown. There was no change in tissue norepinephrine until 3–4 weeks after pacing (*triangles*), even though marked changes in myocardial contractility were observed after 1 day of pacing (*squares*). While plasma norepinephrine was elevated at 1 day after pacing, there was not a progressive rise, despite the progressive decline in LV function. (Reprinted from [19] with permission of The American Society for Clinical Investigation)

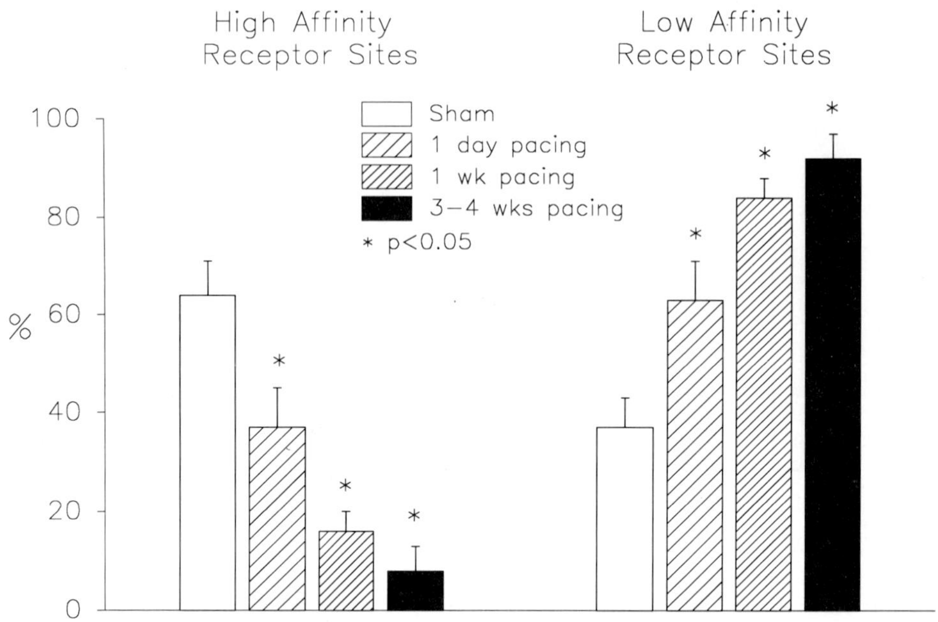

Fig. 4. The average percent of β-adrenergic receptors binding agonist with high and low affinity for hearts from control animals and animals with 1 day, 1 week, and 3–4 weeks' rapid pacing-induced heart failure are shown. There is a progressive and significant increase in low-affinity agonist binding sites, with corresponding loss of high-affinity sites. *Asterisks* denote statistically significant differences from sham. (Redrawn from data contained in [19] with permission of The American Society for Clinical Investigation)

there were no significant differences in the proportion of β_1 to β_2-adrenergic receptors at this point in time compared with sham-operated dogs. After 1 week, and 3–4 weeks of pacing, β_1-adrenergic receptors were depressed significantly as compared to sham-operated dogs (Fig. 3).

Isoproterenol competition curves for sham-operated dogs fit best to a two-site model with 64% ± 7% as high-affinity receptors. After 1 day of pacing, there was a significant loss of high-affinity receptors to 37% ± 8%. At 1 week and 3–4 weeks after pacing, the number of high-affinity sites was further decreased (16% ± 4% and 8% ± 5%, respectively) (Fig. 4).

Adenylyl cyclase activity was depressed significantly after 1 day and further depressed at 1 week and 3–4 weeks of pacing. This included progressive decreases in basal and stimulated activities except for sodium fluoride which was depressed only at 1 week and 3–4 weeks of pacing (Fig. 5).

Studies of $G_{s\alpha}$ reconstituted activity in the LV showed no significant difference in pacing animals as compared to sham-operated control animals (sham-operated: 5.8 ± 0.4; 1 day: 5.5 ± 0.7; 1 week: 6.8 ± 0.4; 3–4 weeks: 5.1 ± 0.7 pmol cyclic AMP/μg per 10 min).

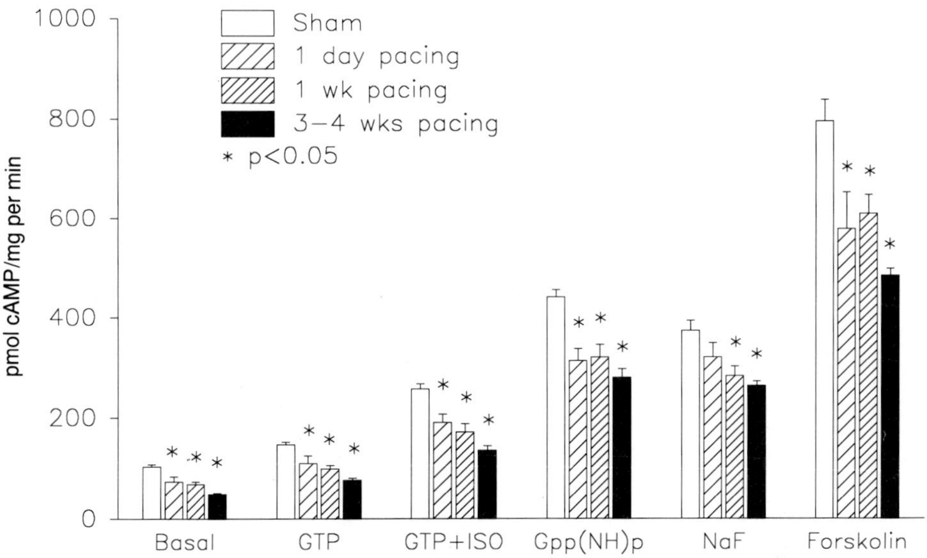

Fig. 5. Adenylyl cyclase activity is shown for basal activity and for maximally stimulated activity using 0.1 m*M* GTP, 0.1 m*M* GTP plus 0.1 m*M* isoproterenol (*ISO*), 0.1 m*M* Gpp(NH)p, 10 m*M* sodium fluoride, and 0.1 m*M* forskolin. Except for sodium fluoride activity, at 1 day of pacing there is a significant decrease in basal and stimulatable adenylyl cyclase activity. This decline in activity continues progressively with increasing duration of rapid ventricular pacing. (Redrawn from data contained in [19] with permission of The American Society for Clinical Investigation)

Immunoblotting of crude cardiac membranes for $G_{i\alpha 2}$ levels showed a significant increase of 44% ± 6% in the animals with 3–4 weeks of pacing-induced failure as compared to sham-operated controls (Fig. 6).

Discussion

During the development of pacing-induced heart failure there is a progressive decline in LV function, with significant decreases in myocardial contractility observed, even at 1 day after pacing, with further progression until frank congestive heart failure develops at 3–4 weeks after pacing. No change in tissue catecholamines were observed until 3–4 weeks after pacing, even though significant changes in myocardial contractility were observed after only 1 day of pacing. Thus, the catecholamine depletion observed in the heart most likely reflects heart failure and not just myocardial dysfunction. However, plasma catecholamines were elevated at 1 day after pacing, and rose further at 3–4 weeks of pacing (Fig. 2). Increases in circulating catecholamines and decreases in myocardial tissue catecholamines are important markers of heart failure, but

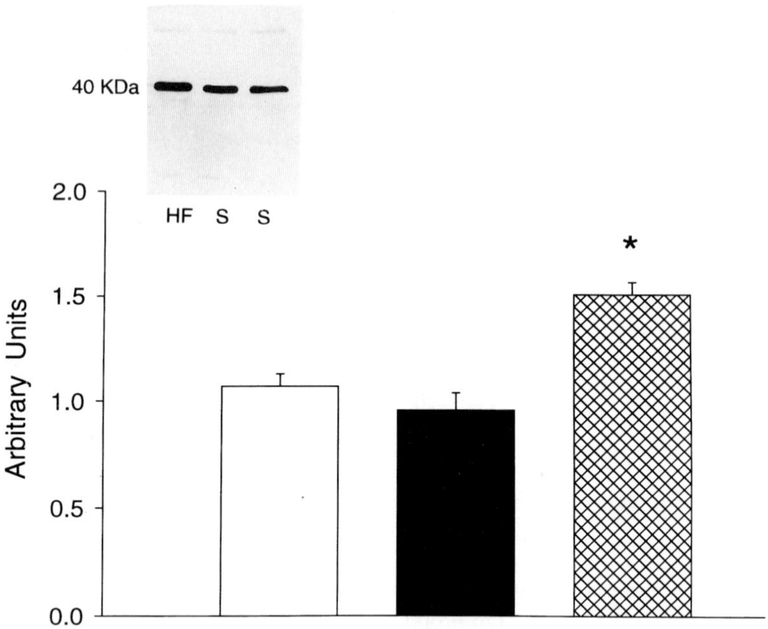

Fig. 6. Relative levels of immunodetectable $G_{i\alpha2}$ are compared in sham-operated animals (*open bar*), 1-day pacing animals (*solid bar*), and 3–4 weeks pacing animals (*cross-hatched bar*). $G_{i\alpha2}$ levels are expressed in arbitrary units. As denoted by the *asterisk*, there was a significant increase ($P < 0.017$) in $G_{i\alpha2}$ levels in 3–4 weeks pacing animals compared with either sham-operated animals or animals after 1 day's pacing. A representative Western blot is shown in the *upper left corner*, depicting enhanced expression of the 40 kDa band, representing $G_{i\alpha2}$ in membranes from the dogs with 3–4 weeks' pacing (*HF*) compared to two of the sham-operated controls (*S*). (Reprinted from [19] with permission of The American Society for Clinical Investigation)

because their regulation is linked to a variety of complex uptake and metabolic mechanisms, their levels cannot predict precise levels of cardiac dysfunction. However, it is possible to conclude from these data that the decline in tissue catecholamines is a result rather than a cause of the heart failure process, whereas the elevated plasma catecholamine levels may actually be important in the pathogenesis of heart failure by inducing desensitization [15,16,24–27]. An important caveat is that the increase in plasma levels of catecholamines may be a marker of altered catecholamine activity that is critical to the desensitization process, but that the actual mechanisms involve alterations in catecholamine levels at the neural-receptor junction, rather than in the systemic circulation.

In this model of heart failure, the rise in plasma catecholamines clearly preceded the down-regulation of β_1-adrenergic receptors by at least 1 week, suggesting that either classical desensitization mechanisms, which occur almost immediately in vitro [28], are not responsible for the down-regulation of β-adrenergic receptors in heart failure, or that desensitization in the intact organism is more complex [29–31]. The complexity may be related to the presence of intact cardiac nerves, in vivo. Because of this, the circulating levels of plasma catecholamines may not provide an accurate index of cardiac sympathetic activity at the sarcolemmal receptor, since neural mechanisms may be more important in the regulation of catecholamine concentration at the receptor site. There are several steps in the process of catecholamine-induced desensitization [29–31]. First, there appears to be a rapid uncoupling of the receptor from activation of adenylyl cyclase, which is in keeping with our observation that the earliest events in the alteration of myocardial β-adrenergic receptor function during the development of pacing-induced heart failure are characterized by uncoupling of the β-adrenergic receptor and reduced adenylyl cyclase activation, rather than β_1-adrenergic receptor down-regulation.

These changes occurred prior to development of heart failure, where LV end-diastolic pressure had not increased significantly, and there were no signs of congestive heart failure. At this time, LV dP/dt was significantly depressed, and responsiveness to sympathomimetic amines was also significantly attenuated [19]. Since adenylyl cyclase stimulation was reduced, this suggests that a defect in the catalytic unit of adenylyl cyclase, however, had occurred at this time. In contrast, there was no change in total β-adrenergic receptor density, no change in $\beta_1:\beta_2$ receptor ratio, and no change in G_s or $G_{i\alpha2}$. These data suggest that the initial changes in β-adrenergic signalling after 1 day of pacing involve a loss of high-affinity β-adrenergic receptors and a defect in the adenylyl cyclase catalytic unit. Since these alterations occurred early and intensified with further progression of the disease, it is interesting to speculate that these mechanisms may be important in the pathogenesis of autonomic dysfunction in heart failure. Interestingly, defects in the message level of isoforms of adenylyl cyclase have been noted in this pacing model of heart failure [32].

Down-regulation of β-adrenergic receptors has been implicated as the dominant mechanism to account for reduced catecholamine responsiveness in heart failure [15,16,24–27]. Since inotropic and chronotropic responses to catecholamines are thought to be mediated through β_1-adrenergic receptor subtype activation, selective down-regulation of β_1-adrenergic receptors would be required for this mechanism to be operative. This has been observed by Bristow et al. [15]. In our studies of pacing-induced heart failure, no significant change in total β-adrenergic receptor density was observed. However, β_1-adrenergic receptor down-regulation was observed at 1 and 3–4 weeks after pacing. At the time that down-regulation of β_1-adrenergic receptors was apparent in dogs, following 1 week and 3–4 weeks of pacing, the β_2-adrenergic receptor subpopulation density was actually increased in this model. The mechanism of the increase in β_2-adrenergic receptors is not known. It remains to be determined if these additional β_2-adrenergic receptors are located on myocytes and are functionally coupled and cause a physiologic action in heart failure.

Another mechanism by which catecholamine responsiveness can be reduced in heart failure may involve the coupling between β-adrenergic receptors and G proteins. It is the high-affinity form of the receptor that is functionally coupled to the GTP-stimulatory protein, G_s, and therefore, represents the most physiological relevant form of the receptor [33,34]. Coupling of the β-adrenergic receptor can be evaluated utilizing agonist-binding techniques [9]. A prior study from our laboratory [9] and others [14] demonstrated uncoupling of the β-adrenergic receptor in heart failure with chronic pressure or volume-overload hypertrophy. However, β-adrenergic receptor coupling has not been assessed in other models of heart failure. A major finding of the studies in pacing-induced heart failure was that the number of β-adrenergic receptors in the high-affinity state decreased progressively in dogs following 1 day, 1 week, and 3–4 weeks of pacing. This appears to be one of the earliest abnormalities in the β-adrenergic receptor signalling pathway that occurs during the development of heart failure. Although prior studies did not assess the relationship between the degree of heart failure and agonist binding, Fowler et al. [35] noted that human myocardial β-adrenergic receptor down-regulation is related to the degree of heart failure, and is associated with specific impairment of the β-agonist-mediated contractile response.

Our study of pacing-induced heart failure did not demonstrate reduced G_s levels in the sarcolemma of animals with pacing-induced heart failure. Feldman et al. [36] also found no reduction in G_s levels in failing human myocardium either by the ADP-ribosylation or by reconstitution assays. G_s has been reported as reduced in the lymphocytes of patients with heart failure using cholera toxin-stimulated labeling [37], and it has been documented that patients who have a low ratio of G_s to G_i in peripheral lymphocytes have more severe hemodynamic abnormality and a worse one-year prognosis than patients with a higher ratio of G_s to G_i [38]. In a prior study on pressure-overload hypertrophy and heart failure, $G_{s\alpha}$ activity was also reduced [39].

While the functional activity of G_s was unchanged after pacing, an increase in $G_{i\alpha2}$ as measured by immunoblotting after 3–4 weeks pacing was observed in the present study. In animal models of heart failure, G_i has been shown to be depressed as measured by pertussis toxin labelling [11]. Another animal study [12] using pertussis toxin labelling as well as immunoblotting has shown an increase in G_i levels. Most human heart failure studies have demonstrated an increase in G_i levels [11,12,36,40,41]. Prior studies [36,40] have suggested that in the late stages of heart failure, an increase in the level of G_i may be responsible for depressed basal and Gpp(NH)p-stimulated adenylyl cyclase activity. While we found that isoproterenol-stimulated adenylyl cyclase was depressed at 1 day, $G_{i\alpha2}$ was not elevated at this point. Therefore, it is unlikely that the increase in G_i is solely responsible for the depressed adenylyl cyclase, and alterations in the catalytic unit of adenylyl cyclase still appear to play an important role.

In summary, abnormalities in β-adrenergic signal transduction with myocardial decompensation and failure involve decreased adenylyl cyclase activity, a specific decrease in β_1-adrenergic receptors, and a loss of high-affinity receptors which are coupled to adenylyl cyclase. Many of these changes actually occur prior to the development of heart failure. Changes occurring at one day after rapid ventricular pacing include increases in plasma catecholamines, uncoupling of the β-adrenergic receptor from adenylyl cyclase, and a decrease in adenylyl cyclase activity. After more prolonged pacing there is a decrease in β_1-adrenergic receptors, decreases in myocardial tissue catecholamines, and increases in $G_{i\alpha 2}$. Therefore, physiological changes in β-adrenergic receptor function during the initial development of heart failure appear to be mediated by the loss of high-affinity β-adrenergic receptors and potentially alterations in adenylyl cyclase activity, and not simply by down-regulation of β-adrenergic receptor density.

Acknowledgment. Supported in part by U.S. Public Health Service Grants HL 38070, HL 37404, and RR 00168

References

1. Francis GS, Cohn JN (1986) The autonomic nervous system in congestive heart failure. Annu Rev Med 37:235–247
2. Thomas JA, Marks BH (1978) Plasma norepinephrine in congestive heart failure. Am J Cardiol 41:233–243
3. Covell JW, Chidsey CA, Braunwald E (1966) Reduction of the cardiac response to postganglionic sympathetic nerve stimulation in experimental heart failure. Circ Res 19:51–56
4. Cohn JN, Levine TB, Olivari MT, Garberg V, Lubra D, Francis GS, Simon AB, Rector T (1984) Plasma norepinephrine as a guide to prognosis in patients with chronic congestive heart failure. New Engl J Med 311:819–823
5. Daly PA, Sole MJ (1990) Myocardial catecholamines and the pathophysiology of heart failure. Circulation 82[Suppl I]:I-35–I-43
6. Chidsey CA, Braunwald E, Morrow AG (1965) Catecholamine excretion and cardiac stores of norepinephrine in congestive heart failure. Am J Med 39:442–451
7. Spann JF, Chidsey CA, Pool PE, Braunwald E (1965) Mechanism of norepinephrine depletion in experimental heart failure produced by aortic constriction in the guinea pig. Circ Res 17:312–321
8. Karliner JS, Barnes P, Brown M, Dollery C (1980) Chronic heart failure in the guinea pig increases cardiac alpha_1- and beta-adrenoceptors. Eur J Pharmacol 67:115–118
9. Vatner DE, Vatner SF, Fujii AM, Homcy CJ (1985) Loss of high affinity cardiac beta adrenergic receptors in dogs with heart failure. J Clin Invest 76:2259–2264
10. Ho K, Lloyd BL, Taylor RR (1981) Cardiac beta-adrenoreceptors in the thyroxine-treated dog. Clin Exp Pharmacol Physiol 8:183–187
11. Calderone A, Bouvier M, Li K, Juneau C, Champlain J, Rouleau J (1991) Dysfunction of the β- and α-adrenergic systems in a model of congestive heart failure: The pacing-overdrive dog. Circ Res 69:332–343

12. Marzo KP, Frey MJ, Wilson JR, Liang BT, Manning DR, Lanoce V, Molinoff PB (1991) β-adrenergic receptor–G protein–adenylate cyclase complex in experimental canine congestive heart failure produced by rapid ventricular pacing. Circ Res 69:1546–1556
13. Fan T-HM, Liang C-S, Kawashima S, Banerjee SP (1987) Alterations in cardiac β-adrenoceptor responsiveness and adenylate cyclase system by congestive heart failure in dogs. Eur J Pharmacol 140:123–132
14. Hammond HK, Roth DA, Insel PA, Ford CE, White FC, Maisel AS, Ziegler MG, Bloor CM (1992) Myocardial β-adrenergic receptor expression and signal transduction after chronic volume-overload hypertrophy and circulatory congestion. Circulation 85:269–280
15. Bristow MR, Ginsburg R, Umans V, Fowler M, Minobe W, Rasmusen R, Zera P, Menlove R, Shah P, Jamieson S, Stinson EB (1986) β_1- and β_2-adrenergic-receptor subpopulations in nonfailing and failing human ventricular myocardium: Coupling of both receptor subtypes to muscle contraction and selective β_1-receptor down-regulation in heart failure. Circ Res 59:297–309
16. Brodde O-E, Zerkowski H-R, Doetsch N, Motomura S, Khamssi M, Michel MC (1989) Myocardial β-adrenergic changes in heart failure: Concomitant reduction in β_1 and β_2-adrenergic function related to the degree of heart failure in patients with mitral valve disease. J Am Coll Cardiol 14:323–331
17. Shannon RP, Komamura K, Stambler BS, Manders WT, Vatner SF (1991) Alterations in myocardial contractility in conscious dogs with dilated cardiomyopathy. Am J Physiol 260:H1903–H1911
18. Komamura K, Shannon RP, Pasipoularides A, Ihara T, Lader AS, Patrick TA, Bishop SP, Vatner SF (1992) Alterations in left ventricular diastolic function in conscious dogs with pacing-induced heart failure. J Clin Invest 89:1825–1838
19. Kiuchi K, Shannon RP, Komamura K, Cohen DJ, Bianchi C, Homcy CJ, Vatner SF, Vatner DE (1993) Myocardial β-adrenergic receptor function during the development of pacing-induced heart failure. J Clin Invest 91:907–914
20. Susanni EE, Manders WT, Knight DR, Vatner DE, Vatner SF, Homcy CJ (1989) One hour of myocardial ischemia decreases the activity of the stimulatory guanine-nucleotide regulatory protein G_s. Circ Res 65:1145–1150
21. Mumby SM, Kahn RA, Manning DR, Gilman AG (1986) Antisera of designed specificity for subunits of guanine nucleotide-binding regulatory proteins. Proc Natl Acad Sci USA 83:265–269
22. Salomon Y, Londos C, Rodbell M (1974) A highly sensitive adenylate cyclase assay. Anal Biochem 58:541–548
23. Peuleur JD, Johnson GA (1977) Simultaneous single isotope radioenzymatic assay of plasma norepinephrine, epinephrine and dopamine. Life Sci 21:625–636
24. Bristow MR, Kantrowitz ME, Ginsburg R, Fowler MB (1985) β-adrenergic function in heart muscle disease and heart failure. J Mol Cell Cardiol 17:41–52
25. Bristow MR, Ginsburg R, Minobe W, Cubicciotti RS, Sageman WS, Lurie K, Billingham ME, Harrison DC, Stinson EB (1982) Decreased catecholamine sensitivity and β-adrenergic-receptor density in failing human hearts. New Engl J Med 307:205–211
26. Dennis AR, Marsh JD, Quigg RJ, Gordon JB, Colucci WS (1989) β-adrenergic receptor number and adenylate cyclase function in denervated transplanted and cardiomyopathic human hearts. Circulation 79:1028–1034

27. Vago T, Bevilacqua M, Norbiato G, Baldi G, Chebat E, Bertora P, Baroldi G, Accinni R (1989) Identification of α_1-adrenergic receptors on sarcolemma from normal subjects and patients with idiopathic dilated cardiomyopathy: Characteristics and linkage to GTP-binding protein. Circ Res 64:474–481
28. Harden TK (1983) Agonist-induced desensitization of the β-adrenergic receptor-linked adenylate cyclase. Pharmacol Rev 35(1):5–32
29. Sibley DR, Lefkowitz RJ (1985) Molecular mechanisms of receptor desensitization using the β-adrenergic receptor-coupled adenylate cyclase system as a model. Nature 317:124–129
30. Benovic JL, Bouvier M, Caron MG, Lefkowitz RJ (1988) Regulation of adenylyl cyclase-coupled β-adrenergic receptors. Annu Rev Cell Biol 4:405–428
31. Su Y-F, Harden TK, Perkins JP (1980) Catecholamine-specific desensitization of adenylate cyclase: Evidence for a multistep process. J Biol Chem 255:7410–7419
32. Ishikawa Y, Katsushika S, Kiuchi K, Shannon RP, Komamura K, Sorota S, Vatner DE, Vatner SF, Homcy CJ (1994) Downregulation of adenylylcyclase Types V and VI mRNA levels in pacing-induced heart failure in dogs. J Clin Invest 93:2224–2229
33. Manalan AS, Besch HR Jr, Watanabe AM (1981) Characterization of $[^3H](\pm)$Carazolol binding to β-adrenergic receptors: Application to study of β-adrenergic receptor subtypes in canine ventricular myocardium and lung. Circ Res 49:326–336
34. DeLean A, Stadel JM, Lefkowitz RJ (1980) A ternary complex model explains the agonist-specific binding properties of the adenylate cyclase-coupled β-adrenergic receptor. J Biol Chem 255:7108–7117
35. Fowler MB, Laser JA, Hopkins GL, Minobe W, Bristow MR (1986) Assessment of the β-adrenergic receptor pathway in the intact failing human heart: progressive receptor down-regulation and subsensitivity to agonist response. Circulation 74: 1290–1302
36. Feldman AM, Cates AE, Veazey WB, Harshberger RE, Bristow MR, Baughman KL, Baumgartner WA, Van Dop C (1988) Increase of the 40 000-mol wt pertussis toxin substrate (G-protein) in the failing human heart. J Clin Invest 82:189–197
37. Horn EM, Chow YK, Neuberg GW, Corwin SJ, Powers ER, Bilezikian JP, Cannon PJ, Steinberg SF (1986) The guanine nucleotide regulatory protein Ns is reduced in congestive heart failure (abstract). Circulation 74[Suppl II]:II-198
38. Horn EM, Gottlieb SS, Morrow B, Bilezikian JP, Packer M (1987) Hemodynamic and prognostic significance of altered lymphocyte guanine nucleotide binding proteins in congestive heart failure (abstract). Circulation 76[Suppl IV]:IV-88
39. Chen L, Vatner DE, Vatner SF, Hittinger L, Homcy CJ (1991) Decreased $G_{s\alpha}$ mRNA levels accompany the fall in G_s and adenylyl cyclase activities in compensated left ventricular hypertrophy. In heart failure, only the impairment in adenylyl cyclase activation progresses. J Clin Invest 87:293–298
40. Böhm M, Gierschik P, Jakobs K-H, Pieske B, Schnabel P, Ungerer M, Erdmann E (1990) Increase of $G_{i\alpha}$ in human hearts with dilated but not ischemic cardiomyopathy. Circulation 82:1249–1265
41. Eschenhagen T, Mende U, Nose M, Schmitz W, Scholz H, Haverich A, Hirt S, Döring V, Kalmár P, Höppner W, Seitz H-J (1992) Increased messenger RNA level of the inhibitory G protein α subunit $G_{i\alpha\text{-}2}$ in human end-stage heart failure. Circ Res 70:688–696

Mechanical Aspects

2.3 Effect of Mild Pressure Overload on Mechanoenergetics of the Rabbit Heart

Martin M. LeWinter, Hitoshi Yaku, and Bryan K. Slinker[1]

Summary. We determined the effect of a mild pressure overload (perinephritic hypertension) on cardiac mechanoenergetics in New Zealand white rabbits ($n = 7$). Results were compared to sham operated controls ($n = 8$) and rabbits rendered hypothyroid ($n = 5$). Using an isovolumically contracting, red blood cell perfused, isolated heart preparation, mechanoenergetics were assessed as the inverse slopes of the V_{O_2}–pressure–volume area relation (contractile efficiency) and the V_{O_2}–stress time integral relation (contractile economy), where V_{O_2} is myocardial oxygen consumption. The energy cost of excitation–contraction coupling was assessed as unloaded V_{O_2} minus basal V_{O_2} per beat. Morphologic measurements demonstrated no significant increase in left ventricular or heart-weight-to-body-weight ratio in pressure overload hearts. In controls, percent V_3 isomyosin was 80% ± 7% (±SD), while in hypothyroid hearts V_3 averaged 100% ± 1% and in pressure overload 98% ± 1% (both $P < 0.01$ *vs* controls). Both efficiency and economy demonstrated trends toward higher values in pressure overload compared to either hypothyroid or control hearts. Considered as a function of percent V_3 isomyosin and compared to control and hormonally modified (hyper- and hypothyroid) hearts, values for efficiency and economy were clearly elevated. In contrast, V_{O_2} used for excitation–contraction coupling was not significantly different among the three groups. Thus, a very mild pressure overload results in increased efficiency and economy. It is proposed that the most likely explanation for this finding is an alteration at the level of the contractile proteins, independent of changes in isomyosin composition.

Key words: Mechanoenergetics—Hypertrophy—Ventricular mechanics—Isomyosins—Contractile proteins

[1]The Cardiology Unit, University of Vermont College of Medicine, Burlington, VT 05401, USA

Introduction

Based on experiments performed in strips of ventricular myocardium, alterations in the mechanics and energetics of contraction have been recognized for some time in patients with dilated cardiomyopathy and in patients and experimental animals with severe mechanical overload [1–9]. Although not uniform, mechanical alterations tend to consist of slowing of contraction and relaxation, with variable force-generating capacity. A consistent mechanoenergetic finding has been increased contractile economy, i.e., a decrease in the energy cost of generating a unit of tension time integral [3,4,8,9]. These alterations in mechanoenergetics have been related to concomitant alterations in both excitation–contraction (E–C) coupling and the composition of the contractile proteins [1–12].

It has been recognized for many years that isomyosin composition is an important determinant of the mechanoenergetic behavior of heart muscle [3,4,8,9,13–15]. This is exemplified by the relationship between contractile economy and isomyosin composition in normals and hormonally modified (hyper- and hypothyroid) hearts [4,8,13]. Hyperthyroid hearts demonstrate larger proportions of the high-ATPase-activity V_1 isomyosin and low economy, while hypothyroid hearts have a high proportion of the slower V_3 isomyosin and high economy. Recently, Hasenfuss et al. [8,9] related contractile economy to isomyosin composition in normal, hormonally modified, mechanically overloaded, and failing myocardium in several species, including humans. With both mechanical overload and failure, increases in contractile economy appeared to be much greater than could be accounted for by changes in isomyosins alone. Although these increases in contractile economy could be partly explained by changes in E–C coupling, after taking these into account, Hasenfuss et al. [8] postulated an alteration at the level of the contractile proteins independent of isomyosin shifts as the mechanism of their findings.

Considerably less mechanoenergetic information is available in hypertrophy and failure in the beating heart. Considering the changes in structure and geometry which occur as the heart remodels in response to chronic stress, it would seem important to achieve an understanding of the effect of hypertrophy and failure at this level. Several investigators have applied the approach originated by Suga et al. [16] for the study of mechanoenergetics in the beating heart to models of hypertrophy and failure. This approach employs isolated, perfused heart preparations in which mechanical unloading is employed to partition myocardial oxygen consumption (V_{O_2}) into mechanical and nonmechanical components. Total mechanical energy output is characterized as pressure–volume area (PVA). The inverse slope of the linear relationship between PVA and mechanical V_{O_2} (mechanical energy output divided by input) is employed as a measure of contractile efficiency. Using this approach, we reported a decrease in contractile efficiency in hearts from rabbits rendered hyperthyroid [17]. We ascribed this change to the major shift of isomyosins from predominantly V_3 to predominantly V_1 which occurs in adult hyperthyroid rabbits.

Izzi et al. [18] used a similar approach in dogs with concentric left ventricular hypertrophy due to pressure overload and did not demonstrate an alteration in contractile efficiency. Wolff et al. [19] studied the pacing tachycardia model of heart failure in dogs and reported increased contractile efficiency. All of the information cited here with respect to alterations in mechanoenergetic behavior of either the beating heart or isolated heart muscle in hypertrophy and/or failure has been obtained under conditions of severe stress. In the present study, we employed a mild pressure overload in an attempt to determine whether such changes require a severe stress or can occur with a very modest hypertrophic stimulus. In order to accomplish this, we used the cellophane-wrap model of perinephritic hypertension in rabbits, which can be manipulated to produce a minimal pressure overload.

Materials and Methods

Experimental Models

We studied hearts from male, New Zealand White rabbits (average weight 3.7 ± 0.32 kg) subjected to hypertension (n = 7) and hypothyroidism (n = 5), and sham operated controls (n = 8). Cellophane-wrap of the kidneys [20] was produced under sterile conditions using a bilateral flank incision. This results in mild to moderate hypertension appearing over several weeks. Hypothyroidism was produced by inclusion of propylthiouracil in the rabbits' drinking water [17]. The cellophane-wrap and sham animals were killed at about six weeks after surgery, while hypothyroid rabbits were killed after 3–4 weeks of propylthiouracil treatment [17]. At the time of death all rabbits were between 6–7 months of age.

Heart Preparation

Isolated hearts were studied using a bovine red blood cell perfused preparation which has been described previously [21]. Briefly, after premedication with Fentanyl (0.044 mg/kg i.m.) and Droperidol (2.2 mg/kg i.m.), each rabbit was anesthetized with ketamine hydrochloride (20 mg/kg i.m.) and xylazine (1 mg/kg i.m.), subjected to a tracheotomy, ventilated with a Harvard respirator, and given heparin (1000 U/kg via the marginal ear vein). Through a midsternal incision the pericardium was incised and a flexible tube (2.5-mm OD, 2-mm ID) introduced into the right ventricle (RV) via the right atrial appendage. Following simultaneous ligation of the pulmonary hili and superior and inferior venae cava, the ascending aorta was cannulated with a rigid plastic tube (4-mm OD, 2.5-mm ID), and perfusion begun. Interruption of coronary flow was less than 15 seconds. The heart was then removed from the chest and hung from the arterial tube.

After a small vent (1-mm OD, 1-cm length) was inserted in the left ventricular (LV) apex, the left atrium was opened widely. All chordae tendineae were cut to allow an LV balloon to fit within the LV chamber. A thin latex balloon (unstressed volume 3 ml) attached to the end of a rigid tube (0.8-mm OD) was inserted into the LV via the mitral orifice and secured by a ligature around the left atrium just above the mitral annulus. The other end of the rigid tube was connected to a Gould P23XL pressure transducer (Gould, Oxnard, Calif., USA), and a 2-ml graduated syringe with a resolution of 0.02 ml was connected to the tube via a stopcock. To minimize the contribution of RV V_{O_2} to total V_{O_2}, the RV was kept collapsed throughout. The heart was placed in a chamber with a water jacket to maintain heart temperature at 35°–37°C.

Coronary flow was measured with timed collections of the coronary venous drainage into a graduated cylinder from the tube introduced in the RV. This does not account for LV Thebesian flow, which is negligible [22]. Coronary arteriovenous O_2 content difference was measured with an A-VOX system, which continuously sampled arterial perfusate and venous effluent. The A-VOX system was calibrated against a Lex-O_2-Con oximeter (Lexington, Waltham, Massachusetts, USA) during each experiment.

A perfusate consisting of bovine red cells suspended in Krebs-Henseleit buffer was used for coronary perfusion of the isolated heart. Fresh whole bovine blood was spun in a refrigerated centrifuge (5°C) at 3500 rpm for 25 min, the plasma was aspirated, and the remaining packed cells mixed with the same volume of buffer and spun at the same rpm for the same time. This washing procedure was performed three times on the first day and once every day thereafter. The buffer had the following composition in m*M*: 108.0 NaCl, 4.0 KCl, 2.5 $CaCl_2$, 1.4 KH_2PO_4, 1.4 $MgSO_4$, 25.0 $NaHCO_3$, 11.0 dextrose, and 10.0 Na-pyruvate (all Sigma). Gentamicin (3 mg/l) was added to the buffer to suppress bacterial growth.

Before each experiment, red cells were suspended to a final hematocrit of 35% in buffer which also included 10 IU/l of insulin. The perfusate was equilibrated with 98% O_2 and 2% CO_2 to achieve a pO_2 of over 100 mmHg and a pCO_2 of around 40 mmHg. pH was adjusted to 7.35–7.45 by adding NaOH. The temperature of the perfusate was maintained at 35°–37°C with water jackets around an oxygenator and a pressurized chamber in the arterial tube. The perfusate was not recirculated.

The heart was paced at approximately 190 beats/min via electrodes attached to the left atrium. Coronary perfusion pressure was kept constant at approximately 80 mmHg with a pressure regulator throughout each experiment.

Experimental Protocol

The same experimental protocol was performed in each group. After reaching stable levels of LV pressure and V_{O_2} under unloaded conditions, LV pressure, coronary flow, and coronary arteriovenous O_2 content difference was measured at 5–8 different LV volumes including V_0 with the LV contracting isovolumically. V_0 is the volume at which isovolumic peak LV pressure was zero. The maximal volume was chosen as the volume at which either LV end-diastolic pressure reached 10 mmHg or peak systolic pressure reached about 100 mmHg. At each ventricular volume, we waited at least 3 minutes to obtain stable, steady-state LV pressure and V_{O_2}.

After these measurements were completed, the heart was arrested by a rapid infusion of 20% KCl solution (0.2 ml per minute) followed by a slower infusion of the same solution (0.03 ml per minute). Fifteen minutes following cardiac arrest produced by the KCl solution, coronary flow and coronary arteriovenous O_2 content difference were measured for two minutes at V_0.

After each experiment, the LV (free wall plus ventricular septum) and RV (free wall) were weighed quickly and tissue samples were taken from the LV lateral free wall (including both endocardium and epicardium) and frozen in liquid nitrogen for myosin isoform measurement.

Data Analysis

Date for LV pressure and coronary arteriovenous O_2 content difference were collected at 5-ms intervals with a personal computer (Gateway 2000, North Sioux City, S.D., USA) and stored on a hard disk for off-line analyses.

V_{O_2} per minute was obtained as the product of coronary flow (ml/min) and coronary arteriovenous O_2 content difference (vol%). Because the measured total V_{O_2} always includes the V_{O_2} of the collapsed RV, we subtracted this value from the total V_{O_2}. V_{O_2} of the collapsed RV was calculated as total V_{O_2} at $V_0 \times$ (RV weight)/(total heart weight). LV V_{O_2} was divided by heart rate to yield V_{O_2} per beat ($ml\,O_2 \cdot beat^{-1}$), and normalized for LV weight to be expressed as $ml\,O_2 \cdot beat^{-1} \cdot 100\,g^{-1}$.

LV chamber contractility was quantified by calculating E_{max} [23]. E_{max} is the maximum value for the instantaneous LV pressure–volume ratio: $P(t)/(V_{iso} - V_0)$, where $P(t)$ is instantaneous pressure, and V_{iso} is isovolumic volume. Linear regression analysis of end-systolic (peak) pressure–volume data was used to dertermine E_{max} and the volume axis intercept (V_0). E_{max} was also normalized for LV weight to give units of $mmHg \cdot ml^{-1} \cdot 100\,g^{-1}$.

LV systolic pressure–volume area (PVA) is an expression of total mechanical energy generated by each contraction and is highly correlated with V_{O_2} per beat [16]. PVA is the area surrounded by the end-systolic and end-diastolic pressure–volume relations and the systolic pressure–volume trajectory in the pressure–volume diagram [16,22]. For isovolumic contractions, PVA is the sum of the triangular area formed by the three straight lines connecting the end-systolic, end-diastolic, and V_0 points and the small area between the straight line connecting V_0 and the end-diastolic points and the nonlinear end-diastolic pressure–volume curve. The triangular area was calculated as $(P_{es} - P_{ed}) \times (V - V_0)/2$, where P_{es} and P_{ed} are end-systolic and end-diastolic pressures, respectively, and V is isovolumic ventricular volume. The additional small area was computed as $P_{ed} \times (V - V_0)/4$ on the assumption that the end-diastolic pressure–volume relation is approximated by a third power function of ($V - V_0$). We neglected PVA below zero, as previously described. PVA was normalized for LV weight and expressed as $mmHg \cdot ml \cdot beat^{-1} \cdot 100\,g^{-1}$.

Contractile efficiency was defined as the energy conversion efficiency from V_{O_2} for mechanical purposes to the total mechanical energy as represented by PVA [16,22]. V_{O_2} (ml O_2) and PVA (mmHg·ml) can be converted to the same units of energy (joules). Therefore, the reciprocal of the slope of the V_{O_2}–PVA relation after conversion to joules represents contractile efficiency. The V_{O_2} axis intercept of the V_{O_2}–PVA relation represents V_{O_2} for nonmechanical energy utilization (i.e., V_{O_2} for E–C coupling and basal metabolism).

Stress time integral (STI) was calculated as the analogue of tension time integral in isolated muscle studies [3,4,8]. STI is the time integral of total ventricular wall force per unit cross-sectional area of the ventricular wall for one cardiac cycle. Total ventricular wall force (F, g) was calculated as 1.36 ($g \cdot cm^{-2} \cdot mmHg^{-1}$) multiplied by the product of ventricular pressure (P, in mmHg) and lumen cross-sectional area, πr_i^2 (cm^2), based on the force–equilibrium equation for a sphere as previously reported by Suga et al. [24], where r_i is the internal radius of the ventricle. Wall stress (S, in $g \cdot cm^{-2}$) was calculated as F divided by the cross-sectional area of the ventricular wall, $\pi(r_0^2 - r_i^2)$ (cm^2), where r_0 is the external radius of the ventricle. Thus, $S = 1.36 \cdot P \cdot r_i^2 (r_0^2 - r_i^2)^{-1}$. The calculated r_i was derived from measured intraventricular volume (V_i, cm^3). r_0 was derived from the external volume of the ventricle [($V_i + V_m$), in cm^3], where V_m is LV weight (g), on the assumption that the specific gravity of muscle is $1\,g \cdot cm^{-3}$. Therefore, $S = 1.36 \cdot V_i^{\frac{2}{3}} \cdot P \cdot [(V_i + V_m)^{\frac{2}{3}} - V_i^{\frac{2}{3}}]^{-1}$. To obtain STI (g·s), S was integrated through one cardiac cycle according to the methods of Gibbs and Gibson [25] and Holubarsch et al. [26].

Contractile economy was calculated as the reciprocal of the slope of the linear V_{O_2}–STI relation, and is an analogue of myothermal economy of the isometric twitch of isolated muscle, representing the energy cost of a unit of STI generation. The V_{O_2} axis intercept of this relation represents V_{O_2} for nonmechanical energy utilization.

Basal V_{O_2} measured following KCl arrest was divided by the heart rate present before cardiac arrest to calculate basal V_{O_2} per beat [17]. This value was subtracted from the unloaded V_{O_2} to calculate V_{O_2} used for E–C coupling.

We analyzed myosin isoform content with pyrophosphate gel electrophoresis using frozen tissue samples obtained from the LV lateral free wall in each group of hearts. This procedure has been described elsewhere [26]. Briefly, cardiac myosin was extracted by homogenization of frozen, powdered tissue in 100 m*M* $Na_4P_2O_7$, 5 m*M* EGTA, 2 m*M* 2-mercaptoethanol, and 0.2 m*M* dichlorvos, pH 8.8 (1:20, w/v) on ice in a glass/glass hand-held homogenizer. Electrophoresis was performed at 84 V (14 V/cm constant voltage) for $18\frac{1}{2}$ hours at 2°C using a Pharmacia electrophoresis chamber (GE-2/4, Pharmacia, Uppsala, Sweden) which circulates the upper and lower chamber buffers [both contained 20 m*M* $Na_4P_2O_7$, pH 8.8, 10% glycerol and 2 m*M* cysteine (freebase)]. Gels were stained overnight in 0.025% Coomassie brilliant blue R-250, 25% isoproanol, and 10% acetic acid, and destained in 10% acetic acid. The destained gels were scanned with a high-resolution laser beam densitometer. Areas for each protein peak were determined by analysis of total peak area using Peakfit curve fitting softwear (Jandel Scientific, Corte Madera, Calif, USA) and fitting with a Gaussian shape.

All data are expressed as mean ± standard deviation. Comparisons of mean values for mechanical and energetic variables between sham, pressure overload, and hypothyroid hearts were performed by analysis of variance. Linear regression analyses were used to fit the V_{O_2}–PVA and V_{O_2}–STI relations and the end-systolic pressure–volume relation in order to obtain E_{max}. Analysis of covariance was performed to evaluate differences in the slopes of V_{O_2}–PVA or V_{O_2}–STI relations and the end-systolic pressure–STI relations between groups. $P < 0.05$ was considered statistically significant.

Results

At the time of sacrifice, mean tail cuff arterial blood pressure in the sham controls and hypothyroid rabbits was similar (69 ± 6.2 and 66 ± 9.8 mmHg). Mean arterial blood pressure was 113 ± 16.9 in pressure overload rabbits, significantly greater than the value in the other two groups ($P < 0.001$). Morphologic characteristics of the three groups are shown in Table 1. Heart weight/body weight and LV weight/body weight ratios were significantly lower in hypothyroid hearts compared to pressure-overload hearts but neither was significantly different compared to control hearts. Percent V_3 isomyosin was 80% ± 7% in control rabbits, 100% ± 1% in hypothyroid rabbits, and 98% ± 1% in pressure overload rabbits. The latter values were significantly different from the controls. Selected mechanical variables are listed in Table 2. Both E_{max} and normalized E_{max} were not significantly different in control and pressure overload rabbits, although there was a trend towards higher values in the pressure overload group. Both E_{max} and normalized E_{max} were significantly reduced in hypothyroid rabbits compared to either control or pressure overload rabbits. T_{max}, the time required to reach maximum pressure under baseline

Table 1. Morphological characteristics.

	Control	Hypothyroid	Pressure overload
Heart weight/body weight (g/kg)	2.3 ± 0.3 (±SD)	2.0 ± 0.1	2.5 ± 0.4*
LV weight/body weight (g/kg)	1.8 ± 0.2	1.5 ± 0.1	1.9 ± 0.4*
LV weight/RV weight (g/g)	3.3 ± 0.4	3.3 ± 0.4	3.7 ± 0.5
% V_3 isomyosin	80 ± 7	100 ± 1**	98 ± 1**

* $P < 0.05$ *vs* hypothyroid.
** $P < 0.001$ *vs* control.
LV, left ventricle.

Table 2. Mechanical variables.

	Control	Hyperthyroid	Pressure overload
E_{max} ($mmHg \cdot ml^{-1}$)	95 ± 15	57 ± 9*	110 ± 11
Normalized E_{max} ($mmHg \cdot ml^{-1} \cdot 100\,g$)	6.6 ± 1.2	3.1 ± 0.6*	8.2 ± 1.1
T_{max} (ms)	125 ± 6	158 ± 17**	126 ± 8
Maximum dP/d*t* ($mmHg \cdot s^{-1}$)	1284 ± 268	1060 ± 103	1276 ± 138

* $P < 0.01$ *vs* control and pressure overload.
** $P < 0.05$ *vs* control and pressure overload.
E_{max}, maximum value of instanteous left ventricular pressure–volume ratio; T_{max}, time required to reach maximum pressure; dP/d*t*, rate of change of pressure.

Table 3. Energetic variables.

	Control	Hypothyroid	Pressure overload
V_{O_2}–PVA Relation slope (10^{-5} ml $O_2 \cdot mmHg^{-1} \cdot ml^{-2}$)	2.6 ± 1.1	2.3 ± 0.7	1.6 ± 0.6*
Intercept (ml $O_2 \cdot beat^{-1} \cdot 100\ g^{-1}$)	0.029 ± 0.005	0.024 ± 0.006	0.030 ± 0.011
Efficiency (%)	30.6 ± 13.7	33.5 ± 16.6	50.4 ± 16.7
V_{O_2}–STI Relation slope (10^{-4} ml $O_2 \cdot g^{-1} \cdot s^{-1} \cdot 100\,g^{-1}$)	2.45 ± 1.00	1.95 ± 0.38	1.69 ± 0.73
Intercept (ml $O_2 \cdot beat^{-1} \cdot 100\ g^{-1}$)	0.029 ± 0.004	0.023 ± 0.006	0.029 ± 0.001
Economy ($10^4\,g \cdot s \cdot ml\,O_2^{-1} \cdot 100\,g$)	0.49 ± 0.21	0.53 ± 0.13	0.73 ± 0.35

* $P < 0.05$ *vs* control.
V_{O_2}, myocardial oxygen consumption; PVA, pressure–volume area; STI, stress time integral.

Table 4. Energetic variables.

	Control	Hypothroid	Pressure overload
Unloaded V_{O_2}(ml $O_2 \cdot beat^{-1} \cdot 100\,g^{-1}$)	0.028 ± 0.006	0.024 ± 0.005	0.029 ± 0.011
Basal V_{O_2} (ml $O_2 \cdot min^{-1} \cdot 100\,g^{-1}$)	1.11 ± 0.32	1.29 ± 0.23	1.19 ± 0.33
E–C coupling V_{O_2} (ml $O_2 \cdot beat^{-1} \cdot 100\,g^{-1}$)	0.023 ± 0.005	0.022 ± 0.007	0.024 ± 0.006

E–C, excitation–contraction.

conditions, was similar in control and pressure overload hearts, but significantly increased in hypothyroid hearts. LV maximum dP/d*t* tended to be lower in hypothyroid hearts compared to control or pressure overload, but this difference was not statistically significant. Energetic variables related to the V_{O_2}–PVA and V_{O_2}–STI relations are summarized in Table 3. The slope of the V_{O_2}–PVA relation was significantly reduced in mild pressure overload hearts compared to control hearts, but not significantly different compared to hypothyroid hearts. The slope was not significantly different between control or hypothyroid hearts. There was a trend toward a reduced intercept of this relation in hypothyroid hearts, but this was not significant. Although there was a substantial increase in

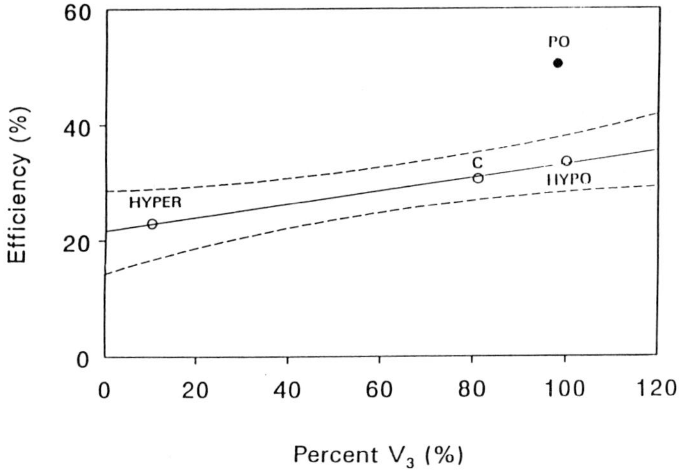

Fig. 1. Contractile efficiency as a function of percent V_3 isomyosin in hyperthyroid (*HYPER*), sham control (*C*), hypothyroid (*HYPO*), and pressure overload (*PO*) hearts. Line and 95% confidence intervals were obtained by linear regression analysis

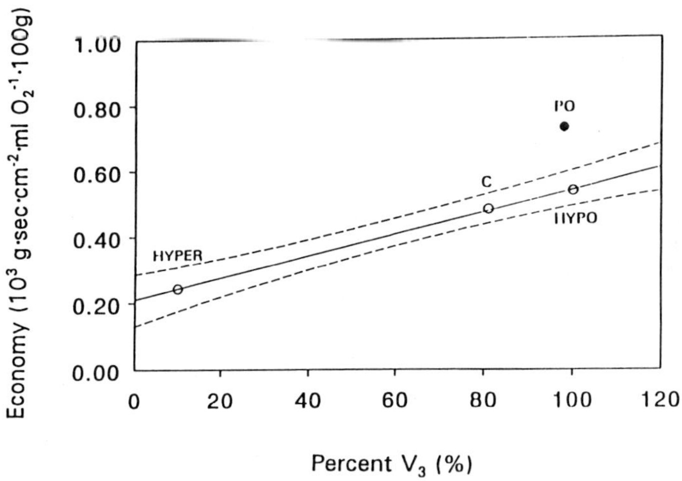

Fig. 2. Contractile economy as a function of percent V_3 isomyosin

average contractile efficiency in pressure overload hearts, this trend did not achieve statistical significance compared to control or hypothyroid hearts. The slope of the V_{O_2}–STI relation tended to be lower in both pressure overload and hypothyroid hearts, but neither was significantly different compared to control hearts. Similarly, economy tended to be higher in the pressure overload hearts but this also was not significantly different compared to the other two groups. As expected, intercept values for the V_{O_2}–STI relation were virtually identical to those of the V_{O_2}–PVA relation. Results of unloaded V_{O_2} and basal V_{O_2} are shown in Table 4. Unloaded V_{O_2} tended to be slightly lower in hypothyroid hearts, but there were no significant differences amongst any of the groups. Similarly, basal V_{O_2} was not significantly different in any of the groups. E–C coupling V_{O_2}, determined by subtracting basal V_{O_2} from unloaded V_{O_2}, was also similar in each group.

In an attempt to differentiate the effects of isomyosin composition from other potential influences on contractile efficiency and economy, we plotted efficiency and economy data as a function of percent V_3, as shown in Figs. 1 and 2. In these analyses, we included data we had previously obtained in hyperthyroid hearts [17]. As can be seen in these figures, efficiency and economy in the hyperthyroid, control, and hypothyroid hearts have a linear relationship with percent V_3 isomyosin. In contrast, efficiency and economy in pressure overload hearts appear to be increased out of proportion to changes in isomyosin composition, despite the fact that when compared statistically to control and hypothyroid hearts, the changes in pressure overload hearts did not quite reach statistical significance. Thus, by determining the correlation between efficiency and economy over a wide range of isomyosin composition in control and hormonally modified hearts, the increased efficiency and economy in pressure overload hearts is even more apparent.

Discussion

The most important finding of this study was that an extremely mild pressure-overload stress resulted in increases in contractile efficiency and economy which appear to be in excess of those which might be expected from the modest isomyosin shift (from 80% V_3 in control to 100% in pressure overload) which was observed. This point is further borne out by the higher efficiency and economy in pressure-overload compared to hypothyroid hearts (which had identical isomyosin composition), although this difference did not achieve significance using a standard analysis of variance approach. In this case, the pressure-overload stimulus was so mild that there was no statistically significant increase in left ventricular mass. Indeed, the only objective evidence of pressure overload was the difference in measured blood pressure and the aforementioned, small shift in isomyosin composition. In contrast, basal V_{O_2} and calculated V_{O_2} used for E–C coupling were not altered in pressure-overload hearts compared to either hypothyroid or control hearts. These results therefore suggest that the increased efficiency and economy were due to an alteration at the level of the contractile proteins as opposed to a change in E–C coupling or as a manifestation of structural abnormalities related to left ventricular hypertrophy.

In isolated muscle myothermal studies, similar results with respect to alterations in contractile economy have been noted in hyperthyroid and hypothyroid hearts [3,4,26]. We previously documented comparable changes in both economy and efficiency in the hormonally modified, isolated, red blood cell perfused rabbit heart [17]. In rabbits, pressure overload has previously been demonstrated to cause increased contractile economy, once again based on the results of isolated muscle, myothermal experiments [3,4,8]. In contrast, Izzi et al. [18] failed to document an increase in contractile efficiency in the isolated canine heart following a period of pressure overload. Recently, Hassenfuss et al. [8] demonstrated a cross-species, linear relationship between contractile economy and the proportion of V_3 isomyosin in normal and hypo- and hyperthyroid hearts. They also demonstrated that with mechanical overload (mitral regurgitation, pressure overload) and in failing myocardium (dilated cardiomyopathy) contractile economy was substantially increased compared to what would be expected based on the linear relation between V_3 isomyosin and economy in normal and hormonally modified hearts [8,9]. This result is obviously very similar to our own. However, in the studies of Hassenfuss and others [1,5–9], the mechanical overload has been severe and in general associated with alterations in E–C coupling. In contrast, in our model of very mild pressure overload, our results once again suggest that there was no major alteration in energy used for E–C coupling. Since hypertrophy was no more than minimal, this leads to our suggestion that the observed changes in mechanoenergetics are best explained by a change at the level of the contractile proteins independent of the modest isomyosin switch which occurred.

Several alterations independent of isomyosin switches have been shown to influence the ATPase activity of the contractile proteins, including induction of different troponin isoforms [27,28] and the extent of myosin light chain phosphorylation [29]. A precise delineation of whether and what sort of contractile protein alterations caused our findings, should be a fruitful area of investigation in future. Our results also suggest that, in contrast to E–C coupling, contractile protein alterations occur early during a mild pressure overload stimulus. Undoubtedly, subsequent alterations in E–C coupling can further modify mechanoenergetic behavior. The notion that contractile protein alterations occur readily in response to changing conditions is supported by the fact that isomyosin composition normally changes simply as a function of age [30]. To our knowledge, this is the first demonstration that a very mild mechanical overload stimulus results in measurable changes in the mechanoenergetic behavior of the ventricle.

Another interesting feature of our results is the fact that the mechanics of contraction were not markedly influenced by the mild pressure overload stimulus, despite the alterations in mechanoenergetic behavior. The hypothyroid hearts displayed typical and previously demonstrated decreases in E_{max} along with slowing of contraction [17]. However, the mild pressure overload hearts were virtually identical to normal hearts with respect to contraction mechanics. In conjunction with our previous suggestion that our results are most consistent with a change at the level of the contractile proteins, this result leads to the speculation that in more severe forms of hypertrophy and failure, changes in contraction mechanics are mainly related to altered E–C coupling rather than contractile protein alterations. Alternatively, since gross structural alterations in the mild pressure overload hearts were not present, it is also possible that the structural alterations which occur in more severe mechanical overload contribute to altered contraction mechanics.

In summary, we have shown that a minimal pressure overload results in measurable increases in contractile efficiency and economy in the isolated, red blood cell perfused rabbit heart. Our results suggest that the mechanism of this change in mechanoenergetic behavior is due to some alteration at the level of the contractile proteins which cannot be explained by isomyosin switches. Our results further indicate that mechanoenergetic alterations typical of pressure overload do not necessarily require the presence of altered E–C coupling and/or major structural changes of the myocardium. Future measurements of myofibrillar ATPase activity along with more detailed analyses of the composition of the contractile proteins in this model should provide insight into the mechanism of these findings.

Acknowledgments. This study was supported by NIH Grant No. HL 45116. We would like to thank Mr. Steven Bell for his technical assistance and Ms. Candace McCarthy for her secretarial help.

References

1. Alpert NR, Mulieri LA (1977) The partitioning of altered mechanics in hyperthyroid heart muscle between the sarcoplasmic reticulum and the contractile apparatus by means of myothermal measurements. Basic Res Cardiol 72:153–159
2. Coughlin P, Gibbs CL (1981) Cardiac energetics in short- and long-term hypertrophy induced by aortic coarctation. Cardiovasc Res 15:623–631
3. Alpert NR, Mulieri LA (1982) Increased myothermal economy of isometric force generation in compensated cardiac hypertrophy induced by pulmonary artery constriction in the rabbit. Circ Res 50:491–500
4. Holubarsch C, Litten RZ, Mulieri LA, Alpert NR (1985) Energetic changes of myocardium as an adaptation to chronic hemodynamic overload and thyroid gland activity. Basic Res Cardiol 80:582–593
5. Gwathmey JK, Morgan JP (1988) Altered calcium handling in experimental pressure overload hypertrophy in the ferret. Circ Res 75:836–834
6. Gwathmey JK, Copelas L, MacKinnon R (1987) Abnormal intracellular calcium handling in myocardium from patients with end-stage heart failure. Circ Res 61: 70–76
7. Katz AM (1990) Cardiomyopathy of overload: A major determinant of prognosis in congestive heart failure. N Engl J Med 322:100–110
8. Hasenfuss G, Mulieri LA, Blanchard EM, Holubarsch C, Leavitt BJ, Ittleman F, Alpert NR (1991) Energetics of isometric force development in control and volume-overload human myocardium. Comparison with animal species. Circ Res 68: 836–846

9. Hasenfuss G, Mulieri LA, Leavitt BJ, Allen PD, Haeberle JR, Alpert NA (1992) Alteration of contractile function and excitation–contraction coupling in dilated cardiomyopathy. Circ Res 70:1225–1232
10. Nagai R, Zarain-Herzberg A, Brandl CJ, Fujii J, Tada M, MacLennan DH, Alpert NR, Periasamy M (1989) Regulation of myocardial Ca^{2+} ATPase and phospholamban mRNA expression in response to pressure overload and thyroid hormones. Proc Natl Acad Sci USA 86:2966–2970
11. Mercadier JJ, Lompre AM (1990) Altered sarcoplasmic reticulum Ca^{2+}-ATPase gene expression in the human ventricle during end-stage heart failure. J Clin Invest 85:305–309
12. Morgan JP (1991) Abnormal intracellular modulation of calcium as a major cause of cardiac contractile dysfunction. N Engl J Med 325:625–632
13. Alpert NL, Mulieri LA (1982) Heat, mechanics, and myosin ATPase in normal and hypertrophied heart muscle. Fed Proc 41:192–198.
14. Kissling G, Rugg H, Malloy L, Jacob R (1982) Alterations in cardiac oxygen consumption under chronic pressure overload. Significance of isoenzyme pattern of myosin. Basic Res Cardiol 77:255–269.
15. Hirzel HO, Tuchschmid CR, Schneider J, Krayenbuehl HP, Schaub MC (1985) Relationship between myosin isoenzyme composition, hemodynamics, and myocardial structure in various forms of human cardiac hypertrophy. Circ Res 57:729–740
16. Suga H (1990) Ventricular energetics. Physiol Rev 70:247–292
17. Goto Y, Slinker BK, LeWinter MM (1990) Decreased contractile efficiency and increased nonmechanical energy cost in hyperthyroid rabbit heart. Circ Res 69:999–1010
18. Izzi G, Zile MR, Gaasch WH (1991) Myocardial oxygen consumption and the left ventricle pressure-volume area in normal and hypertrophic canine hearts. Circulation 84:1384–1392
19. Wolff MR, de Tombe PP, Harasawa Y, Burkhoff D, Bier S, Hunter WC, Gerstenblith G, Kass DA (1992) Alterations in left ventricular mechanics, energetics, and contractile reserve in experimental heart failure. Circ Res 70:516–529.
20. Campbell DJH, Skinner SL, Day AJ (1973) Cellophane perinephritis hypertension and its reversal in rabbits. Circ Res 33:105–114
21. Yaku H, Slinker BK, Myhre ESP, Watkins MW, LeWinter MM (1991) Stability of myocardial oxygen consumption–pressure–volume area relation in red cell-perfused rabbit heart. Am J Physiol 261:H1630–H1635
22. Goto Y, Slinker BK, LeWinter MM (1988) Similar normalized E_{max} and O_2 consumption–pressure–volume area relation in rabbit and dog. Am J Physiol 255: H366–H374
23. Suga H, Sagawa K (1974) Instantaneous pressure–volume relationships and their ratio in the excised, supported canine left ventricle. Circ Res 35:117–126
24. Suga H, Goto Y, Nozawa T, Yasumura Y, Futaki S, Tanaka N (1987) Force-time integral decreases with ejection despite constant oxygen consumption and pressure–volume area in dog left ventricle. Circ Res 60:797–802
25. Gibbs CL, Gibson WR (1970) Energy production in cardiac isotonic contractions. J Gen Physiol 56:732–740
26. Holubarsch C, Goulette RP, Litten RZ, Martin BJ, Mulieri LA, Alpert NR (1985) The economy of isometric force development, myosin isoenzyme pattern, and myofibrillar ATPase activity in normal and hypothyroid rat myocrdium. Circ Res 56:78–86

27. Morimoto S, Ohtsuki I (1987) Ca^{2+} and Sr^{2+}—sensitivity of the ATPase of rabbit skeletal myofibrils: Effect of the complete substitution of troponin C with cardiac troponin C, calmodulin and parvalbumin. J Biochem 101:291–301
28. Dieckman LJ, Solaro RJ (1990) Effect of thyroid states on thin filament Ca^{2+} regulation and expression of troponin I in perinatal and adult rat hearts. Circ Res 67:344–351
29. Margossian SS (1985) Reversible dissociation of dog cardiac myosin light chain 2 and its influence on ATP hydrolysis. J Biol Chem 260:13747–13754
30. Litten RZ, Martin BJ, Buchthal RH, Nagai R, Low RB, Alpert NR (1985) Heterogeneity of myosin isozyme content of rabbit heart. Circ Res 57:406–414

2.4 Mechanisms of Ventricular Reserve Limitation in Cardiac Hypertrophy

David A. Kass[1]

Summary. Ventricular hypertrophy is usually characterized by resting abnormalities of diastolic function with preserved systolic performance. However, there are often profound limitations of both diastolic and systolic functional reserve to physiologic stress. One of the most well studied reserve limitations is to chronotropic stress. Rapid atrial pacing can result in marked elevation of diastolic pressure and stiffness in animal hypertrophy models and in humans with idiopathic asymmetric hypertrophy presenting with chest pain syndrome. In other patients with severe hypertrophy and congestive failure symptoms, diastolic function does not deteriorate with rapid pacing, suggesting that underlying etiology and severity of disease are important factors to this response. Systolic reserve limitations to pacing stress are also found in both animal and human hypertrophy. Raising heart rate from 80 to 160 min−1 increases end-systolic elastance by nearly 100% in normal humans, while it is virtually unchanged in hypertrophied hearts. Mechanisms that may underlie the loss of contractile reserve to chronotropic challenge are abnormal subendocardial perfusion, altered calcium cycling, and changes in myofilament proteins. Each mechanism is reviewed. In addition to chronotropic reserve limitations, the hypertrophied heart has limited preload and inotropic reserve due to increased end-systolic chamber stiffness. A high end-systolic stiffness results in minimal augmentation of pump function (i.e., cardiac output) when contractility is increased. Furthermore, such a heart is highly sensitive to preload change, with marked alterations in systolic pressure generation and thus wall stress resulting from relatively small changes in chamber diastolic filling. Current and future therapeutic approaches to this disorder need to consider all of these reserve limitation mechanisms.

[1] Division of Cardiology, 538 Carnegie Bldg., Johns Hopkins Medical Institutions, Baltimore, MD 21287, USA

Key words: Hypertrophy—Contractility-reserve—Pressure-volume relations—Pacing—Diastole—Excitation-contraction coupling—End-systolic elastance

Introduction

Ventricular hypertrophy, whether evolving in response to chronic pressure overload or as a genetic abnormality, is typically characterized by resting diastolic dysfunction and apparent preservation of systolic performance. The left ventricle has a reduced cavity size with a thickened wall, and the myocardium contains increased collagen and fibrous tissue, often with fiber disarray[1–3]. These changes contribute to elevated diastolic pressures and delayed early diastolic filling [3–5]. In addition to structural changes, calcium handling is abnormal with left ventricular hypertrophy (LVH), most notably affecting sarcoplasmic reticular calcium sequestration and sarcolemmal calcium entry [6–9]. This can delay relaxation and lead to higher levels of intracellular calcium. Both changes further exacerbate diastolic failure. Lastly, there is loss of normal coronary flow reserve which is thought to result in endocardial hypoperfusion under stress[10,11]. Recent studies have also reported that high energy phosphate metabolism[12] and mechanical function[13] of the subendocardium is itself abnormal with LVH, independent of coronary flow.

In contrast to diastole, resting systolic abnormalities are rarely observed in animal models or humans with LVH. As a consequence of the thickened wall and reduced chamber volumes, ejection fraction and other ejection indices are usually preserved if not supranormal [3,14–17]. Isovolumic contractile indexes such as the maximal rate of pressure rise are also normal in most studies [15,16,18]. In forms of the disease with asymmetric septal involvement, systolic outflow obstruction can play a role in limiting flow and increasing metabolic demand [11]. However, whether or not this accelerates the progression to contractile failure is unclear.

Despite such baseline abnormalities, many patients (and most animal models) with LVH are asymptomatic at rest, but have marked limitations of reserve function. Recent studies have started to focus on the pathophysiology of this functional reserve limitation, and this forms the subject of this review. I have placed a major emphasis on the response of the hypertrophied heart to pacing tachycardia, as this form of stress has been most extensively studied in preparations ranging from isolated myocytes to intact humans. Limitations of preload and contractile reserve are also addressed, particularly as they are influenced by increased basal systolic stiffness of the hypertrophied heart.

Chronotropic Reserve Limitations

Diastole

The influence of rapid atrial pacing on diastolic (and systolic) ventricular mechanics in a conscious animal model of hypertrophy was first systematically

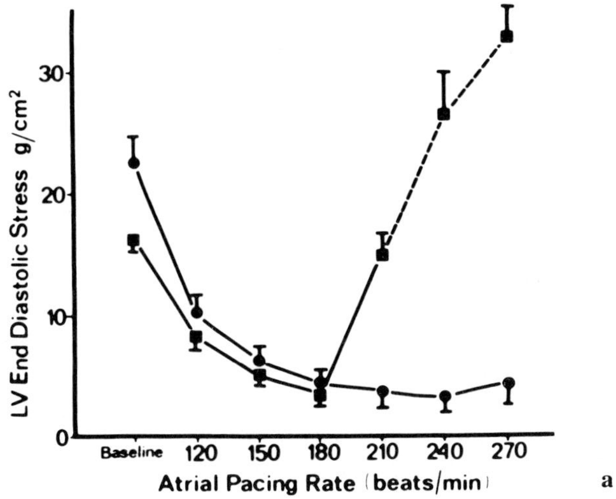

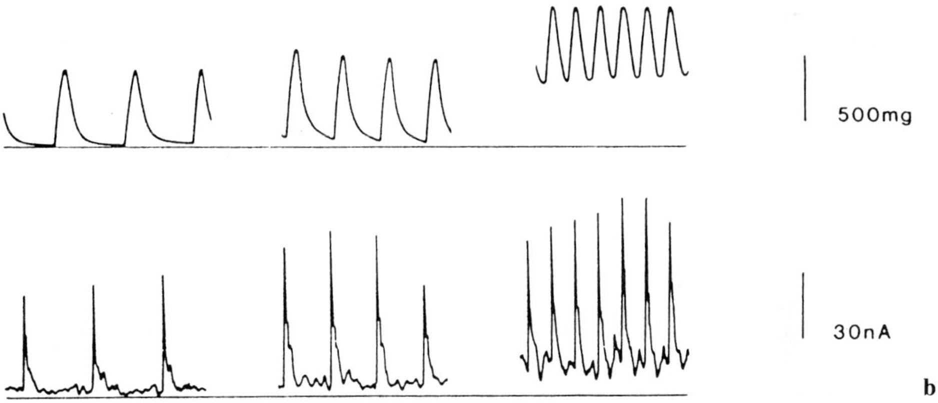

Fig. 1. **a** Influence of rapid atrial pacing on ventricular diastolic stress in canine model of chronic pressure-overload hypertrophy. There is marked disproportionate rise in stress in the left ventricular hypertrophy (LVH) animals (*squares*) at fast pacing rates. *Circles*, controls. (From [15] with permission) **b** Increasing stimulation frequency raises both rest tension (*bottom*) and calcium (*top*) levels in isolated trabecula from end-stage hypertrophied human heart. (From [7] with permission)

evaluated in a relatively recent study by Fujii et al. [15]. These investigators induced pressure overload LV hypertrophy by banding the ascending aorta of 8- to 10-week-old puppies. After 1–2 years of growth, the animals had significant LVH with a 70% increase in LV mass. They were then instrumented for conscious study and exposed to incremental atrial pacing (baseline of 90 up to maximal pacing rate of 240 min^{-1}). Both diastolic and systolic abnormalities were observed. The dominant diastolic abnormality was a marked rise in end-diastolic pressure (LVEDP) and wall stress at pacing rates exceeding 180 min^{-1}

(Fig. 1a). Chamber diastolic stiffness increased by nearly 50% in the LVH group, in contrast to no change in controls. This corroborated results of prior studies which had reported elevated LVEDP during pacing in association with a reduced ratio of endocardial/epicardial flow and increased lactate extraction [10,19]. Subsequent data from isolated muscle strips obtained from human explant hearts with end-stage hypertrophic cardiomyopathy also found that increased stimulation frequency led to marked elevations of diastolic tension and resting calcium [7] (Fig. 1b).

Comparable studies of the effects of pacing on diastole in human subjects are fewer. Pasternac et al. [20], in 1982, reported on a small group ($n = 4$) of hypertrophic cardiomyopathy (HCM) patients who underwent atrial pacing. Increasing heart rate from 72 to $133\,\text{min}^{-1}$ led to only a small change in LVEDP (from 17 to 19.5 mmHg), although there was evidence of increased lactate production. Cannon et al. [11] reported results on 20 patients with HCM, all presenting with a primary complaint of chest pain. In their study, increasing heart rate from 82 to $147\,\text{min}^{-1}$ resulted in an increase in LVEDP from 16 mmHg to 28 mmHg. Furthermore, this elevation of LVEDP persisted for 10 s after terminating pacing. These data also demonstrated a rise in lactate extraction and blunting of coronary flow reserve, suggesting that abnormalities of myocardial supply/demand balance contributed to the pressure elevation.

More recently, we undertook an investigation of pacing-induced hemodynamic dysfunction in a group of patients with concentric LVH [21]. Unlike prior human studies, we measured continuous pressure–volume loops and relations at each incremented pacing rate, and employed a multicycle analysis of diastolic cardiac function. This approach could better separate components of active and passive chamber properties from altered loading conditions induced by pacing.

Ten patients with LVH (maximal diastolic wall thickness of about 2 cm) were compared to eight control patients. Seventy percent of the LVH patients were referred for evaluation of congestive heart failure symptoms. The control group presented with atypical chest pain or headache/dizziness and early borderline hypertension. These latter subjects had normal hearts by echocardiography, electrocardiography, and ventriculography. All study patients had normal epicardial coronary angiography. To perform pressure–volume analysis in humans, we utilized the conductance catheter method [22,23]. This technique provides continuous on-line pressure–volume (PV) loops, and systolic and diastolic relations can be derived by varying chamber filling by transient balloon catheter obstruction of inferior vena cava inflow. For the study, baseline PV loops and relations were recorded at sinus rhythm; then, heart rate was incremented at steps of 25–30 beats/min using right atrial pacing. At each pacing rate, data were recorded after several minutes' stabilization, including steady-state PV loops, and repeat assessment of PV relations (balloon occlusion of inferior vena cava).

At baseline, abnormalities were only demonstrated in diastole. End-diastolic pressure was higher (20.2 ± 6.2 *vs* 12.3 ± 4.9 mmHg), the time constant of isovolumic relaxation was longer (52.6 ± 13.9 *vs* 40.8 ± 10.6 ms), and chamber compliance was lower (3.2 ± 0.7 *vs* 5.1 ± 2.3 ml/mmHg) in the LVH group compared to controls (all $P < 0.05$). Resting heart rate, cardiac output, vascular resistance, ejection fraction, systolic pressures, and dP/dt_{max} were similar in the two groups.

Given these baseline diastolic abnormalities, one might predict that a reduction of diastolic filling period due to rate increase would disproportionately compromise chamber filling and thus ejection in LVH hearts. This would be

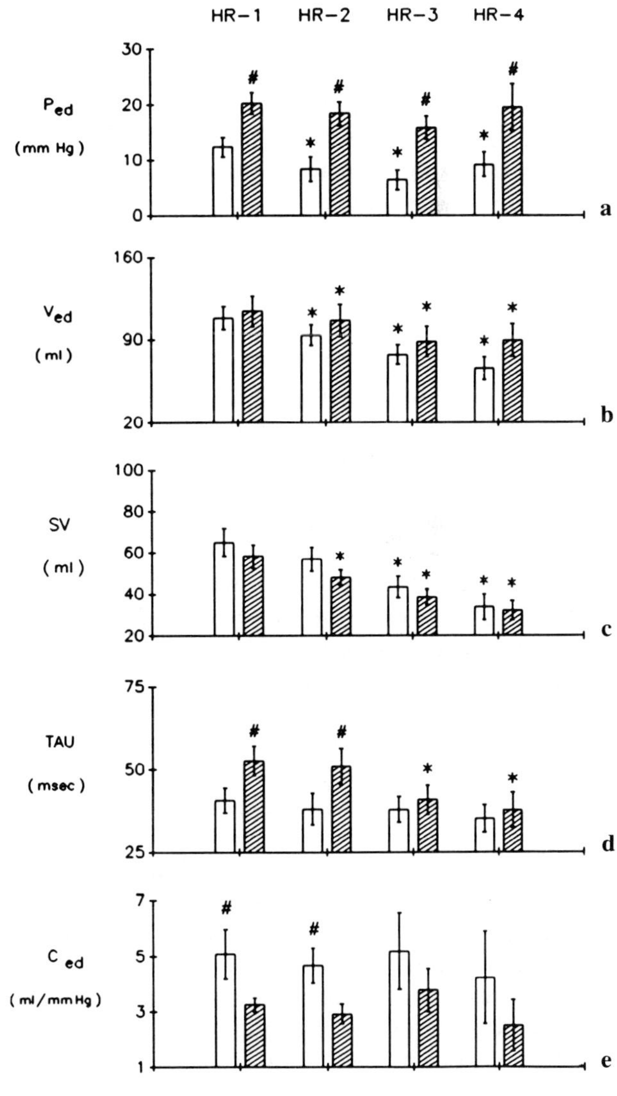

Fig. 2a–e. Effect of incremental atrial pacing on net chamber filling and diastolic properties in patients with concentric nonobstructive LVH. **a** end-diastolic pressure (P_{ed}; mmHg); **b** end-diastolic volume (V_{ed}; ml); **c** stroke volume (*SV*; ml); **d** relaxation time constant (*TAU*; ms); and **e** passive chamber compliance (C_{ed}; ml/mmHg). #, $P < 0.05$ Controls versus LVH; *, $P < 0.05$ versus control. Heart rates are: HR-1 (70 min^{-1}), HR-2 (100 min^{-1}), HR-3 (125 min^{-1}), HR-4 (155 min^{-1}). *Shaded bars*, LVH patients; *open bars*, control patients

worsened if there was further deterioration of diastolic function with pacing, as previously found in hypertrophied dog and human hearts [11,15]. Surprisingly, however, this was not observed in this study. There was also no disproportionate rise in end-diastolic pressure at faster pacing rates in the LVH subjects (Fig. 2a). As shown in Fig. 2b and 2c, neither net chamber filling (end-diastolic volume [EDV]) nor ejection (stroke volume) were significantly lower at faster rate in the LVH group.

How may these results be reconciled with the diastolic dysfunction found at rest? Part of the explanation can be found in the isovolumic relaxation and compliance data, shown in Fig. 2d and 2e. While relaxation was prolonged in LVH subjects at baseline, it shortened disproportionately more in these patients as heart rate was increased, eventually eliminating the disparity. Although chamber compliance did not demonstrate a similar improvement with faster pacing rate, it also did not fall (i.e., stiffer chamber) as had been observed in animals [15].

These diastolic responses are at odds with earlier results from the supra-aortic banded or perinephritic hypertension models [10,15,24]. Basal prolongation of relaxation time is widely observed with animal and human LVH [13,25], although its response during rapid pacing has not been prreviously reported. Interestingly, in one study of human *dilated* cardiomyopathy, isovolumic relaxation also quickened at faster pacing rates more in congestive heart failure (CHF) hearts than in controls [26]. One potentially important difference between prior animal data and our clinical results lies in the systolic loads. Peak systolic pressures were similar between control and LVH patients (137 ± 16 mmHg for controls, *vs* 150 ± 29 for LVH; P = NS). This contrasts to the animal studies where LV pressure is typically 50%–100% higher in the LVH group compared to controls [10,15,24]. Such pressure loads themselves delay relaxation, increase diastolic pressures, and raise stiffness [27], and thereby could importantly contribute to an abnormal pacing response. To date, there are no intact animal data in which persistent hypertrophy has been studied in the absence of such disparate elevated systolic loads.

The etiology of hypertrophy in humans and its clinical presentation may also dictate the precise nature of pacing-induced diastolic abnormalities. In the earlier study of Cannon et al. [11], all subjects presented with a chief complaint of chest pain, and virtually all developed their typical pain during atrial pacing. In contrast, the LVH group in our study had a higher baseline LVEDP, but the dominant symptom was exertional dyspnea and paroxysmal marked pulmonary edema. None of these patients developed chest pain with rapid pacing.

To summarize, while animal models and some prior clinical studies have demonstrated marked increases in ventricular diastolic pressure with rapid pacing, this response does not necessarily characterize many patients with symptomatic LVH. The etiology and symptomatology of the LVH, the co-existence of cavity obstruction and chest pain, and the presence or absence of marked elevations of systolic load (as in LVH from aortic stenosis or severe hypertension) are all likely to influence the hemodynamic response to pacing stress. As a consequence, as we found in our study, diastolic reserve function may be better than it would seem based on baseline abnormalities.

Systole

In isolated muscle strips of end-state hypertrophied hearts, developed tension declines as stimulation frequency increases [7]. This has been also demonstrated in isolated cell preparations from hypertrophied guinea pig ventricles [28] and in muscle strips from failing human myocardium [29]. In intact conscious dogs, rapid pacing both disproportionately lowers peak systolic pressure and fractional shortening, as well as the velocity of circumferential fractional shortening [15].

A major limitation of virtually all prior pacing studies in intact animals and humans has been a reliance on measures of cardiac function that do not adequately differentiate between primary chamber abnormalities and alterations due to rate-related changes in filling volumes and arterial pressures. Ideally, one assesses contractile function using measures that can reasonably separate out these factors. One paradigm for such analysis was presented by Freeman et al., in a pressure–volume relation study of the effects of incremental heart rate in intact conscious dogs [30]. We recently used the same approach to provide an in-depth and systematic evaluation of the hemodynamic responses to pacing tachycardia in patients with and without left ventricular hypertrophy [21].

Four different load-independent assessments of systolic function were measured at each of four different atrial pacing rates. Two indexes, the slopes of the end-systolic pressure–volume relation (E_{es}) and stroke work–end-diastolic volume relation (M_{sw}) were obtained by analysis of multiple pressure–volume loops during transient preload reduction [31,32]. Two other measures, maximal power and the maximal rate of pressure rise, both divided by end-diastolic volume, were derived from beats at the resting filling volume [33]. Results are shown in Fig. 3. All three ejection phase indexes (E_{es}, M_{sw}, and $Power_{mx}/EDV$) demonstrated a marked blunting in the magnitude of contractile augmentation at faster pacing rates in LVH subjects. Intriguingly, there was no such disparity between control and LVH subjects in the isovolumic phase index — $dP/dt_{mx}/EDV$.

This disparity between reduced ejection phase but not isovolumic phase contractile function with incremental pacing in LVH has been observed in animal hypertrophy studies [15,34], although not specifically highlighted. For example, Fujii et al. [15] reported that while the velocity of circumferential shortening and the shortening fraction were significantly reduced in LVH dogs with rapid pacing, the change in LV dP/dt_{mx} was not significantly different. A similar finding was reported in LVH dogs undergoing treadmill exercise [24]. Our data are the first to show this disparity in intact human LVH. This difference between ejecting and isovolumic contractile function appears some-

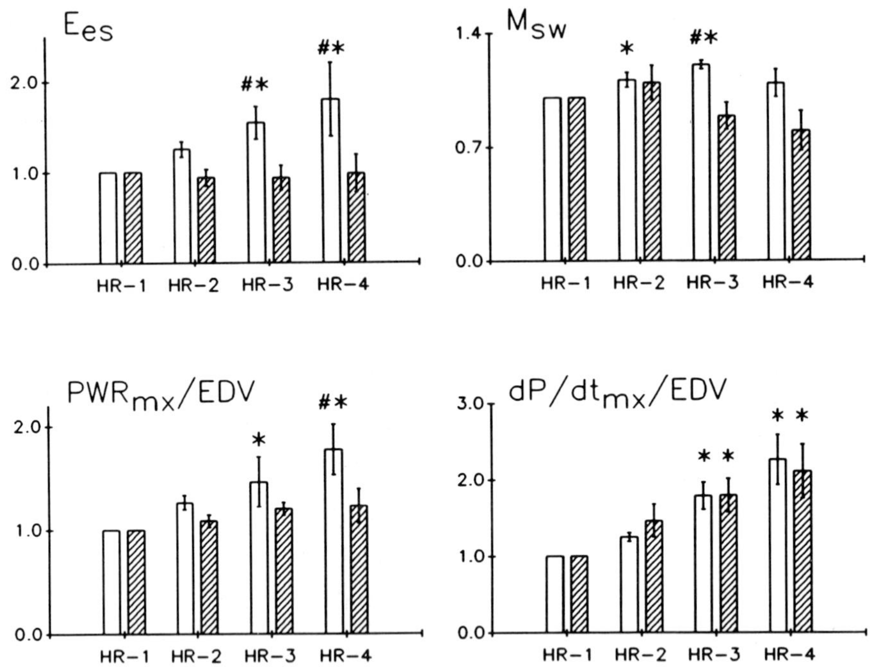

Fig. 3. Effect of incremental atrial pacing on chamber contractile function. Four in exes are displayed. Ejection phase indexes include: E_{es}, end-systolic elastance (mmHg/ml); M_{sw}, slope of stroke-work–end-diastolic volume relation (mmHg); and PWR_{mx}/EDV, maximal ventricular power divided by end-diastolic volume (watts/ml × 10^2). The isovolumic phase index is $dP/dt_{mx}/EDV$, (mmHg·s^{-1}·ml^{-1}). Symbols and heart rates are same as for Fig. 2

what unique to hypertrophic cardiomyopathy, as it is not observed during pacing stress in subjects with dilated cardiomyopathy [26].

Mechanisms of Diminished Chronotropic Reserve

There are several potential explanations for a decline in ejection function with rapid pacing in LVH. These include abnormal endocardial flow reserve with development of ischemia, altered calcium cycling, and changes in myofilament or structural proteins involved in shortening.

There is considerable evidence to support a role of subendocardial ischemia in limiting pacing reserve function with LVH, both in animal and human models. In dogs with chronically banded aortas, rapid-pacing-induced abnormalities in chamber systolic function are associated with a fall in endocardial/epicardial flow ratio from 1.1 to 0.85 [15]. Studies have also shown that endocardial shortening is most reduced in this setting [19]. Heterogeneity of the response among experimental animals has further supported a linkage between reduced endocardial/epicardial flow ratio, increased lactate uptake, and diastolic dysfunction [10]. For example, Bache et al. [10] reported a marked increase in LVEDP only in those animals which also displayed a reduced endocardial/epicardial flow ratio and increased lactate uptake. Interestingly, this did not correlate with higher LV mass or systolic load. Cannon and colleagues found in humans a blunting of great cardiac vein reserve with rapid pacing that correlated with the rise in LVEDP [35]. More recent data have shown abnormal basal high-energy phosphate metabolism, as demonstrated, for example, by a 32% reduction in phosphocreatine (CP) to ATP ratio versus controls [12]. These abnormalities were not corrected by adenosine-induced increases in coronary flow. With rapid atrial pacing, diastolic pressure also rose markedly with LVH, concomitant with worsening of both midwall and subendocardial CP/ATP ratio, as well an increased ratio of inorganic phosphate to total ATP.

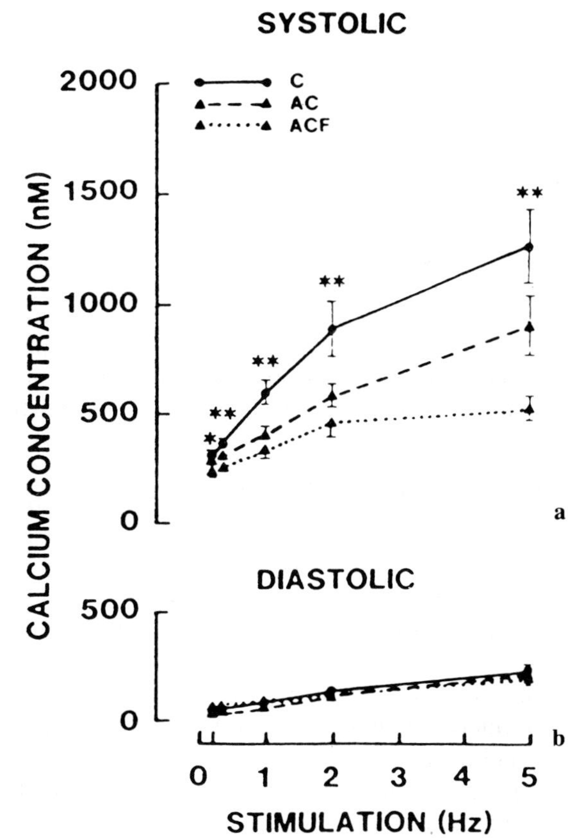

Fig. 4a,b. Incremental pacing rate in isolated hypertrophied (*ACF*, *AC*) versus normal (*C*) myocytes from guinea pig. Calcium transients are reduced at faster stimulation rates in the most hyperrophied cells. (From [28] with permission)

These data provide considerable support to the notion that endocardial ischemia can be an important contributor to LVH dysfunction with rapid pacing. However, there has always been a mechanistic "chicken–egg" ambiguity in these data, in that the rise in diastolic pressure itself may contribute to the fall in endocardial flow and ischemia. In fact, whether or not diastolic dysfunction is always required in order to observe limited systolic reserve to chronotropic stimuli was until recently unresolved. Our clinical LVH study [21] showed for the first time that such a linkage was not required, in that there was no demonstrable deterioration of diastolic function with pacing despite markedly blunted systolic reserve.

A second mechanism for loss of pacing reserve relates to abnormal calcium cycling in hypertrophied myocardium. Studies of isolated hypertrophic myocytes have shown reduced peak-systolic Ca^{2+} transients with faster stimulation rates [28,36] (Fig. 4). In addition, there is abnormal sarcoplasmic reticular uptake of Ca^{2+} [8], and evidence for an increase in sarcolemmal calcium influx [37]. These changes have been implicated in underlying enhanced post-extrasystolic potentiation of hypertrophied muscle [8], and prolonged and abnormal Ca^{2+} transients and relaxation delay [38]. In human LVH studies, prolonged isovolumic relaxation and diminished early maximal filling velocity have been generally ascribed to altered Ca^{2+} handling [4]. We recently reported that post-pacing potentiation is also increased, supporting greater calcium influx [21]. However, this potentiation decayed much more rapidly in LVH hearts than in controls, suggesting an abnormality of sarcoplasmic reticulum Ca^{2+} uptake. Thus, in addition to suboptimal endocardial flow and ischemia, abnormalities in Ca^{2+} handling also likely contribute to functional reserve limitations in LVH.

Another potential contributor to reduced chronotropic reserve are alterations in the myofilament proteins themselves that could limit rapid velocity of shortening. The reduction of ejection-phase contractile indexes despite preservation of isovolumic contractile function suggests that the hypertrophied heart may have increased deactivation accompanying shortening, or an increased internal ventricular resistance [39,40]. Increased myocardial viscosity [41], which is more commonly linked with late diastolic dysfunction, could contribute to reduced ejection function. In some species, myosin isoform changes with hypertrophy parallel the shift from fast to slow twitch behavior [42]. Although this does not appear identically in humans [43], an alternative change in myofilament proteins may still contribute to slowing of crossbridge cycling kinetics with LVH, and thus to a suboptimal contractile response during shortening.

Preload and Inotropic Reserve: Role of End-systolic Stiffness

The preceding discussion dealt with the hemodynamics and mechanisms underlying limited chronotropic reserve in LVH. This was chosen as it is the most common method by which the LVH heart has been stressed in isolated tissues, whole animals, and intact humans. However, clearly there are other very important cardiovascular reserve mechanisms invoked during exercise and other stresses, and these too are limited by LVH. In particular, the fact that the LVH heart often displays a steep end-systolic pressure–volume relation (high E_{es}) [16,21,44] itself impacts on these important reserve mechanisms.

In patients with idiopathic asymmetric hypertrophic cardiomyopathy, the slope of the end-systolic pressure–volume relation (ESPVR) is nearly three times normal ($E_{es} = 6.7 \pm 2.8$) compared to controls (2.3 ± 1.5) [44]. Patients with concentric hypertrophy due to hypertension have an intermediate slope (4.2 ± 3.8) [21]. A higher E_{es} does not necessarily belie enhanced contractile state of the myocytes, since much of this stiffness may be due to chamber geometric changes, fibrosis, and other structural alterations within the myocardium. However, it does have direct implications regarding cardiovascular reserve capacity.

An example of how a steep ESPVR limits preload reserve is shown in Fig. 5a. Pressure–volume loops for a patient with marked idiopathic hypertrophic

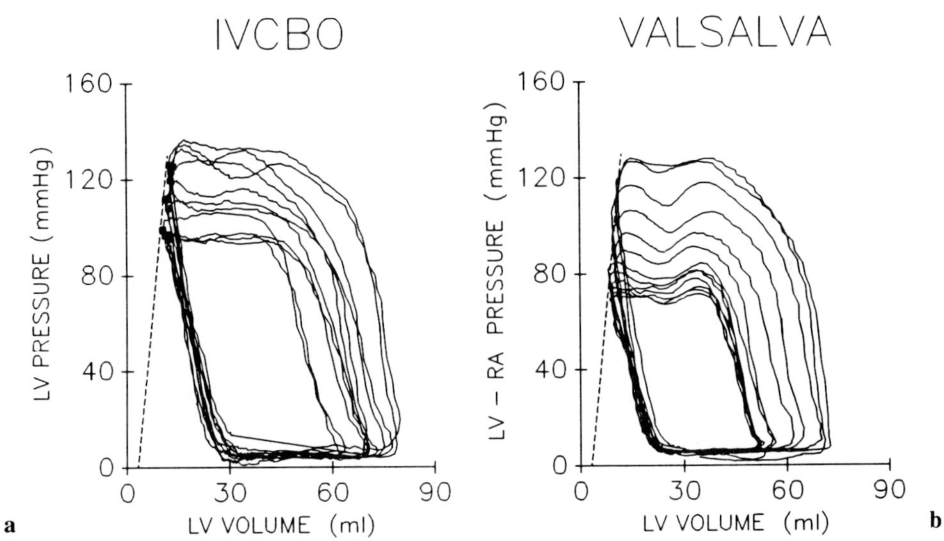

Fig. 5. Increased basal systolic stiffness limits preload reserve adaptation. **a** Transient lowering of chamber filling by balloon occlusion of the inferior vena cava (*IVCBO*) in a patient with hypertrophic cardiomyopathy induced a marked decline in systolic chamber pressure due to the steep end-systolic pressure–volume relation (ESPVR). As shown in the **b**, this has physiologic significance, as a similar pressure decline occurred when the patient performed a Valsalva maneuver. These changes were not associated with increased outflow obstruction, but could be directly related to the steep ESPVR. Thus, systolic stiffening (steep ESPVR) compromises the cardiac adaptive capacity to changes in preload volume. *RA*, right atrial (pressure)

cardiomyopathy are shown, obtained by transient balloon occlusion of the inferior vena cava (IVCBO). There is a steep decline in systolic pressure for the induced fall in preload volume. This can be clinically reduced, as shown in Fig. 5b, where the same patient performed a Valsalva maneuver. In normal subjects, reduced preload during Valsalva results in relatively small arterial pressure changes, which are usually compensated by reflex activation. In contrast, the HCM patient displayed a marked fall in systolic pressure and stroke volume during Valsalva.

Patients with HCM often experience presyncope with isometric exercise or Valsalva maneuvers [3]. This has been primarily ascribed to enhanced outflow obstruction with reduced chamber volumes. However, a high end-systolic chamber elastance itself results in a greater decline in developed systolic pressure for a given change in preload volume, and this probably is an important contributor to preload sensitivity in this disorder. The steep ESPVR also means that *increasing* preload will result in a disproportionately greater rise in chamber workload and thus myocardial oxygen demand. In hypertrophied hearts in which baseline metabolism and coronary flow reserve are abnormal [11,45], this stresses the heart when volume is recruited to invoke the Frank-Starling mechanism.

A steep baseline ESPVR aslo limits the effectiveness of increments in contractile function on improving forward pump function. Figure 6 displays computer model generated pressure–volume loops from a normal subject (Fig. 6a) and one with chronic LVH (Fig. 6b). In both examples, beats are shown before

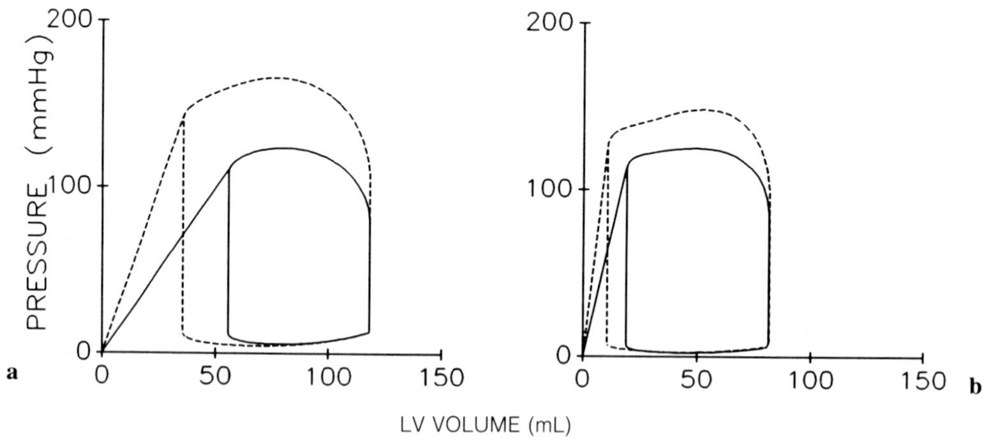

Fig. 6. Increased basal systolic stiffness limits contractile reserve with LVH. Computer model pressure–volume loops for "normal" patient (**a**) and LVH patient (**b**). Baseline loops (*solid lines*) are shown with matched stroke volumes, but a steep ESPVR for the LVH patient. When contractility is increased (twofold rise in slope of ESPVR), there is a much greater increment in pump function when the baseline slope is not already very high (i.e., **a**)

and after a 100% increase in inotropic state (doubling of E_{es}), holding preload volume, heart rate, and arterial impedance loading constant. There is much less of a rise in stroke volume (and thus cardiac output) due to the contractile increase when E_{es} starts out very high (i.e., Fig. 6b).

This result is predicted from coupling equations that have been previously presented [33]. Based on the simple time-varying elastance model, stroke volume (SV) can be written as:

$$SV = E_{es}/(E_{es} + E_a) \cdot (V_{ed} - V_o),$$

where E_a is the arterial load parameter (effective arterial elastance), V_{ed} is end-diastolic volume, and V_o the volume-axis intercept of the ESPVR. From this expression, the percent increment in SV following a pure doubling of E_{es} can be shown to be equal to:

$$\% \uparrow SV = 100/(1 + 2\alpha).$$

where α is the ratio of E_{es}/E_a. For any given value of arterial loading (E_a), the higher the baseline (higher α) E_{es}, the smaller the increment in SV when E_{es} is doubled.

An analogous expression can be derived for the present increase in systolic pressure if afterload resistance is doubled. This is given by:

$$\% \uparrow P_{es} = 100/(1 + 2/\alpha)$$

As E_{es} rises ($\uparrow \alpha$), the increase in P_{es} also rises considerably. This contributes to the outstripping of myocardial demand from supply when vascular resistance is increased.

This analysis places the benefits of negative inotropic treatment for LVH in a somewhat new light. Both calcium-channel and β blockers are commonly used in treating LVH, and are recognized to have negative inotropic effects. We recently confirmed that both lower E_{es} by an average of 30% when used at routine clinical doses [47]. This reduces α, lowering the gain relating change in chamber filling or arterial resistance, to systolic pressures, workload, or stroke volume. It also enhances the reserve capacity in response to inotropic stimulation during stress. In addition to benefits on diastolic function of these agents [17,25], these systolic effects are also likely very important in explaining their clinical utility.

Conclusions

Ventricular hypertrophy is associated with abnormalities of ventricular diastolic and systolic function at rest, and most impressively, by a reduced capacity to respond to increased demand. Abnormal functional reserve manifests itself by limitations in the cardiac response to changes in heart rate, ventricular accommodation to preload and arterial load variation, and minimal hemodynamic benefits from augmented contractility. As these are the three major mechanisms by which stress demands are met, it is not surprising that many patients develop exertional fatigue and dyspnea. Ongoing investigations of the precise cellular and molecular mechanisms underlying limited reserve, and the capacity of existing and novel therapies to improve them, will hopefully result in improved clinical outcome in this common disorder.

References

1. Factor SM, Butany J, Sole MJ, Wigle ED, Williams WC, Rojkind M (1991) Pathologic fibrosis and matrix connective tissue in the subaortic myocardium of patients with hypertrophic cardiomyopathy. J Am Coll Cardiol 17:1343–1351
2. Weber KT, Janicki JS, Schroff SG, Pick R, Chen RM, Bashey RI (1988) Collagen remodeling of the pressure-overloaded, hypertrophied nonhuman primate myocardium. Circ Res 62:757–765
3. Maron BJ, Bonow RO, Cannon RO III, Leon MB, Epstein SE (1987) Hypertrophic cardiomyopathy: Interrelations of clinical manifestations, pathophysiology, and therapy. N Engl J Med 316:780–789
4. Lorell BH, Grossman W (1987) Cardiac hypertrophy: the consequences for diastole. J Am Coll Cardiol 9:1189–1193
5. Bonow RO (1992) Left ventricular diastolic dysfunction as a cause of congestive heart failure. Mechanisms and Management. Ann Intern Med 117:502–510
6. Gwathmey JK, Morgan JP (1985) Altered calcium handling in experimental pressure-overload hypertrophy in the ferret. Circ Res 57:836–843
7. Gwathmey JK, Warren SE, Briggs GM, Copelas L, Feldman MD, Phillips PJ, Callahan M Jr, Schoen FJ, Grossman W, Morgan JP (1991) Diastolic dysfunction in hypertrophic cardiomyopathy. J Clin Invest 87:1023–1031
8. de la Bastie D, Levitsky D, Rappaport L, Mercadier J-J, Marotte F, Wisnewsky C, Brovkovich V, Schwartz K, Lompre A-M (1990) Function of the sarcoplasmic reticulum and expression of its Ca2+-ATPase gene in pressure overload-induced cardiac hypertrophy in the rat. Circ Res 66:554–564
9. Ito Y, Suko J, Chidsey CA (1974) Intracellular calcium and myocardial contractility v. calcium uptake of sarcoplasmic reticulum fractions in hypertrophied and failing rabbit hearts. J Mol Cell Cardiol 6:237–247
10. Bache RJ, Arentzen CE, Simon AB, Vrobel TR (1984) Abnormalities in myocardial perfusion during tachycardia in dogs with left ventricular hypertrophy: metabolic evidence for myocardial ischemia. Circulation 69:409–417
11. Cannon RO III, Dilsizian V, O'Gara PT, Udelson JE, Tucker E, Panza JA, Fananapazir L, McIntosh CL, Wallace RB, Bonow RO (1992) Impact of surgical relief of outflow obstruction on thallium perfusion abnormalities in hypertrophic cardiomyopathy. Circulation 85:1039–1045
12. Zhang J, Merkle H, Hendrich K, Garwood M, From AHL, Ugurbil K, Bache RJ (1993) Bioenergetic abnormalities associated with severe left ventricular hypertrophy. J Clin Invest 92:993–1003
13. Hittinger L, She YT, Patrick TA, Hasebe N, Komamura K, Ihara T, Manders WT, Vatner SF (1992) Mechanisms of subendocardial dysfunction in response to exercise in dogs with severe left ventricular hypertrophy. Circ Res 71:423–434

14. Mirsky I, Aoyagi T, Crocker VM, Fujii AM (1990) Preload dependence of fiber shortening rate in conscious dogs with left ventricular hypertrophy. J Am Coll Cardiol 15:899
15. Fujii AM, Gelpi RJ, Mirsky I, Vatner SF (1988) Systolic and diastolic dysfunction during atrial pacing in conscious dogs with left ventricular hypertrophy. Circ Res 62:462–470
16. Alyono D, Ring WS, Crumbley AJ, Schneider JR, O'Connor MJ, Parrish D, Bache RJ, Anderson RW (1984) Global left ventricular contractility in three models of hypertrophy evaluated with E_{max}. J Surg Res 37:48–54
17. Bonow RO, Ostrow HG, Rosing DR, Cannon RO III, Lipson LC, Maron BJ, Kent KM, Bacharach SL, Green MV (1983) Effects of verapamil on left ventricular systolic and diastolic function in patients with hypertrophic cardiomyopathy: pressure–volume analysis with a nonimaging scintillation probe. Circulation 68: 1062–1073
18. Matsuno Y, Morioka S, Murakami Y, Kobayashi S, Moriyama K (1988) Left ventricular end-systolic wall stress–dimension relationship in unanesthetized dogs with perinephritic hypertension. Jpn Circ J 52:1370–1376
19. Nakano K, Corin WJ, Spann JF Jr, Biederman RWW, Denslow S, Carabello BA (1989) Abnormal subendocardial blood flow in pressure overload hypertrophy is associated with pacing-induced subendocardial dysfunction. Circ Res 65:1555–1564
20. Pasternac A, Noble J, Streulens Y, Elie R, Henschke C, Bourassa MG (1982) Pathophysiology of chest pain in patients with cardiomyopathies and normal coronary arteries. Circulation 65:778
21. Liu CP, Ting CT, Lawrence W, Maughan WL, Chang MS, Kass DA (1993) Diminished contractile response to increased heart rate in intact human left ventricular hypertrophy: systolic versus diastolic determinants. Circulation 88(Pt. 1): 1893–1906
22. Kass DA, Midei M, Graves W, Brinker JA, Maughan WL (1988) Use of a conductance (volume) catheter and transient inferior vena caval occlusion for rapid determination of pressure–volume relationships in man. Cath Cardiovasc Diag 15: 192–202
23. Baan J, Van der Velde ET, de Brun HG, Smeenk GJ, Koops J, van Dijk AD, Temmerman D, Senden J, Buis B (1984) Continuous measurement of left ventricular volume in animals and humans by conductance catheter. Circulation 70: 812–823
24. Hittinger L, Shannon RP, Kohin S, Manders WT, Kelly P, Vatner SF (1990) Exercise-induced subendocardial dysfunction in dogs with left ventricular hypertrophy. Circ Res 66:329–343
25. Lorell BH, Paulus WJ, Grossman W, Wynne J, Cohn PF (1982) Modification of abnormal left ventricular diastolic properties by nifedipine in patients with hypertrophic cardiomyopathy. Circulation 65:499–507
26. Feldman MD, Alderman JD, Aroesty JM, Royal HD, Ferguson JJ, Owen RM, Grossman W, McKay RG (1988) Depression of systolic and diastolic myocardial reserve during atrial pacing tachycardia in patients with dilated cardiomyopathy. J Clin Invest 82:1661–1669
27. Gelpi RJ, Pasipoularides A, Lader AS, Patrick TA, Chase N, Hittinger L, Shannon RP, Bishop SP, Vatner SF (1991) Changes in diastolic cardiac function in developing and stable perinephritic hypertension in conscious dogs. Circ Res 68:555–567

28. Siri FM, Krueger J, Nordin C, Ming Z, Aronson RS (1991) Depressed intracellular calcium transients and contraction in myocytes from hypertrophied and failing guinea pig hearts. Am J Physiol 261:H514–H530
29. Mulieri LA, Hasenfuss G, Leavitt B, Allen PD, Alpert NR (1992) Altered myocardial force–frequency relation in human heart failure. Circulation 85:1743–1750
30. Freeman GL, Little WC, O'Rourke RA (1987) Influence of heart rate on left ventricular performance in conscious dogs. Circ Res 61:455–464
31. Suga H, Sagawa K, Shoukas AA (1973) Load independence of the instantaneous pressure–volume ratio of the canine left ventricle and effects of epinephrine and heart rate on the ratio. Circ Res 32:314
32. Glower DD, Spratt JA, Snow ND, Kabas JS, Davis JW, Olsen CO, Tyson GS, Sabiston DC, Rankin JS (1985) Linearity of the Frank-Starling relationship in the intact heart: the concept of preload recruitable stroke work. Circulation 71: 994–1009
33. Kass DA, Maughan WL, Guo ZM, Kono A, Sunagawa K, Sagawa K (1987) Comparative influence of load versus inotropic states on indexes of ventricular contractility: Experimental and theoretical analysis based on pressure–volume relationships. Circulation 76:1422–1436
34. Taylor PB, Helbing RK, Rourke S, Churchill D (1989) Effect of catecholamine-induced cardiac hypertrophy on the force–interval relationship. Can J Physiol Pharmacol 67:40–46
35. Cannon RO III, Rosing DR, Maron BJ, Leon MB, Bonow RO, Watson RM, Epstein SE (1985) Myocardial ischemia in patients with hypertrophic cardiomyopathy: contribution of inadequate vasodilator reserve and elevated left ventricular filling pressures. Circulation 71:234–243
36. Bailey BA, Houser SR (1992) Calcium transients in feline left ventricular myocytes with hypertrophy induced by slow progressive pressure overload. J Mol Cell Cardiol 24:365–373
37. Keung EC (1989) Calcium current is increased in isolated adult myocytes from hypertrophied rat myocardium. Circ Res 64:753–763
38. Bentivegna LA, Ablin LW, Kihara Y, Morgan JP (1991) Altered calcium handling in left ventricular pressure-overload hypertrophy as detected with aequorin in the isolated, perfused ferret heart. Circ Res 69:1538–1545
39. Suga H, Yamakoshi K (1977) Effects of stroke volume and velocity of ejection on the end-systolic pressure of canine left ventricle: End-systolic volume clamping. Circ Res 40:445–450
40. Schroff SG, Janicki JS, Weber KT (1985) Evidence and quantification of left ventricular systolic resistance. Am J Physiol 249:H358–H370
41. de Tombe PP, ter Keurs HE (1992) An internal viscous element limits unloaded velocity of sarcomere shortening in rat myocardium. J Physiol (London) 454: 619–642
42. Alpert NR, Mulieri LA (1982) Increased myothermal economy of isometric force generation in compensated cardiac hypertrophy induced by pulmonary artery constriction in the rabbit. Circ Res 50:491–500
43. Mercadier JJ, Bouveret P, Gorza L, Shiaffino S, Clark WA, Zak R, Swynghedauw B, Schwartz K (1983) Myosin isoenzymes in normal and hypertrophied human ventricular myocardium. Circ Res 53:52–62
44. Jeremy RW, Fletcher PJ, Thompson J (1989) Coronary pressure–flow relations in hypertensive left ventricular hypertrophy. Circ Res 65:224–236

45. Pak PH, Kass DA (1993) Diastolic interdependence in hypertrophic cardiomyopathy (abstract). Circulation 88:I-345
46. Kass DA, Wolff MR, Ting CT, Liu CP, Lawrence W, Chang MS, Maughan WL (1993) Diastolic compliance of hypertrophied ventricle is not acutely altered by pharmacologic agents influencing active processes. Ann Intern Med 119:466–473

2.5 Coronary Circulation in Patients with Pressure-Overloaded Left Ventricular Hypertrophy

FUMIHIKO KAJIYA and AKIHIRO KIMURA[1]

Summary. Pressure-overloaded left ventricular hypertrophy is the major risk factor causing adverse cardiovascular events, including myocardial ischemia and heart failure. The aim of this study was to investigate the characteristics of phasic blood flow pattern in patients with pressure-overloaded left ventricular (LV) hypertrophy, i.e., hypertension and pure aortic valve stenosis. Coronary blood flow velocity measurements were performed by a 20-MHz Doppler catheter or by a 20-MHz 80-channel Doppler velocimeter. The coronary circulation of pressure-overloaded LV hypertrophy was characterized by (1) enhanced systolic retrograde flow, (2) delayed early diastolic coronary inflow, and (3) increased blood flow in mid-to-late diastole. The vascular and perivascular histological changes with increased systolic vascular compression and impaired LV relaxation may affect the phasic coronary flow pattern, i.e., increased systolic retrograde flow and delayed early diastolic inflow. These flow changes may result in decreased coronary flow reserve and subendomyocardial ischemia in the patients with pressure-overloaded left ventricular hypertrophy.

Key words: Essential hypertension—Aortic stenosis—Coronary blood velocity—Doppler catheter—Slosh phenomenon—Coronary flow reserve

Introduction

Pressure-overloaded left ventricular (LV) hypertrophy is generally regarded as a compensatory process that normalizes LV systolic wall stress (force/unit area) during chronic hemodynamic perturbation, due to pressure overload [1,2]. Despite normalization of systolic wall stress, abnormalities of myocardial

[1] Department of Medical Engineering and Systems Cardiology, Kawasaki Medical School, 577 Matsushima, Kurashiki, Okayama, 701-01 Japan

perfusion, especially in the subendocardium, occur in the absence of occlusive coronary artery disease, causing exertional angina pectoris [3]. The increased vulnerability of the hypertrophied ventricle to ischemia is explained by a decreased coronary vasodilating capacity; i.e., decreased coronary flow reserve [4]. Some plausible mechanisms for decreased coronary flow reserve have been proposed: (a) pathological changes in the coronary vascular bed and/or interstitial tissue, (b) dysfunction of coronary microcirculation, and (c) hemodynamic and cardiomechanical effects on coronary circulation. The pathological changes include decreased capillary density [5], an increased wall-to-lumen ratio in the coronary resistance vessels [6], arteriolar rarefaction [7], and perivascular and interstitial tissue fibrosis [8]. Along with the microcirculatory dysfunction, impaired endothelial cell and smooth muscle cell functions may develop with cardiac hypertrophy. The alterations of mechanical function of the hypertrophied heart include increased extravascular compression during systole and impaired refilling of vessels during diastole.

Although there have been several animal models of pressure-overload LV hypertrophy, either induced by banding of the ascending aorta, artificial aortic valve stenosis, or renovascular hypertension, or using the spontaneous hypertensive rat, studies of coronary hemodynamics of the human hypertrophied heart have been limited. The aim of this study was to investigate the characteristics of phasic blood flow pattern in patients with pressure-overloaded LV hypertrophy, i.e., hypertensive LV hypertrophy and pure aortic valve stenosis.

Methods

Group 1: Patients with Essential Hypertension and Normal Controls Without LV Hypertrophy

Twenty-three patients aged 37 to 71 years (58 ± 8 years; 19 males and 4 females) with untreated essential hypertension who complained of chest pain were studied [9]. Hypertension was defined as a history of raised blood pressure (values of more than 160/95 mmHg), a sustained blood pressure increase documented during hospital admission, and a mean arterial pressure of more than 110 mmHg at the time of cardiac catheterization. None of the patients had a history of previous myocardial infarction, nor did they have valvular heart disease. All the hypertensive patients had sinus rhythm without atrioventricular block or bundle branch block on electrocardiograms. The Romhilt-Estes electrocardiographic hypertrophy score was 6.2 ± 1.8.

A total of 13 patients aged 48 to 69 years (a mean age of 57 years; 9 males and 4 females), suffering from long-lasting atypical chest pain which was not sensitive to glyceryl trinitrate, served as normal controls. These patients had no LV hypertrophy nor any abnormalities in hemodynamic data. No abnormalities were found either in electrocardiograms or in ^{201}thallium myocardial perfusion imaging (at rest and during exercise).

All patients with essential hypertension and normal controls underwent coronary angiograms with a standard Judkins catheter before and after acetylcholine administration at a rate of 5 mg/s for approximately 20 s into the ostium of the left coronary artery through the catheter. Angiographic findings were interpreted and discussed by three physicians specializing in cardiovascular disease. These physicians agreed that none of the patients had any visible coronary artery stenosis or coronary spasms. For contrast ventriculography, 35–40 ml of iopamidole was injected into the left ventricle. A single plane cineangiocardiogram was obtained at 60 frames per second on a 30° right anterior oblique projection. The same physicians also agreed that the left ventricular functions of the studied patients were normal; i.e., an ejection fraction greater than 50% with no abnormalities in regional wall motion. The absence of abnormality in regional wall motion was also supported by two-dimensional echocardiography (SSH-160A, Toshiba, Tokyo, Japan).

Group 2: Patients with Chronic Pure Aortic Valve Stenosis

Six patients (4 men and 2 women, a mean age of 60 years) with chronic pure aortic stenosis were studied during open heart surgery before and after aortic valve replacement with a St. Jude Medical prosthetic valve [10]. A cardiac catheterization study was performed before operation, and absence of coronary artery disease and abnormal LV regional wall motion were confirmed by coronary angiography and left ventriculogram in all patients.

These investigations were approved by the human subjects committee of Kawasaki Medical School and informed written consent was obtained from all patients studied.

Blood Flow Velocity Measurements for Group 1

Coronary blood flow velocity measurements were performed by a No. 3F 20-MHz Doppler catheter (model DC101, Millar Instruments, Houston, TX, USA) which was discussed in our previous papers [11]. The catheter was advanced through a standard guiding catheter (Softip PTCA guiding catheter, No. 8F, Schneider, Minneapolis, Minn., USA) into a coronary artery. The Doppler catheter was selectively positioned in about the proximal one-third of the left anterior descending coronary artery (LAD; segment 6 or 7 of the AHA classification) and range gated until a high-quality phasic signal of blood flow velocity was obtained.

Measurements of the LAD flow velocities were performed under control conditions and after the injection of papaverine hydrochloride (6–12 mg) into the artery through the Doppler catheter. The coronary flow reserve was evaluated as the ratio of the maximum value of the mean flow velocities to the resting mean flow velocity. Among blood velocity variables, we especially noted the time after the beginning of diastole to peak velocity (time for diastolic rise; TDR) and the mid-to-late diastolic deceleration rate ($\Delta V/\Delta T$, see

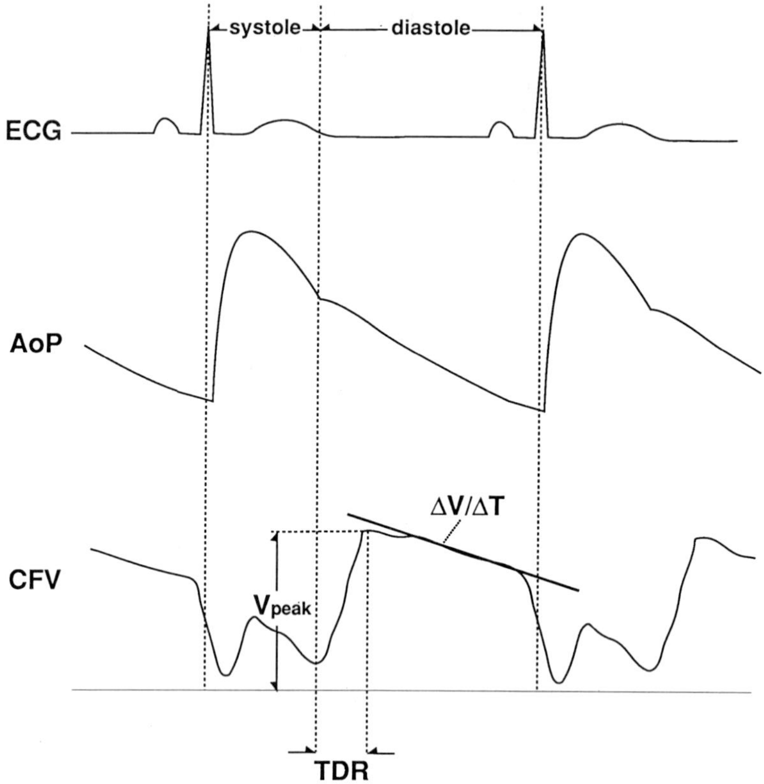

Fig. 1. Schematic illustration of the phasic blood velocity waveform in the left anterior descending coronary artery (LAD) and variables extracted from the waveform. *AoP*, aortic pressure; *CFV*, coronary flow velocity; *TDR*, time for diastolic rise of the LAD flow; V_{peak}, diastolic peak velocity; $\Delta V/\Delta T$, mid-to-late diastolic velocity deceleration rate of the LAD flow

Fig. 1). The $\Delta V/\Delta T$ was normalized by the peak velocity (V_{peak}) as $\Delta V/\Delta T \cdot V_{peak}$). The coronary flow was recorded simultaneously with aortic pressure by a Millar SPC484-A pressure transducer (Millar Instruments) and a lead II electrocardiogram. Hemodynamic data were averaged for five consecutive heart beats.

Blood Flow Velocity Measurements for Group 2

We measured the blood velocity in the LAD (segment 6 or 7) in the patients with aortic stenosis using 20-MHz 80-channel Doppler velocimeter developed in our laboratory [12]. A specially designed probe holder made of silicon rubber was used to place the transducer at a 60° angle on the LAD without dissection of the vessels. Also, the operator followed cardiac motion carefully with his fingers. The Doppler signals were analyzed by a fast Fourier transform (FFT) or a zero-cross method, both in real time. When 30 to 45 minutes had elapsed after discontinuation of the cardiopulmonary bypass after aortic valve replacement and when a steady hemodynamic state had been achieved, measurements of the flow velocity in the LAD were performed. The peak systolic retrograde flow velocity, the early diastolic inflow (TDR), and peak diastolic anterograde flow velocity were read from the envelope in the FFT display before and after aortic valve replacement.

Results

Phasic Pattern of Coronary Blood Flow Velocities in Patients with Essential Hypertension and Aortic Stenosis

Figure 2a shows a representative tracing of the coronary blood velocity waveform in normal controls, and Fig. 2b shows that in hypertensive left ventricular hypertrophy (S is systole and D is diastole). The velocity waveform of hypertrophied heart was characterized, firstly, by the existence of systolic retrograde flow (arrow), which may be squeezed-out from deeper myocardial vessels, and secondly, by delayed early diastolic inflow, i.e., the time-delay from the beginning of diastole to the peak flow (TDR). The mean values of TDR in the patients with hypertensive left ventricular hypertrophy and in normal controls were 145 ± 56 ms and 66 ± 15 ms, respectively ($P < 0.001$). Absolute flow is greater in hypertrophy due to the increase in heart mass as already well documented.

Figure 3 shows representative tracings of coronary blood velocity in a patient with aortic valve stenosis before and after the valve replacement. As in hypertensive LV hypertrophied patients, greater systolic retrograde flow and delayed early diastolic filling (TDR) are the main characteristics of coronary flow in patients with aortic stenosis. By aortic valve replacement (Fig. 3b), systolic retrograde flow was decreased and the delayed early diastolic flow (prolongation of TDR) was improved. The late systolic retrograde flow (Fig. 3b, arrow) may be related to the closure insufficiency of the artificial valve. The change in the systolic retrograde flow following valve replacement is summarized in Fig. 4. After aortic valve replacement, peak systolic retrograde flow decreased by about 50% compared with before valve replacement. These results indicate that systolic retrograde flow in aortic stenosis is caused by the high LV pressure, since it is decreased significantly after the removal of high LV pressure by the valve replacement without any histological recovery.

Figure 5a summarizes the TDR in the hypertrophy groups and the control group. The TDR of aortic stenosis (AS) and of hypertension (HT) were significantly longer than that in the control group by about 150% and 100%, respectively. There was not a statistically significant difference of TDR between

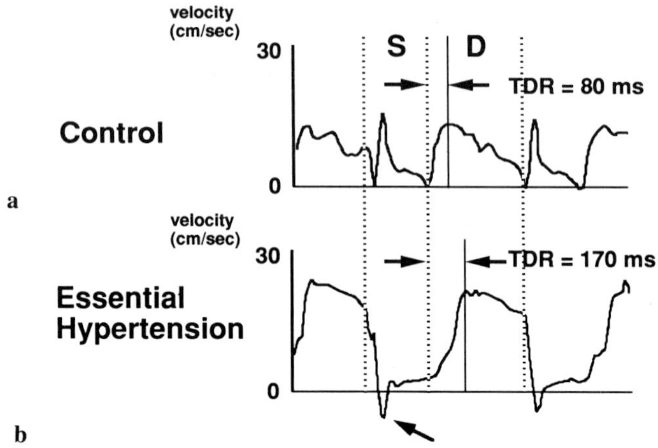

Fig. 2. a A representative tracing of the coronary flow velocity waveform from normal controls. **b** The waveform of a patient with hypertensive left ventricular hypertrophy. The velocity waveforms of LV hypertrophy were characterized by the existence of systolic retrograde flow (*arrow*) and delayed early diastolic inflow (*TDR*). *S*, systole; *D*, diastole. This figure was originally presented by Tadaoka et al. [9] and is reprinted by permission of the British Cardiac Society

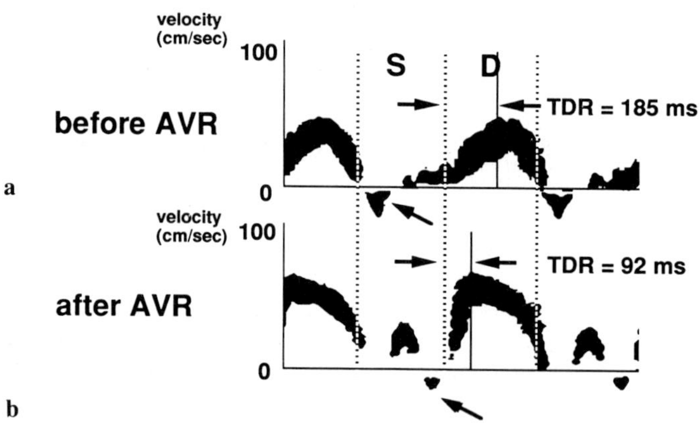

Fig. 3a,b. Representative tracings of coronary blood velocity waveforms in a patient with pure aortic valve stenosis before (**a**) and after (**b**) the valve replacement (*AVR*). As in hypertensive LV hypertrophied patients, increased systolic retrograde flow and delayed early diastolic filling (*TDR*) are the main characteristics of coronary flow in patients with pure aortic stenosis. By aortic valve replacement, systolic retrograde flow was decreased and the delayed early diastolic flow (prolongation of TDR) was improved. (From [10] with permission)

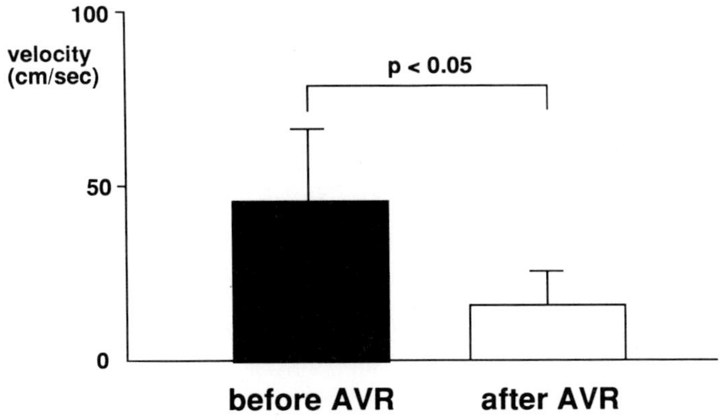

Fig. 4. Systolic retrograde flow before and after aortic valve replacement (*AVR*). After aortic valve replacement, the peak systolic retrograde flow decreased by about 50% compared with that before valve replacement

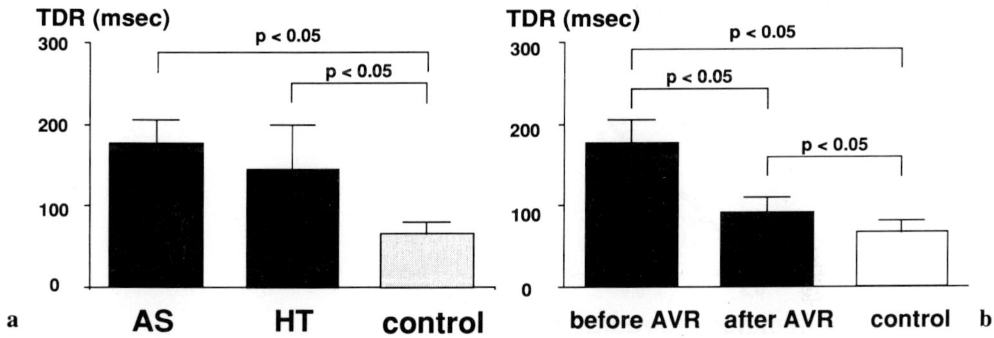

Fig. 5a,b. TDR values in the hypertrophy groups and the control group. **a** TDR's of aortic stenosis (*AS*) and hypertension (*HT*) were significantly longer than that of the control group by about 150% and 100%, respectively, but there was no statistically significant difference between AS and HT. **b** TDR values in patients with aortic stenosis were shortened significantly by valve replacement (*AVR*), but were still longer than that in the control group

AS and HT. Figure 5b shows TDR values in patients with aortic stenosis before and after valve replacement (AVR) with reference to the control group. The TDR value was improved significantly by valve replacement ($P < 0.05$), but it was still longer than that in the control group ($P < 0.05$).

The relationship between TDR in pressure-overloaded LV hypertrophy groups and the LV relaxation time constant is shown in Fig. 6a. The TDR shows a significant positive correlation with the LV relaxation time constant;

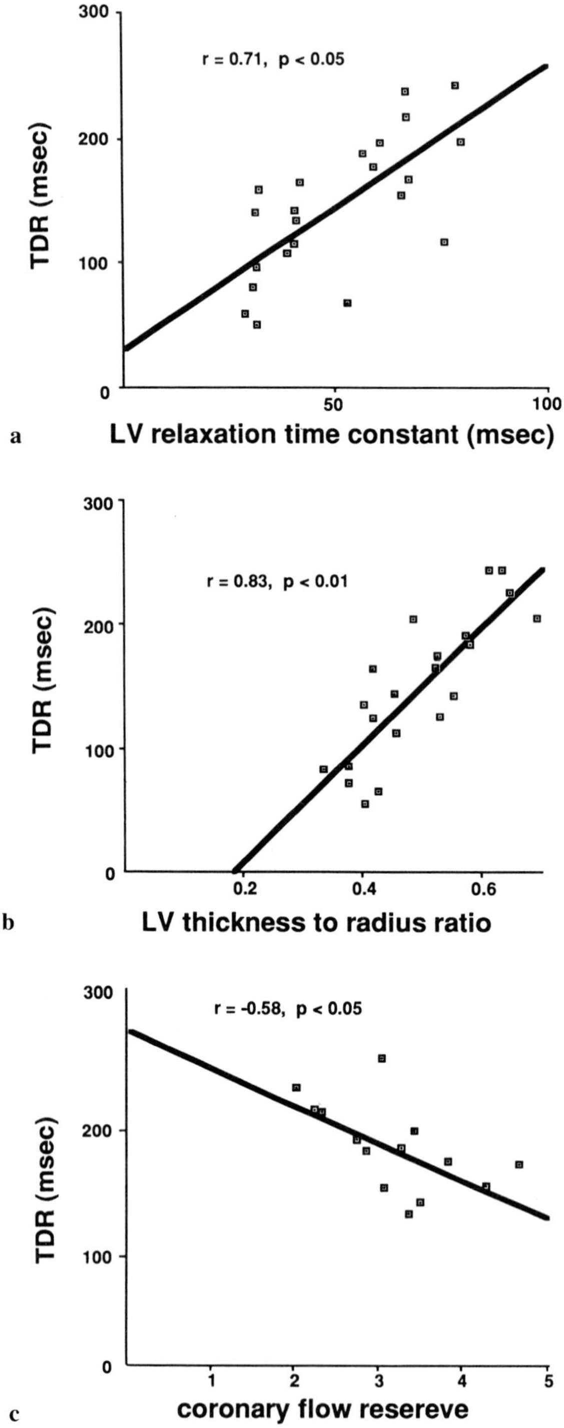

Fig. 6a–c. Correlation analysis between TDR and other variables. TDR shows a significant positive correlations with the LV relaxation time constant (**a**) and with LV wall thickness (**b**), and a negative correlation with coronary flow reserve (**c**). (From [9] with permission)

i.e., the longer the TDR, the greater the LV relaxation time constant (r = 0.71, $P < 0.05$). TDR also shows a significant positive correlation with LV wall thickness (Fig. 6b, r = 0.83, $P < 0.01$) and a negative correlation with coronary flow reserve (Fig. 6c, r = −0.58, $P < 0.05$).

The values of $\Delta V/(\Delta T \cdot V_{peak})$ in patients with hypertensive LV hypertrophy and in normal controls were $1.26 \pm 0.61\,s^{-1}$ and $3.03 \pm 1.18\,s^{-1}$, respectively ($P < 0.001$). In patients with hypertensive left ventricular hypertrophy, $\Delta V/(\Delta T \cdot V_{peak})$ correlated well with the degree of hypertrophy (r = 0.75, $P <$ 0.01), with the TDR (r = 0.82, $P < 0.01$), and with the coronary flow reserve (r = 0.68, $P < 0.01$).

Discussion

Major findings of our present clinical studies are that the coronary circulation of pressure-overloaded LV hypertrophy is characterized by (1) enhanced systolic retrograde flow, (2) delayed early diastolic coronary inflow, and (3) increased blood flow in mid-to-late diastole. Both systolic retrograde flow and delayed early diastolic inflow may cause the underperfusion of subendomyocardium in pressure-overloaded LV hypertrophy. On the other hand, the increase in blood flow during mid-to-late diastole may partly compensate the reduction of coronary inflow by these two mechanisms.

Our conclusions depend mainly upon factors (1) and (2), and take into account the phasic nature of systolic retrograde flow and diastolic flow in patients with pressure-overloaded LV hypertrophy.

Phasic Nature of Systolic Retrograde Flow in Patients with Pressure-Overloaded LV Hypertrophy

Although systolic retrograde flow has been observed both in patients and in animals with hypertension, aortic stenosis, or hypertrophied cardiomyopathy, its quantitative description with pathophysiological interpretation has been hampered so far. Recent reports from our laboratory indicated that, in dogs, the systolic retrograde flow increased with the severity of stenosis in the coronary artery, and this caused the reduction of endomyocardial flow [13,14]. In other words, when coronary artery stenosis increases, a substantial amount of blood which enters into the myocardium during diastole, flows backward to epicardial vessels from intramyocardial vessels during systole. This transmural to-and-fro blood flow movement may be called the "slosh phenomenon" [13]. Thus, the increase of stenotic severity of coronary artery augments sloshing, resulting in subendocardial underperfusion. The increase in slosh in coronary artery stenosis is mainly attributable to a decrease in the post-stenotic pressure which acts as back-pressure against retrograde flow, and to an increase in compliance of epicardial arteries due to the post-stenotic intravascular pressure reduction.

In pressure-overloaded LV hypertrophy, a sloshing phenomenon similar to the one in coronary artery stenosis occurs with the increase in the systolic retrograde flow. This implies that the extravascular compressive force acting on intramyocardial vessels cannot be reduced by cardiac hypertrophy, which may normalize LV systolic wall stress. Thus, the augmented systolic retrograde flow is probably caused by an increase in extravascular compression force due to high LV pressure. In fact, the systolic retrograde flow is decreased by the removal of high LV pressure by aortic valve replacement in patients with pure aortic stenosis, indicating the importance of increased LV pressure as a cause of systolic retrograde flow. Along with other causes of increased systolic retrograde flow, hypertrophied myocytes with an increased interstitial collagen content may squeeze intramyocardial vasculature more vigorously, propelling blood in intramyocardial vessels to epicardial arteries during systole (Fig. 7b). We conclude that the augmentation of the slosh phenomenon may contribute to subendocardial vulnerability to ischemia in patients with pressure-overloaded LV hypertrophy.

Phasic Nature of Diastolic Flow in Patients with LV Hypertrophy

Prolonged early diastolic inflow (elongation of TDR) is an important characteristic of the coronary flow waveform in patients with LV hypertrophy caused either by essential hypertension [9] or by chronic pure aortic stenosis [10]. The delayed TDR implies a decreased early diastolic inflow. Three main reasons for the delayed TDR in pressure-overloaded LV hypertrophy may be as follows. First, if the extravascular compressive force increases in the microvessels during systole, vascular resistance at end-systole increases by decreasing vascular diameter, which may impede the early diastolic refilling [15]. Second, the impaired LV relaxation in pressure-overloaded LV hypertrophy may relate to the delayed TDR. Our previous findings that the TDR was shortened when the impairment of relaxation was ameliorated by verapamil in patients with hypertensive LV hypertrophy may support the contribution of impaired relaxation to the delayed TDR [9]. Third, pathological changes in pressure-overloaded LV hypertrophy, such as hypertrophied myocytes, arterial wall thickening, and an increase in interstitial collagen may cause the delayed early diastolic coronary refilling (Fig. 7b). The third mechanism is consistent with the present result that the delayed TDR was still observed after aortic valve replacement, since the hemodynamics can be improved but the histological changes cannot be remodeled immediately after valve replacement.

Decreased Coronary Flow Reserve in Pressure-Overloaded LV Hypertrophy

It is well known that coronary vasodilating capacity (coronary flow reserve) especially in the subendomyocardium is impaired in pressure-overloaded LV hypertrophy [4]. Some plausible mechanisms were mentioned in the Introduc-

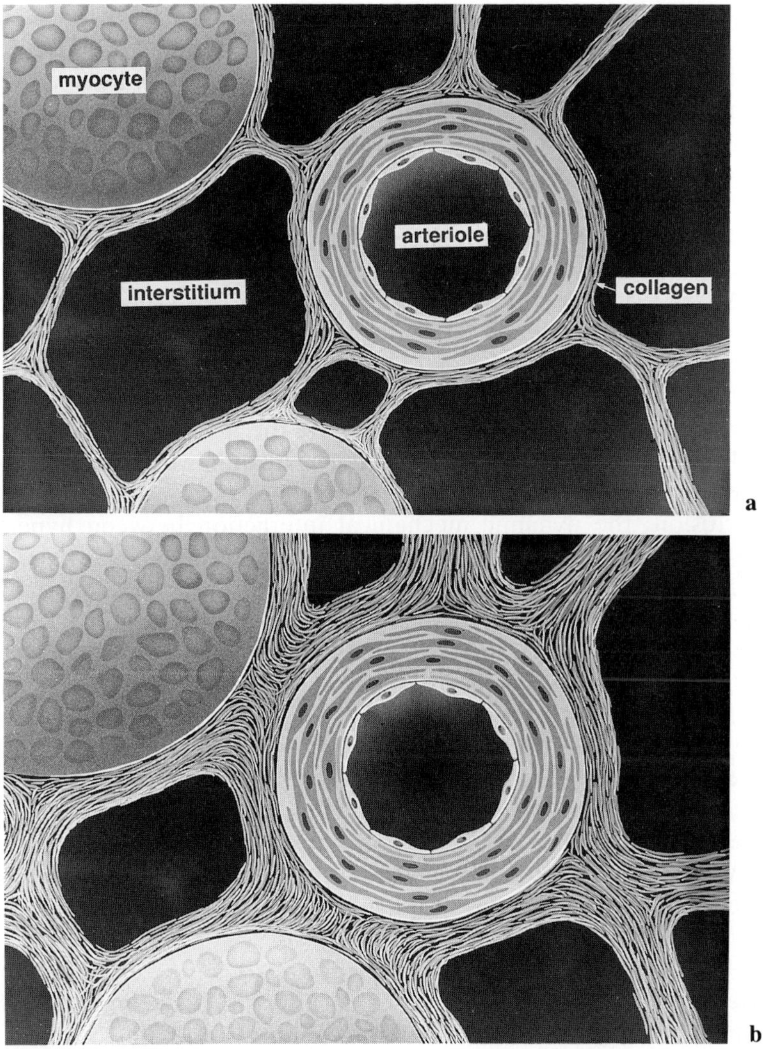

Fig. 7a,b. Schematic drawings of possible relations between intramyocardial resistance vessels and myocytes, collagen fibers, and interstitium in normal (**a**) and hypertrophied (**b**) hearts. Compared with the normal heart, the hypertrophied heart is characterized by an increase in the volume fraction of collagen associated with (1) interstitial fibrosis, (2) vascular fibrosis, and (3) microscopic scarring that follows myocyte necrosis. The interstitial fibrosis in a hypertrophied heart may be closely associated with abnormalities in its stiffness and in its pumping and relaxation functions, which may reduce the coronary flow reserve directly. The perivascular fibrosis and medial thickening of coronary resistance vessels may affect vasodilator reserve directly with impaired functions of vascular smooth muscle cells and endothelial cells tion. In this study, we demonstrated that the delayed TDR correlated well with the coronary flow reserve. Although it is difficult to discuss the causal relationship on the basis of a correlation analysis alone, the delayed TDR may be an important mechanism for decreasing the coronary flow reserve. The increased systolic retrograde flow in pressure-overloaded LV hypertrophy may also cause the reduction of coronary flow reserve by increasing the coronary slosh phenomenon, especially in subendomyocardium.

The other important hemodynamic change in pressure-overloaded LV hypertrophy is the decrease in the mid-to-late diastolic deceleration rate of the velocity $\Delta V/(\Delta T \cdot V_{peak})$ [16]. The value of $\Delta V/(\Delta T \cdot V_{peak})$ correlated inversely with the coronary flow reserve. Since the TDR is delayed and systolic retrograde flow increased in pressure-overloaded LV hypertrophy, the blood flow in the later part of diastole may increase to compensate for the delayed TDR and increased systolic retrograde flow, to maintain the myocardial flow per unit LV mass [16]. Our study supports that this mechanism is working in the pressure-overloaded hypertrophied heart.

In conclusion, the dynamic mechanical interaction between hypertrophied myocytes surrounded by increased interstitial connective tissue, and intramyocardial coronary vessels under high LV pressure is the fundamentally important factor in reducing intramyocardial coronary perfusion in pressureoverloaded LV hypertrophy (Fig. 7). In most cases of hypertensive LV hypertrophy, the number of microvessels decreases and the vascular wall-to-lumen ratio increases. The function of vascular endothelial cells and smooth muscle cells may also be impaired. These vascular and perivascular histological changes with increased systolic vascular compression and impaired LV relaxation affect the phasic coronary flow pattern, i.e., increased systolic retrograde flow and delayed early diastolic inflow. These flow changes may result in decreased coronary flow reserve and subendomyocardial ischemia in patients with pressure-overloaded left ventricular hypertrophy.

Acknowledgments. We thank Dr. Takashi Fujiwara, Dr. Schin-ichiro Tadaoka, Dr. Toshitami Sawayama, Dr. Yoshifumi Wada, Dr. Masami Goto, Dr. Yasuo Ogasawara, and Dr. Katsuhiko Tsujioka for their excellent work and also Osamu Hiramatsu and Hiroyuki Tachibana for their technical support for the experiments. The authors acknowledge the support of grants from the Kawasaki Medical School Grant for Project Research in Japan (No. 1-102).

References

1. Hood WP, Rackley CE, Rolett E (1968) Wall stress in the normal and hypertrophied left ventricle. Am J Cardiol 22:550–558
2. Gunther S, Grossman W (1979) Determinants of ventricular function in pressure overload hypertrophy in man. Circulation 59:679–688

3. Goodwin JR (1973) Hypertrophic disease of the myocardium. Prog Cardiovasc Dis 16:199–238
4. Bache RJ (1988) Effects of hypertrophy on the coronary circulation. Prog Cardiovasc Dis 31:403–440
5. Tomanek RJ, Palmer PJ, Peiffer GL, Schreiber KL, Eastham CL, Marcus ML (1986) Morphometry of canine arteries, arterioles and capillaries during hypertension and left ventricular hypertrophy. Circ Res 58:38–46
6. Folkow B (1982) Physiological aspects of primary hypertension. Physiol Rev 62:347–504
7. Hutchins PM, Darnell AE (1974) Observations of a decrease number of small arterioles in spontaneously hypertensive rats. Circ Res 34 and 35[Suppl I]:I-161–I-165
8. Weber KT, Brilla CG (1991) Pathological hypertrophy and cardiac interstitium. Fibrosis and renin-angiotensin-aldosterone system. Circulation 83:1849–1865
9. Tadaoka S, Wada Y, Kimura A, Yada T, Tamura K, Hasegawa K, Nezuo S, Sawayama T, Tsujioka K, Kajiya F (1991) Effect of left ventricular hypertrophy secondary to systemic hypertension on left coronary flow dynamics. Cardiovasc Res 25:955–964
10. Fujiwara T, Nogami A, Masaki H, Yanaka H, Matsuoka S, Yoshida H, Fukuda H, Katsumura T, Kajiya F (1989) Coronary flow velocity waveforms in aortic stenosis and the effects of valve replacement. Ann Thorac Surg 48:518–522
11. Tadaoka S, Kagiyama M, Hiramatsu O, Ogasawara Y, Tsujioka K, Wada Y, Sawayama T, Kajiya F (1990) Accuracy of 20-MHz Doppler catheter coronary artery velocimetry for measurement of coronary blood flow velocity. Cathet Cardiovasc Diagn 19:205–213
12. Kajiya F, Ogasawara Y, Tsujioka K, Nakai M, Goto M, Wada Y, Tadaoka S, Matsuoka S, Mito K, Fujiwara T (1986) Evaluation of human coronary blood flow with an 80-channel 20-MHz pulsed Doppler velocimeter and zero-cross and fourier transform methods during cardiac surgery. Circulation 74[Suppl 3]:III-53–III-60
13. Kimura A, Hiramatsu O, Yamamoto T, Ogasawara Y, Yada T, Goto M, Tsujioka K, Kajiya F (1992) Effect of coronary stenosis on phasic pattern of septal artery in dogs. Am J Physiol 262:H1690–H1698
14. Goto M, Flynn AE, Doucette JW, Kimura A, Hiramatsu O, Yamamoto T, Ogasawara Y, Tsujioka K, Hoffman JIE, Kajiya F (1992) Effect of intracoronary nitroglycerin administration on phasic pattern and transmural distribution of flow during coronary artery stenosis. Circulation 85:2296–2304
15. Hoffman JIE, Spaan JAE (1990) Pressure-flow relations in coronary circulation. Physiol Rev 70:331–390
16. Tadaoka S, Kimura A, Yada T, Tsujioka K, Nezuo S, Sawayama T, Kajiya F (1993) Decreased mid-to-late diastolic decay of diastolic coronary artery flow velocity in pressure-overloaded left ventricular hypertrophy. Heart Vessels 8:91–97

Morphological Aspects

2.6 Morphology of Left Ventricular Hypertrophy in the Human

Masami Imakita and Chikao Yutani[1]

Summary. The hypertrophied heart typically exhibits various changes in architecture as well as in histology, according to the cause and stage of hypertrophy. The macroscopic and histologic changes in hypertrophied hearts are briefly described. The various dimensions of the autopsied hearts, width of myocytes, contents of myocytes, and extent of fibrosis were compared between one group of patients who seemed to have hypertrophied hearts secondary to arterial hypertension in adaptive growth or a prolonged state of successful adaptation, and a second group of patients who appeared to have almost normal hearts. There were significant differences in heart weight, the length of the inflow portion of the left ventricle, the wall thickness of the left ventricle and interventricular septum, the width of myocytes, and the extent of fibrosis.

Key words: Cardiac hypertrophy—Left ventricle—Architecture—Histology—Morphometry—Morphology

The heart may respond to various stimuli by an increase in functioning myocardial mass [1]. The causes of cardiac hypertrophy include an increase in preload, impairment of the pump function, an increased afterload, and idiopathy. The term "cardiac hypertrophy" traditionally has meant that the increase in the mass of the heart is a consequence of an increase in the size of its constituent cells [2,3]. However, the hypertrophied heart exhibits architectural changes and is different from an enlarged copy of the original one. Also, it is now recognized that cardiac hypertrophy involves an increase in the numbers of various types of connective cells and deposition of increased amounts of connective tissue proteins in the interstitial spaces, as well as an increase in the size of cardiac muscle cells [4]. Furthermore, it has been reported that in certain instances, cardiac muscle cells increase in number [5].

[1]Department of Pathology, National Cardiovascular Center, 5-7-1 Fujishirodai, Suita, Osaka, 565 Japan

Macroscopic Changes

Left ventricular hypertrophy can be defined as an increase in the functioning myocardial mass of the left ventricle. It is said that the only convincing method for the accurate assessment of ventricular hypertrophy is weighing of the separated ventricles using a technique based on that of Fulton [6]. However, cardiac hypertrophy conventionally refers to heart weights exceeding the accepted limits of normal for age, sex, and body weight [7]. There is the following guide for normal heart weight: adult male heart weight, 0.45% of body weight, average 300 g, range 250–350 g; adult female heart weight, 0.40% of body weight, average 250 g, range 200–300 g [8].

Classically, two types of ventricular hypertrophy are recognized: concentric and eccentric (Fig. 1). Concentric hypertrophy is usually associated with conditions that cause an increase in afterload, such as aortic stenosis and systemic hypertension. In pure concentric hypertrophy of the left ventricle, the ventricular wall shows an increase in thickness, but the short axis chamber diameter does not become significantly larger. The wall thickness generally increases 25% to 75%, and the left ventricle appears as a thick ring surrounding a small chamber on transverse section. The heart with concentric hypertrophy shows an elongated contour with an increased base-apex length. Eccentric hypertrophy is associated with dilated cardiomyopathies and with conditions that cause volume overload, such as mitral regurgitation. In pure eccentric hypertrophy, both the thickness of the left ventricular wall and the short axis diameter of the ventricle increase proportionately. The heart with eccentric hypertrophy shows a globular configuration with increased base-apex and short-axis dimensions.

There is another type of cardiac hypertrophy, asymmetric hypertrophy, which is usually seen in hypertrophic cardiomyopathy [9]. In hypertrophic cardiomyopathy, the ventricular septum is thicker than the left ventricle free wall which is also thick, whereas the ventricular septum in the usual type of hypertrophy becomes thickened to the same extent as the free walls of the ventricles.

In left ventricular hypertrophy, the architecture of the left ventricle may change conspicuously, and the posterior and superior walls show the most marked changes in contour [2] (Figs. 2, 3). The posterior and superior walls of the left ventricle become bowed and elongated beyond the mitral ring, and because of their elongation, the mitral valve becomes tilted so that it lies more nearly parallel with the plane of the aortic valve. The outward bulge of myocardium about the mitral ring is more exaggerated beyond the margin of the mitral ring than normal. Also, the bulging of the myocardial wall into the lumen along the left ventricular outflow tract becomes conspicuous and may impede the aortic flow. The trabeculae corneas and papillary muscles are elongated and very prominent. In hearts with eccentric hypertrophy, the portion of the left ventricular chamber which lies in front of the anterior mitral valve is much more dilated than is the portion behind this valve. The apical

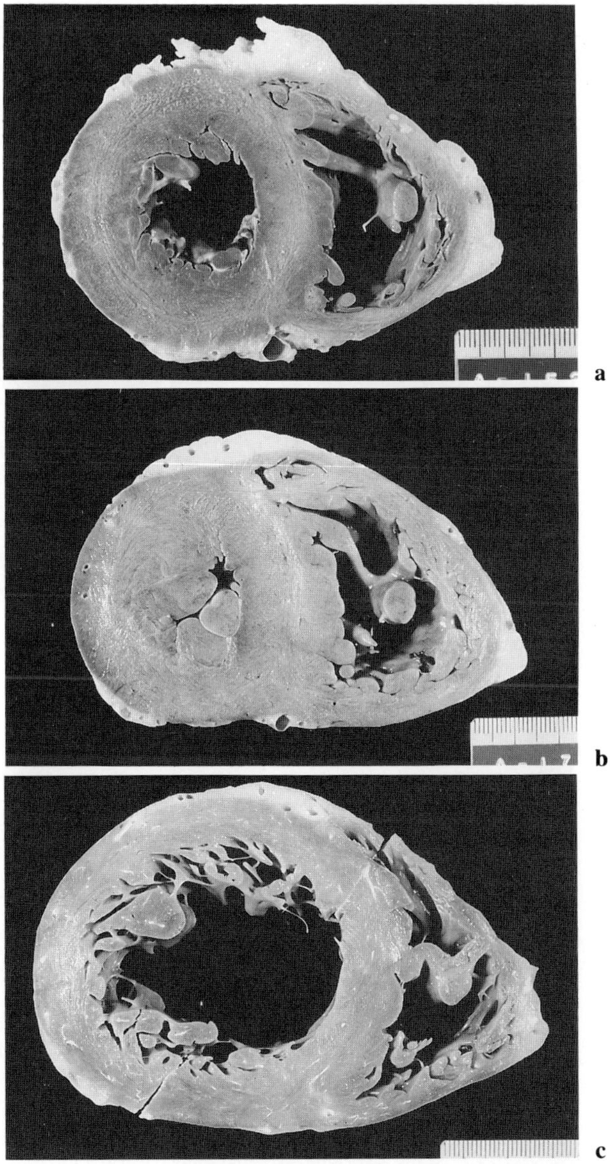

Fig. 1a–c. Transverse slices of hearts. **a** The almost normal heart from a 66-year-old woman. **b** The hypertrophied heart from a 63-year-old man. **c** The hypertrophied and dilated heart from a 49-year-old man

portion of the chamber also becomes dilated and papillary muscles appear to originate higher on the posterior wall of the heart than normally. Papillary muscles may show tapering and blend imperceptibly into chordae. The mitral valve is often elongated.

Table 1 shows various measurements (mean ± SD) in 10%-formalin-fixed, autopsied hearts from two groups (n = 21). Group 1 was composed of 12

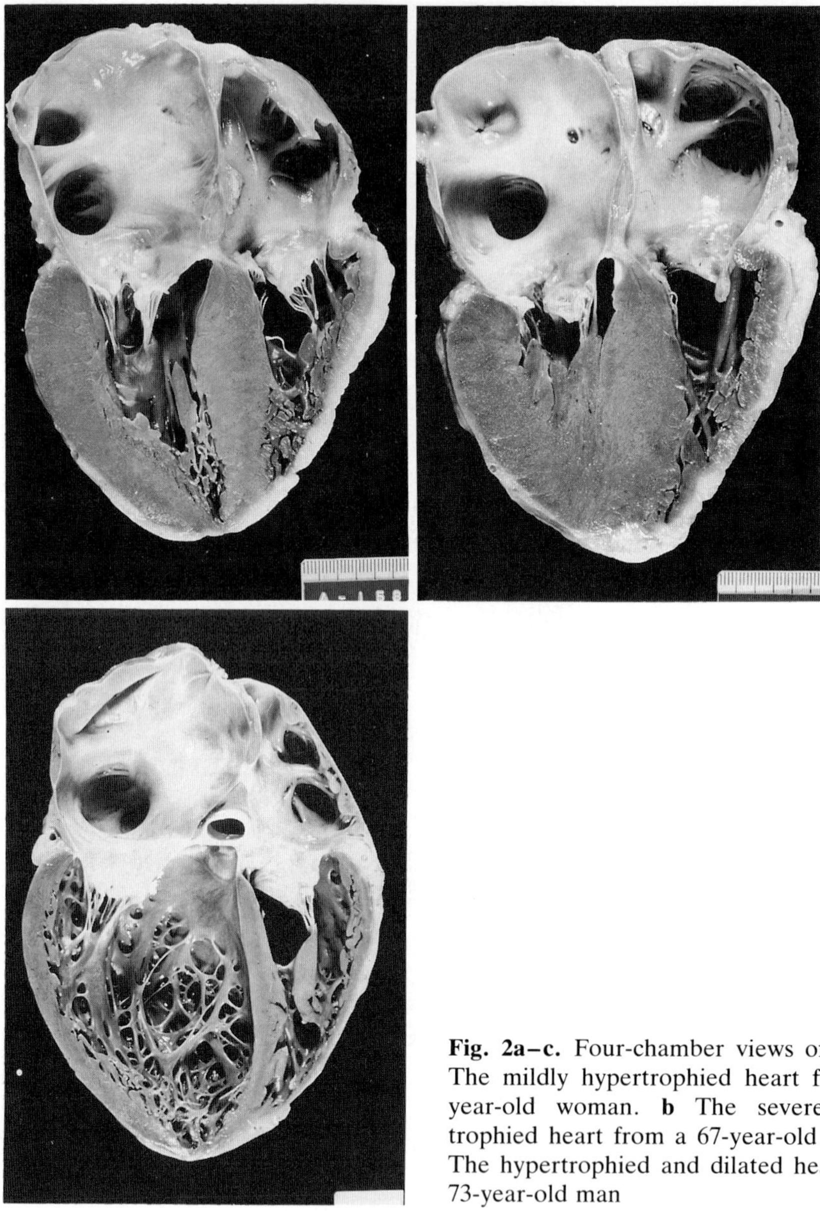

a b c

Fig. 2a–c. Four-chamber views of hearts. **a** The mildly hypertrophied heart from a 59-year-old woman. **b** The severely hypertrophied heart from a 67-year-old woman. **c** The hypertrophied and dilated heart from a 73-year-old man

patients (5 men and 7 women) who had a history of hypertension. Group 2 comprised 9 patients (5 men and 4 women) who had no history of hypertension. All patients died a noncardiac death at fifth to seventh decades and had no history of ischemic heart disease, heart failure, diabetes mellitus, or

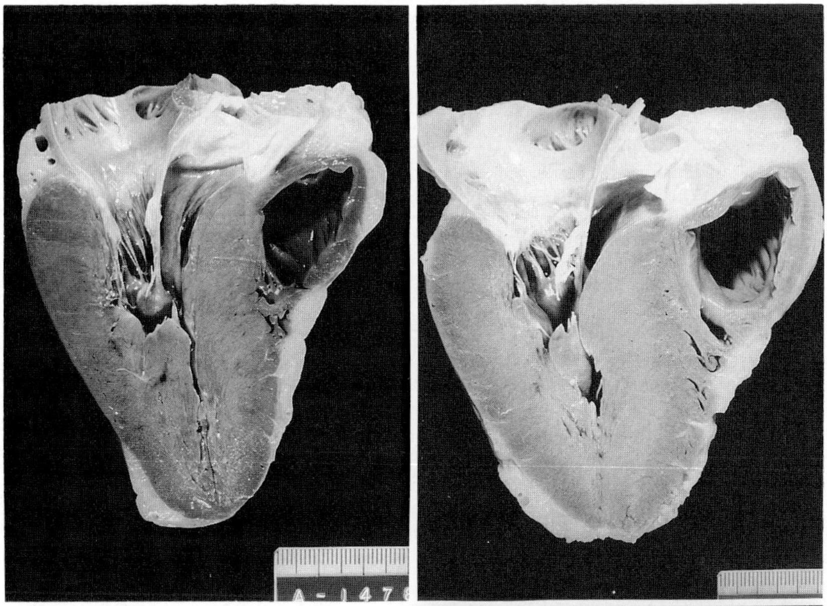

a b

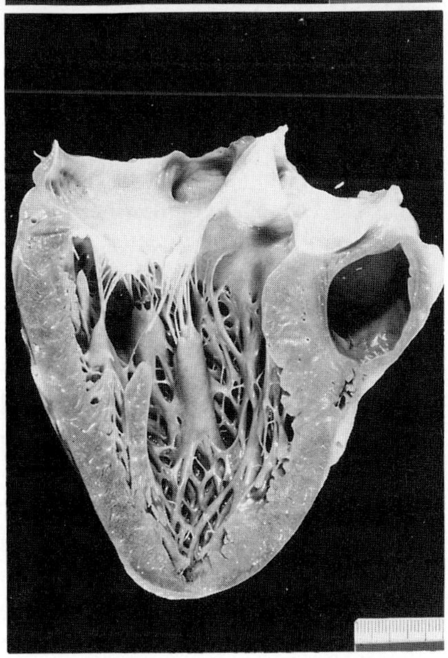

c

Fig. 3a–c. Left ventricular long-axis views of hearts. **a** The almost normal heart from a 53-year-old man. **b** The hypertrophied heart from a 59-year-old woman. **c** The hypertrophied and dilated heart from a 49-year-old man

hyperlipidemia. All hearts of group 1 were greater in weight than hearts of group 2, and the average heart weight showed a significant difference between the groups. The average circumference of aortic valve in group 1 was significantly greater than that of group 2, but the circumferences of other cardiac valves did not show a significant difference between both groups. Although

Table 1. Dimensions of heart (mean ± SD).

	Group 1 (hypertension +)	Group 2 (hypertension −)
Age (year)[1]	53 ± 8.5	62 ± 4.5
Male/female	5/4	5/7
Heart weight (g)[1]	285 ± 29	385 ± 34
Circumference of valves (cm)		
Tricuspid valve	9.2 ± 1.20	9.4 ± 1.39
Pulmonary valve	6.0 ± 0.91	6.0 ± 0.88
Mitral valve	8.1 ± 0.59	7.7 ± 0.60
Aortic valve[1]	5.9 ± 0.59	7.0 ± 0.63
Length of ventricles (cm)		
RV inflow portion[2]	5.3 ± 0.45	5.9 ± 0.77
RV outflow portion[3]	7.4 ± 0.39	7.3 ± 0.82
LV inflow portion[1,2]	6.1 ± 0.72	7.0 ± 0.79
LV outflow portion[3]	7.3 ± 0.57	7.8 ± 0.7
LV inner perimeter[4]	5.7 ± 1.02	5.8 ± 0.57
Thickness of wall (mm)		
RV	2.7 ± 0.42	2.7 ± 0.36
LV anterior wall[1]	12.7 ± 1.06	15.7 ± 2.11
LV lateral wall[1]	13.2 ± 1.01	15.8 ± 1.87
LV posterior wall[1]	13.1 ± 1.46	15.7 ± 1.75
Interventricular septum[1]	13.4 ± 1.51	16.4 ± 1.81

RV, right ventricle; LV, left ventricle.
[1] $P < 0.05$ when tested by two-tailed Student's *t*-test.
[2] Length of inflow portion: apex to atrioventricular valve annulus.
[3] Length of outflow portion: apex to semilunar valve annulus.
[4] LV inner perimeter: at the level of tip of papillary muscle.

these significant differences are thought to be mainly due to arterial hypertension, greater aging in group 1 might contribute to increase in heart weight and circumference of aortic valve [10–12]. The average length from apex to mitral annulus was significantly longer in group 1 than in group 2, whereas the average inner perimeter of the left ventricle at the level of the tip of the papillary muscles did not show a significant difference between two groups. This result reflected the elongated contour in concentric hypertrophy. The average wall thicknesses of left ventricle and interventricular septum in group 1 were significantly greater than those in group 2. However, some hearts of group 2 had thicker ventricular walls than some of group 1, in spite of the smaller heart weight. The condition in which the heart stopped, in systole or in diastole, probably affected the wall thickness. Although the average surface areas of anterior and posterior leaflets of the mitral valve did not show a significant difference between the groups, the surface areas of both leaflets in group 1 tended to be greater than those in group 2.

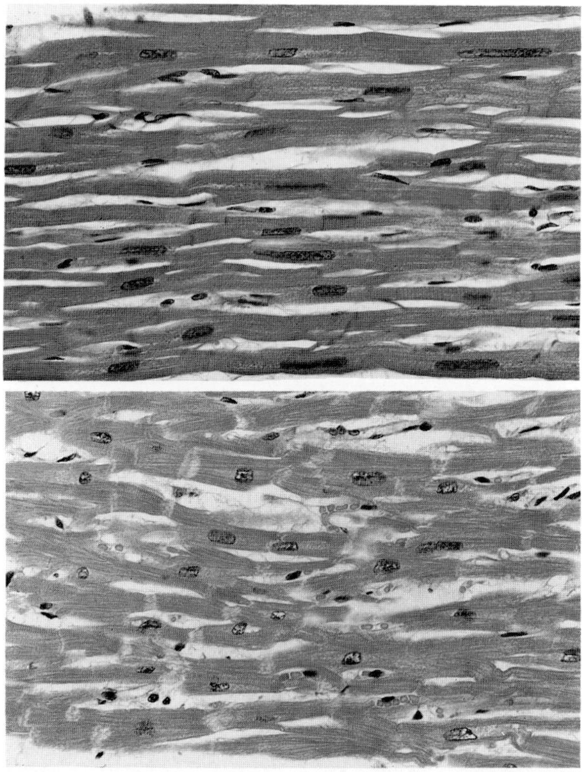

a

b

Fig. 4a,b. Histology of almost normal and hypertrophied hearts under the same magnification. **a** The normal myocardial cells are cylindrical or Y-shaped and have an elongated nucleus. (Hematoxylin-eosin ×350) **b** The hypertrophied muscle cells show a more irregular and less cylindrical shape than the normal cells, and their nuclei are enlarged and rectangular in shape. (Hematoxylin-eosin ×350)

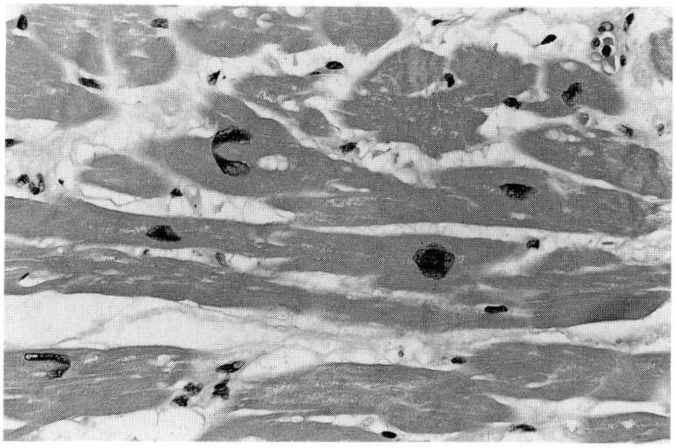

Fig. 5. Histology of the heart from 54-year-old man with dilated cardiomyopathy. The nuclei of myocardial cells show bizarre shapes and a pronounced degree of enlargement. (Hematoxylin-eosin ×350)

Histology

In the hypertrophic heart, longitudinal sections of myocardial fibers are wider than those of normal fibers, and also there are increases in the transverse diameters of the muscle cells. The diameter of a normal myocardial cell is 12 ±

2 μm in the right ventricle and 14 ± 2 μm in the left ventricle. On the basis of average cellular diameter, hypertrophy may be graded as mild (16–20 μm), moderate (21–25 μm), or marked (more than 25 μm) [13]. Usually, myocardial cells do not show uniform hypertrophy, and there are marked variations in the diameters of myocardial cells. The normal myocardial cell is cylindrical, often Y-shaped, and has an elongated nucleus. Hypertrophied muscle cells show a more irregular and less smoothly cylindrical shape than normal cells. The nuclei of hypertrophic muscle cells are enlarged and show a rectangular outline in longitudinal section (Fig. 4). Also, hypertrophic myocardial fibers may have a variety of nuclear shapes which include horseshoe, staghorn, and dumbbell shapes, eccentric location, double nuclei, groups of small nuclei set close together in a row, and nuclei with deep longitudinal grooves. The nuclei in hearts of patients with cardiomyopathy usually exhibit bizarre shapes and pronounced degrees of enlargement (Fig. 5). The increase in nuclear basophilia is considered to be related to polyploidy. The cytoplasm of hypertrophied cardiac muscle cells may not show any abnormal features, and myofibrillar changes are very difficult to detect by light microscopy. In hearts with long-

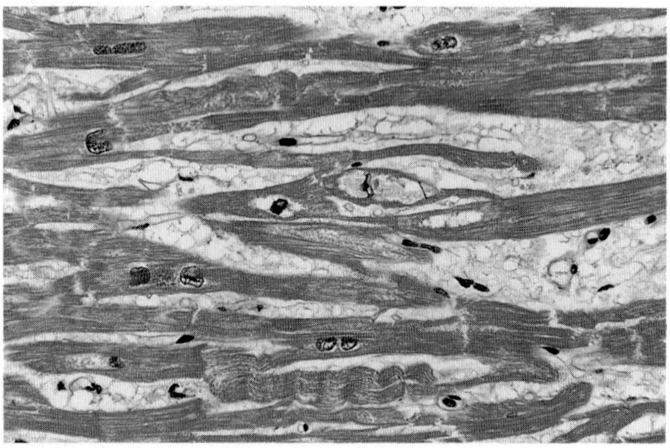

Fig. 6. Histology of the hypertrophied heart. Some myocardial cells show degenerative changes such as increased pigment adjacent to the nuclear poles, and basophilic degeneration. A myocardial cell has double nuclei. (Hematoxylin-eosin ×350)

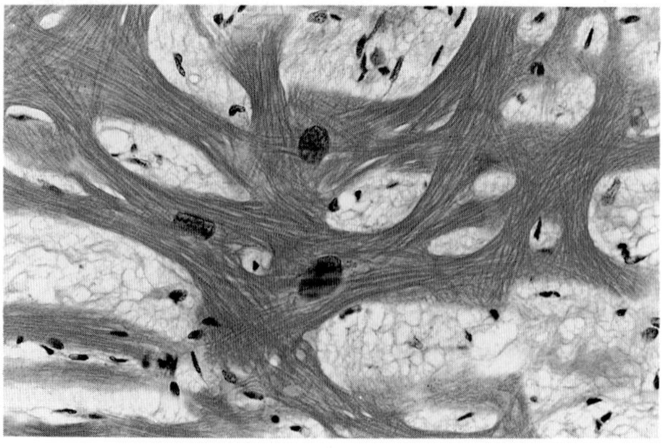

Fig. 7. Histology of the hypertrophic cardiomyopathy. The myocardial cells show severe hypertrophy with nuclear enlargement and myocyte disarray. (Hematoxylin-eosin ×350)

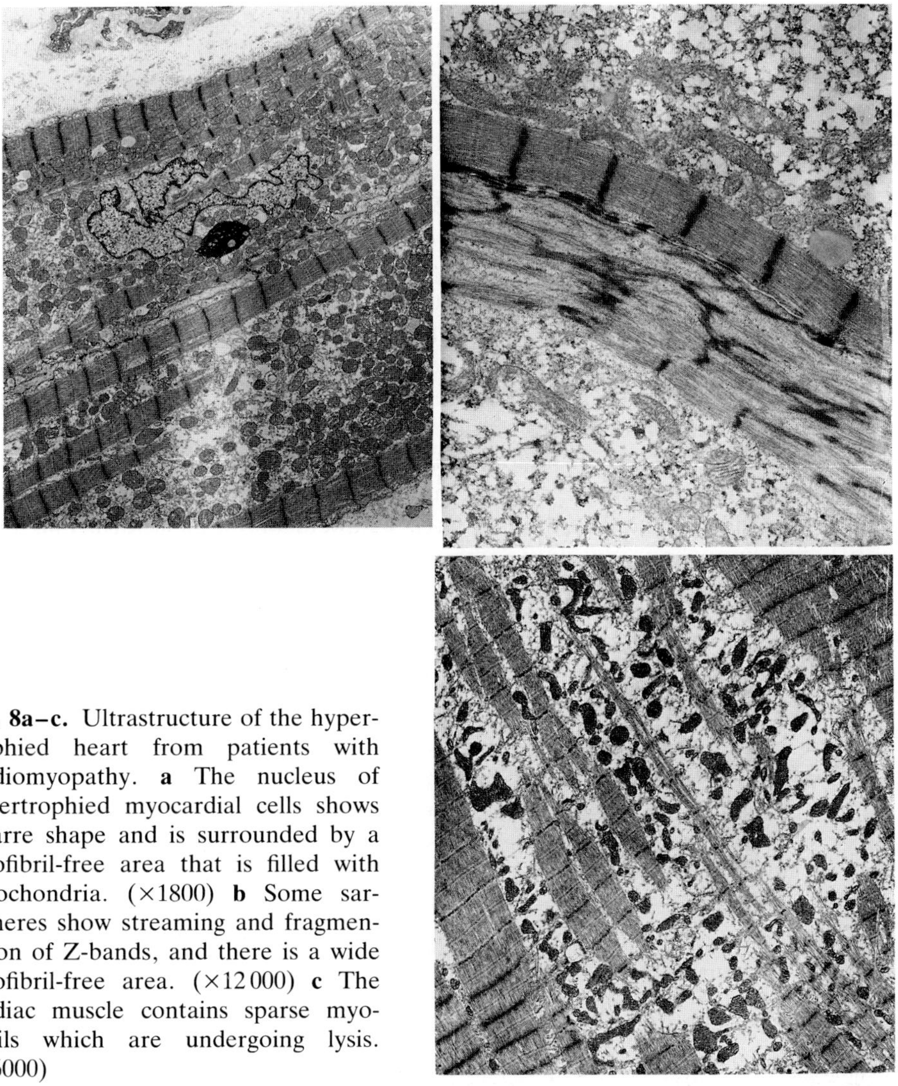

a b c

Fig. 8a–c. Ultrastructure of the hypertrophied heart from patients with cardiomyopathy. **a** The nucleus of hypertrophied myocardial cells shows bizarre shape and is surrounded by a myofibril-free area that is filled with mitochondria. (×1800) **b** Some sarcomeres show streaming and fragmentation of Z-bands, and there is a wide myofibril-free area. (×12000) **c** The cardiac muscle contains sparse myofibrils which are undergoing lysis. (×6000)

standing hypertrophy, some degenerative changes may be seen in myocardial fibers. These comprise vacuolization, increased pigment adjacent to the nuclear poles, basophilic and fatty degeneration, and coagulation and clumping of myofibrils (Fig. 6). In the usual type of hypertrophy, the orderly arrangement of cardiac muscle cells is maintained, but this arrangement is abnormal in hypertrophic cardiomyopathy (Fig. 7). The endocardial thickening and diffuse interstitial fibrosis develop gradually.

Ultrastructurally, the hexagonal array of the myofilaments, the dimensions of the sarcomeres, and the diameter of the thick and thin filaments are similar in normal and hypertrophied muscle cells [14]. Therefore, hypertrophy is not mediated by alterations in size of the contractile elements. However, hypertrophied muscle cells show various ultrastructural changes according to the cause and stage of the hypertrophy (Fig. 8). The ultrastructural changes in hypertrophied cardiac muscle cells have been described as correlating with three phases of cardiac hypertrophy: adaptive growth, a prolonged state of successful adaptation, and failure [4,15].

In the adaptive phase of hypertrophy, cardiac muscle cells show enlargement accompanied by the addition of large numbers of compact myofibrils and mitochondria, but no evidence of degeneration. Nuclei are enlarged and irregular in shape with coiled, ribbon-like nucleoli. There is an increased number of free ribosomes and of cisterns of rough surfaced endoplasmic reticulum in the perinuclear area. The Golgi complexes are enlarged and the intercellular junctions show increased width and extent of folding.

In the prolonged state of adaptation, the changes found in the first stage of hypertrophy tend to become less prominent. Muscle cells are characteristically larger than normal and contain greater numbers of mitochondria and myofibrils, but may show few or no abnormalities in their organelles. Intramitochondrial glycogen, various nuclear abnormalities, and abnormal multiple intercalated disks may be observed.

The late stage of hypertrophy is characterized by degenerative changes in the muscle cells and by interstitial fibrosis. Mildly altered cells are either normal in size or hypertrophied, and show a variable degree of focal myofibrillar loss with preferential loss of thick filaments and mild proliferation of sarcoplasmic reticulum or other organelles. Z-band material may show streaming, streaking, clumping, and fragmentation. Moderately and severely degenerated cells are either normal in size or atrophied and show further progression of the changes that are present in mild degeneration. There are extensive myofibrillar lysis and loss of T tubules, and the myofibril-free areas of these cells are filled with cytoplasmic organelles such as sarcoplasmic reticulum, glycogen, or mitochondria which underwent proliferation. Moderately and severely degenerated cells were present in areas of fibrosis, had thickened basement membranes, and had lost their intercellular connections.

Morphometric Analysis

Although the various changes just mentioned are present in the hypertrophied heart, one may feel that there is little evidence on microscopic examination to confirm the grossly obvious changes and to correlate the structural changes with cardiac function. The mean myocardial fiber diameter may be different in various diseases. Also the amount of fibrillar collagen, its distribution in the myocardium, and intramyocardial arteriole wall thickening can differ with various disease states despite a similar increment in myocytic diameter. Quantitative observations on human hypertrophied hearts, although relatively small in number, showed the increases of myocytic diameter and fibrous content.

Table 2. Morphometric data of heart (mean ± SD).

	Group 1 (hypertension +)	Group 2 (hypertension −)
Width of myocyte (μm)		
RV*	13.3 ± 0.91	15.8 ± 1.65
LV anterior wall*	15.0 ± 0.82	20.3 ± 1.76
LV lateral wall*	15.7 ± 0.82	21.2 ± 1.57
LV posterior wall*	15.7 ± 0.89	21.0 ± 1.56
Interventricular septum*	14.8 ± 1.07	20.2 ± 0.86
Content of myocyte (%)		
RV	77.3 ± 8.34	74.7 ± 8.17
LV anterior wall*	80.9 ± 5.38	75.6 ± 4.81
LV lateral wall	80.3 ± 7.52	76.6 ± 4.91
LV posterior wall	78.8 ± 5.21	75.4 ± 6.68
Interventricular septum	77.0 ± 5.73	75.4 ± 3.42
Content of fibrosis (%)		
RV	1.08 ± 0.65	1.09 ± 0.41
LV anterior wall*	0.64 ± 0.29	1.53 ± 0.72
LV lateral wall*	0.84 ± 0.62	1.50 ± 0.62
LV posterior wall*	0.99 ± 0.49	1.66 ± 0.56
Interventricular septum	1.17 ± 0.73	1.58 ± 0.66

RV, right ventricle; LV, left ventricle.
* $P < 0.05$ when tested by two-tailed Student's t-test.

The morphometric analysis of cardiac hypertrophy has been performed to elucidate the difference of cardiac hypertrophy in various disease states such as volume- and pressure-overload [16–19], and the myocardial structural changes after aortic valve replacement [20,21], and to correlate structural changes with reduced cardiac function [22] and tolerance to ischemia [23]. Table 2 shows the quantitation of myocardial fiber hypertrophy and contents of myocyte and fibrosis in the same autopsied hearts as those used in Table 1. The following method was used in this morphometric analysis. A transverse slice from the middle third of the heart was routinely processed. Each paraffin-embedded slice was sectioned at a thickness of 6 μm, and these sections were stained with elastic van Gieson, Masson's trichrome, and hematoxylin-eosin. The diameters of ventricular myocytes were determined by measuring the distance across the nuclei on longitudinally cut myocytes. At least 200 myocytes were measured in each of the following regions of the hearts: anterior, lateral, and posterior walls of left ventricle, interventricular septum, and right ventricle. Using the well-established point-counting method, the contents of myocyte, fibrosis, and other tissues were determined from 30 random fields in each region of the autopsied heart at a higher magnification with a grid of 100 points. The average diameters of myocardial fiber were significantly greater in all regions of group 1 than in corresponding regions of group 2. The average diameters in all regions of the left ventricle and interventricular septum of group 1 showed a similar increase and reflected the nature of concentric hypertrophy. Although the average contents of myocytes in all areas except the anterior wall of the left ventricle showed no significant difference between group 1 and group 2, the average contents of fibrosis in the left ventricle of group 1 increased significantly when compared with that of group 2. These data appeared to be similar to those from other studies and suggested that there is an increase in the content of fibrosis even in hearts which seemed to be in adaptive growth and a prolonged state of successful adaptation.

References

1. Messerli FH (1983) Clinical determinants and consequences of left ventricular hypertrophy. Am J Med 75:51–56
2. Grant RP (1953) Architectonics of the heart. Am Heart J 46:405–431
3. Hutchins GM, Bulkley BH, Moore GW, Piasio MA, Lohr FT (1978) Shape of the human cardiac ventricles. Am J Cardiol 41:646–654
4. Ferrans VJ (1984) Cardiac hypertrophy: morphological aspect. In: Zak R (ed) Growth of the heart in health and disease. Raven, New York, pp 187–239
5. Linzbach AJ (1960) Heart failure from the point of view of quantitative anatomy. Am J Cardiol 5:370–382
6. Hangartner JRW, Marley NJ, Whitehead A, Thomas AC, Davis MJ (1985) The assessment of cardiac hypertrophy at autopsy. Histopathology 9:1295–1306
7. Zeek PM (1942) Heart weight. 1. The weight of the normal human heart. Arch Pathol 34:820–832
8. Silver MM (1983) Gross examination and structure of the heart. In: Silver MD (ed) Cardiovascular pathology, vol 1. Churchill Livingstone, pp 1–30
9. Roberts WC, Ferrans VJ (1975) Pathologic anatomy of the cardiomyopathies. Idiopathic dilated and hypertrophic types, infiltrative types, and endomyocardial disease with and without eosinophilia. Hum Pathol 6:287–342
10. Eckner FAO, Brown BW, Davidson DL, Glagov S (1969) Dimensions of normal human hearts. After standard fixation by controlled pressure coronary perfusion. Arch Pathol 88:497–507
11. Krovetz LJ (1975) Age-related changes in size of the aortic valve annulus in man. Am Heart J 90:569–574
12. Silver MA, Roberts WC (1985) Detailed anatomy of the normally functioning aortic valve in hearts of normal and increase weight. Am J Cardiol 55:454–461
13. Edwards WD (1987) Applied anatomy of the heart. In: Brandenburg RO, Fuster V, Giuliani ER, McGoon DC (eds) Cardiology. Fundamentals and practice. Year Book Publishers, Chicago, London, pp 47–112
14. Richter GW, Kellner A (1963) Hypertrophy of the human heart at the level of fine structure. An analysis and two postulates. J Cell Biol 18:195–206
15. Marron BJ, Ferrans VJ, Roberts WC (1975) Ultrastructural features of degenerated cardiac muscle in patients with cardiac hypertrophy. Am J Pathol 79:387–434
16. Fuster V, Danielson MA, Rob RA, Broadbent JC, Brown AL Jr, Elveback R (1977) Quantitation of left ventricular myocardial fiber hypertrophy and interstitial

tissue in human hearts chronically increased volume and pressure overload. Circulation 55:504–508

17. Schaper J (1983) Hypertrophy in the human heart: evaluation by qualitative and quantitative light and electron microscopy. In: Alpert NR (ed) Perspective in cardiovascular research, vol 7, Myocardial hypertrophy and failure. Raven, New York, pp 177–196
18. Tanaka M, Fujiwara H, Onodera T, Wu DJ, Matsuda M, Hamashima Y, Kawai C (1987) Quantitative analysis of narrowing of intramyocardial small arteries in normal hearts, hypertensive hearts, and hearts with hypertrophic cardiomyopathy. Circulation 75:1130–1139
19. Schwartzkopff B, Frenzel H, Dieckerhoff J, Betz P, Flasshove M, Schulte HD, Mundhenke M, Motz W, Strauer BE (1992) Morphometric investigation of human myocardium in arterial hypertension and valvular aortic stenosis. Eur Heart J 13[Suppl D]:17–23
20. Schwarz F, Flameng W, Schaper J, Hehrlein F (1979) Correlation between myocardial structure and diastolic properties of the heart in chronic aortic valve disease: effects of corrective surgery. Am J Cardiol 42:895–903
21. Krayenbuehl HP, Hess OM, Monrad ES, Schneider J, Mall G, Turina M (1989) Left ventricular myocardial structure in aortic valve disease before, intermediate, and late after aortic valve replacement. Circulation 79:744–755
22. Schaper J, Schaper W (1983) Ultrastructural correlates of reduced cardiac function in human heart disease. Eur Heart J 4[Suppl A]:35–42
23. Ferreira R, Milei J, Forcada P, Beigelman R, Molteni L, Cutrin JC (1992) The hypertrophied myocardium and coronary disease. Structural changes in patients submitted to aortocoronary bypass surgery. Int J Cardiol 36:203–212

2.7 Interstitial Collagenase Activation Initiates Left Ventricular Remodeling

Calvin Eng, Robert H. Charney, Francis M. Siri, and Mengjia Zhao[1]

Summary. The extracellular collagen matrix of the heart serves an important role in maintaining the configuration and dimensions of the heart. The myocardium undergoes an expansion and dilatation process as a result of nonlethal ischemic injury (stunning) which is due to extensive alterations and degradation of the matrix. This acute remodeling process of the heart involves in situ activation of latent procollagenase in the cardiac interstitium. The present study documented a twofold increase in collagenolytic activity of cardiac lymph from stunned myocardium. There was also a two- to threefold increase in cardiac lymph flow rate during the course of the stunning protocol, a result compatible with the intracellular and extracellular edema noted on ultrastructural studies of stunned myocardium. Possible mechanisms of ischemia-induced activation of latent interstitial collagenase are reviewed.

Key words: Collagenase—Collagen—Myocardial ischemia—Cardiac remodeling—Cardiac lymph

Introduction

The process whereby the heart undergoes macroscopic change in dimension and remodeling must involve the extracellular collagen matrix and the predominant enzyme which degrades collagen, collagenase. We have shown that substantial damage to the extracellular collagen matrix occurs in stunned myocardium [1,2]. This translated into dilatation and expansion of the reperfused region of the heart. Although there was a modest 10% loss of hydroxy-

[1] Cardiology Section, Veteran's Administration Medical Center, 130 W. Kingsbridge Rd., Bronx, New York 10468, and the Mount Sinai School of Medicine, New York, NY, USA

proline content in the stunned myocardium, the ultrastructural picture indicated extensive alterations and degradation of the matrix, with remnant matrix left in situ [1]. Tissue homogenates from the stunned myocardium had 73% greater collagenase activity than those from the normal region of the heart [2]. This was the presumed basis for the acute ischemic remodeling of the ventricle.

For events and processes that occur in the cardiac interstitium, it would be highly desirable to isolate and compartmentalize the experimental measurements to the interstitium. Tissue homogenate data would only provide a nonspecific assessment. Purified tissue extract measurements are also not anatomically specific. The interstitium is composed of the extracellular "gel," matrix, and residential cells such as fibroblasts, macrophages, and mast cells. These structural and cellular components are bathed in the extracellular fluid. Depending on the experimental conditions, this extracellular fluid may contain expressed proteins, enzymes, growth factors, as well as a host of other substances (e.g., peroxides and oxygen-derived free radicals). Access to this extracellular fluid can be gained by collecting lymphatic fluid draining the organ. With some minor anatomic variations, the lymphatic system draining the heart converges into main trunks entering a cardiac lymph node in the mediastinum. Lymph fluids accessed in this manner have demonstrated the early appearance of cardiac enzymes and cytokines during myocardial infarction [3–6]. The following initial study was performed to quantitate lymph flow hemodynamics during a multiple coronary occlusion-reperfusion stunning protocol as well as to assess directly the collagenolytic activity in cardiac lymph.

Methods

Animal Preparation

Six mongrel dogs of both sexes with a mean weight of 25.9 kg (range 22–30 kg) were anesthetized with pentobarbital (30 mg/kg i.v.). After intubation, the animals were placed on an intermittent positive pressure respirator with oxygen supplementation. A midline thoracotomy was performed to expose the heart, great vessels, and the mediastinum. The pericardium was opened and the heart was suspended in a pericardial cradle. Evans Blue dye, 0.05 ml, was injected directly into a region near the apex of the left ventricle. After approximately 10 min, the mediastinum was dissected to expose the cardiac lymphatic system (containing blue dye) located between the superior vena cava and the right brachiocephalic artery. The inferior base of the cardiac lymph node was tied off with several (4-0) silk sutures resulting in distension of the lymphatics. Several drops of 2% lidocaine were also topically applied on the area of interest. The largest lymphatic was identified, the soft tissue underneath was dissected free, and a silk ligature was placed around the vessel. Approximately one half of the lymphatic was cut transversely with microsurgical scissors. A tapered end of polyethylene tubing (PE60) was inserted into the lymphatic, and secured in place with the ligature. The tubing was approximately 60 cm long, and the other end was placed at heart level for continuous lymph fluid collection.

The proximal left circumflex coronary artery was dissected free for coronary occlusion with a snare during the ischemia protocol. Pairs of ultrasonic crystals (1.5 mm in diameter) connected to an ultrasonic dimension system (Scheussler and Associates, Cardiff by the Sea, CA, USA) were implanted in the endocardial region at midventricle, in both the left anterior descending and the left circumflex coronary artery perfusion regions.

Cardiac lymph was collected for 15 min in a continuous and sequential manner in pre-tared 1.5-ml polypropylene Eppendorf centrifuge tubes. The collections were performed with the tubes on ice. After each collection period, the tube was capped, externally wiped dry, and reweighed. The scale used was accurate to 1 μg. Lymph flow rate was calculated and expressed in grams per hour. In four experiments, after reweighing, the tubes were centrifuged for 10 min at 8000 × g in a microcentrifuge (Eppendorf 5415C) at 4°C. The supernatant was decanted and transferred to a fresh tube which was then frozen in dry ice–acetone and stored at −70°C.

Control cardiac lymph was collected for 30 min (two 15-min collections) during stable hemodynamics. A multiple occlusion ischemia-reperfusion stunning protocol was then initiated where 5 min of coronary occlusion was followed by 10 min of reperfusion. This procedure was repeated 12 times [1,2]. Lymph collections were made continuously for each occlusion and reperfusion cycle of 15 min.

Collagenase Assay

Acid-soluble ^{3}H-collagen (rat type I) with a specific activity of 0.26 mCi/mg (New England Nuclear, NET-660, Boston, MA, USA) was used to measure collagenolytic activity of the cardiac lymph. Ten microliters of the labeled soluble collagen (0.06 mCi/ml) was incubated with 80 μl of calcium buffer (20 m*M* Tris-HCl, pH7.6, 5 m*M* $CaCl_2$) at 4°C for 2 h in a 1.5-ml polypropylene microcentrifuge tube. After fibril formation, 10 μl of cardiac lymph was added. The tubes were capped and incubated at 37°C for 23 h with gentle agitation in a temperature-controlled water bath. After incubation, the samples were centrifuged at 12 000 g for 10 min at 4°C. A 10 μl aliquot of the supernatant, representing lymph collagenolytic activity, was counted in a liquid scintillation counter. Ten microliters (100 μg) of bacterial collagenase (Sigma, Type 1A, St. Louis, MO, USA) was then added to the reaction tube, and allowed to stand for 24 h at room temperature. A 10 μl aliquot of this supernatant, representing complete collagenolysis, was counted, These data were used to determine the individual amount of collagen in each reaction tube. Collagenolytic activity in the lymph fluid was calculated and expressed in units/ml of lymph fluid, where one unit of activity liberated 1 μg of collagen/h at 37°C. Collagenolytic activity was also expressed in units/100 mg of protein in the lymph fluid. Total protein content of the lymph fluid was determined calorimetrically using a biuret reagent reaction and protein standards (Sigma).

Data Analysis

Summary data are expressed as mean ± SEM. One-way analysis of variance with repeated measures was utilized to assess the data. Post hoc Newman-Keuls testing was performed after significant F values. A $P < 0.05$ was considered significant.

Results

In the six experiments, the control (C) lymph flow rate was 2.376 ± 0.575 g/h (mean ± SEM; range: 0.412–4.376). The lymph flow rate during the stunning protocol is summarized in Fig. 1. The flow rate increased after the sixth reperfusion period, rising to a value of 5.130 ± 0.836 g/h (range: 3.408–8.932) at the end of the protocol. The latter three flow values were significant compared to control and the sixth reperfusion period [one-way analysis of variance (ANOVA) with repeated measures].

In four of the six experiments, the cardiac lymph was assessed for collagenolytic activity. Samples from baseline control, the seventh reperfusion period, and 15 min after the final reperfusion period were assayed for protein and collagenase activity. The latter two periods were chosen to assess the

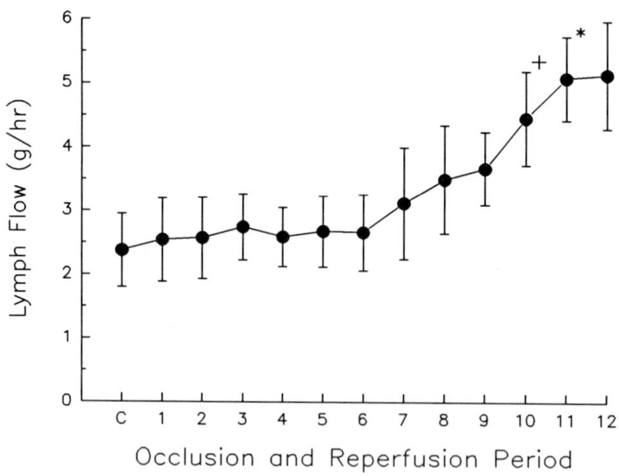

Fig. 1. Lymph flow during the stunning protocol ($n = 6$). Timed collections of 15 min duration were performed during control and 12 occlusion and reperfusion periods. Lymph flow rate begins to increase by the seventh occlusion and reperfusion period. The lymph flow rate at the end of the protocol was twice the rate of the control and during the first six periods. *Error bars* represent standard error of the mean. Analysis of variance with repeated measures was performed on the data with Newman-Keuls post hoc testing. *, $P < 0.001$ compared to control, and $P < 0.005$ compared to period #6. ', $P < 0.025$ compared to control, and $P < 0.05$ compared to periods #6

Table 1. Lymph flow and biochemical measurements.

Experiment number[a]	Lymph flow (ml/h)	Collagenase activity[b] (units/ml)	Lymph protein (g/100 ml)	Collagenase activity[b] (units/100 mg)	Collagenase flux[b] (units/h)	Protein flux (mg/h)
I-A	0.706	78.360	4.040	193.960	55.322	0.285
I-B	2.748	88.180	3.638	242.386	242.319	1.000
I-C	8.932	133.570	2.291	583.021	1193.047	2.046
II-A	2.704	66.860	5.146	129.926	180.789	1.391
II-B	3.386	87.170	4.121	211.526	295.158	1.395
II-C	3.408	93.850	3.899	240.703	319.841	1.329
III-A	2.662	82.490	5.053	163.250	219.588	1.345
III-B	6.776	85.130	3.120	272.853	576.841	2.114
III-C	8.720	124.540	2.641	471.564	1085.989	2.303
IV-A	2.704	87.900	4.498	195.420	237.682	1.216
IV-B	3.288	105.900	3.330	318.018	348.199	1.095
IV-C	3.528	110.030	3.445	319.390	388.186	1.215

[a] Experiments I, II, III, and IV. A, control; B, reperfusion #7; C, final reperfusion.
[b] One unit of collagenase activity = 1 μg of collagen liberated/hour at 37°.

activity at approximately the midpoint and end of the protocol. The results are tabulated in Table 1. Control collagenolytic activity was 78.9 ± 4.5 units/ml or 170 ± 15 units/100 mg protein. At the seventh reperfusion period, activity was 91.6 ± 4.8 units/ml or 261 ± 23 units/100 mg protein. Fifteen minutes after the final reperfusion period, collagenolytic activity was 115.5 ± 8.7 units/ml or 404 ± 77 units/100 mg protein. The latter values were significantly increased compared to baseline, $P < 0.01$ (one-way ANOVA with repeated measures). Collagenolytic activity in the lymph fluid increased significantly when normalized to either lymph volume or protein content. There was a progressive decline in lymph protein content during the stunning protocol: from 4.68 ± 0.26 g/100 ml at control to 3.55 ± 0.22 ($P < 0.03$ compared to control) at the seventh reperfusion period, and 3.07 ± 0.37 ($P < 0.01$ compared to control) at the end of the protocol.

The "flux" or production of collagenase activity in the lymph fluid was calculated as the product of the lymph flow rate (ml/h) and the collagenase activity (units/ml). Collagenolytic flux showed a progressive increase from 173.3 ± 41.1 units/h at baseline control, to 365.6 ± 73.6 at the seventh reperfusion period, and 746.8 ± 228.2 units/h during the final reperfusion period. This trend did not achieve statistical significance; $P < 0.07$. Total protein "flux" in the lymph fluid was 1.059 ± 0.261 mg/h at baseline control, 1.401 ± 0.252 mg/h at the seventh reperfusion period, and 1.723 ± 0.267 mg/h at the final reperfusion period. These changes were not statistically significant.

Discussion

The present results provide further evidence that the elevated collagenolytic activity found in tissue homogenates of stunned myocardium [2] arises from the interstitium. Lymphatic fluid collagenolytic activity increased progressively during the stunning protocol, reaching a level approximately twice control baseline values. This was the case when collagenolytic activity was expressed either in units/ml of lymph fluid or units/100 mg of protein in the lymph fluid. The protein content of the lymph fluid decreased progressively during the ischemia-reperfusion protocol. This result is compatible with greater permeability of the ischemic vasculature. Ultrastructural findings of both intracellular and extracellular edema have been observed in stunned myocardium [1]. The product of the lymph flow rate and the protein content gives a measure of protein "flux" or production at given periods of the stunning protocol (Table 1). Protein "flux" did not significantly change during the course of the study, suggesting that the increase in lymph flow rate was predominantly due to increased vascular permeability to water. In contrast, the flux or production of collagenolytic activity showed a progressive increase, which did not achieve statistical significance ($P < 0.07$). If this result is confirmed with a greater number of experiments, it would suggest either a greater proportion of the procollagenase was activated during the protocol or that a time-dependent exogenous source of collagenase was contributing to the results. Based on the results of our previous study [2], the latter explanation would seem unlikely.

The lymph flow rate accurately reflects the hemodynamics during the particular collection period. Because of the slow flow rates, this is not the case for collagenolytic activity or any biochemical measurements of the lymph fluid. The transit time of the lymph fluid through the finite length of the collection tubing can be estimated, however. For PE60 tubing (i.d. = 0.03 in) of 60-cm length, approximately 8 min are required to reach the collection tube. Since each collection period was 15 min, the biochemical results would at most be shifted to one earlier time period.

In the study of Charney et al. [2], tissue homogenate collagenolytic activity was greater in the postischemic region as compared to the nonischemic region. However, after maximal activation of collagenase using aminophenylmercuric acetate there were no differences between the ischemic and nonischemic regions. In addition, cathepsin G and elastase levels were not different between the two regions. These results indicated that exogenous sources of protease were not a factor. Thus, the ischemic degradation of matrix was felt to be due to activation of preexisting latent collagenase in this model of sublethal ischemic injury. In ischemic models such as myocardial infarction, where infiltration of leukocytes is predominant, leukocyte collagenase, cathepsin G, and elastase would play a major role in matrix degradation. The neutral proteases cathepsin G and elastase can directly degrade fibrillar collagen even without participation of collagenase. In the following discussion, attention is directed at the activation of in situ latent collagenase under conditions where exogenous sources of protease are not involved. Such conditions are probably relevant in most cases of myocardial remodeling where an inflammatory response is not observed.

Activation of Collagenase

It is generally felt that interstitial collagenase exists in a latent or zymogen form. Immunohistochemical methods using antibodies to collagenase have demonstrated extensive localization in the interstitium of many organs including the heart [7]. The presumption is that the extracellular collagenase is predominantly inactive. Thus, fibroblast cell cultures or neutrophils are readily stimulated to secrete inactive procollagenase. Activation of the procollagenase is then achieved by use of a variety of known agents. The in vivo events which lead up to activation of collagenase have not been well defined. Certain in vitro activators of collagenase are probably not of physiological relevance: trypsin, aminophenylmercuric acetate, N-ethylmaleimide, sodium dodecyl sulfate, and thiocyanates. Potential physiologically relevant activators might include: plasmin, kallikrein, oxidized glutathione, hypochlorous acid, and tryptase. The molecular mechanism by which these agents activate collagenase has been reviewed [8,9]. In general, these agents produce an initial cleavage of the procollagenase molecule. By an apparent autocatalytic process, an additional segment is cleaved resulting in a partially active enzyme. This activity is produced by release of a cysteine residue that is in contact with a zinc structure located in the active site of the enzyme. The partially active collagenase can undergo additional autocatalytic cleavage resulting in a maximally active enzyme. This process is apparently slow. Alternatively, stromelysin, another matrix metalloproteinase, can directly cleave the partially active collagenase to produce the maximally active form.

Interstitial Collagenase Activation During Ischemia-Reperfusion

The setting of ischemia followed by reperfusion presents unique considerations for possible activation of procollagenase in the cardiac interstitium. Plasmin is a potent activator of collagenase. The inactive proenzyme, plasminogen, is found in most body fluids. Although it is generally felt that the fibrinolysis system is depressed in clinical ischemic syndromes, this assumption has not been well defined experimentally. Interstitial residential cells such as macrophages and fibroblasts can be stimulated to secrete plasminogen activators of the urokinase type. Alternatively, tissue-type plasminogen activator, produced by vascular endothelial cells, may diffuse back into the interstitial space. The combination of plasminogen and the potential release of activator during ischemia-reperfusion could thus be an important mechanism for ischemic degradation of matrix. This sequence of events needs to be explored experimentally. It is also of interest that the urokinase-type plasminogen activator, a serine protease in its own right, can directly cleave and activate type IV collagenase [10].

Intracellular glutathione participates importantly in maintaining cellular tolerance of oxidative stress. Numerous ischemia-reperfusion studies of the heart and other organs have indicated both a reduction of the reduced form of glutathione and release of the oxidized form of glutathione upon reperfusion. Assuming a myocyte source of the oxidized glutathione, its measurable increase in the venous effluent suggests that concentrations in the interstitium, which the substance must traverse in order to reach the vascular space, must be considerable. Thus, oxidized glutathione activation of latent interstitial collagenase may be a serious consideration in postischemic reperfusion settings. Caulfield and Wolkowicz [11] showed that perfusion of the isolated rat heart with oxidized glutathione resulted in marked ultrastructural loss of the collagen matrix. These results were also observed with in vivo intravenous infusions of oxidized glutathione.

Keller et al. [12] studied reoxygenation injury in an isolated perfused rat heart preparation. After 60 min of hypoxia, reoxygenation resulted in a marked release of myeloperoxidase in the coronary effluent. Since the crystalloid perfusate was cell free, the source of the myeloperoxidase was intrinsic. Immunohistochemical methods indicated that the residential mast cells were the source of the enzyme. Treatment with a mast cell degranulation inhibitor significantly attenuated the release of myeloperoxidase during reoxygenation. With a mast cell source of release, the local concentration of myeloperoxidase in the cardiac interstitium must have been several-fold greater than the impressively high levels measured in the coronary effluent. The particular relevance of myeloperoxidase in the cardiac interstitium is that this enzyme catalyzes the production of hypochlorous acid, with hydrogen peroxide as substrate. Numerous studies of ischemia-reperfusion in the heart have found the production of oxygen-derived free radicals upon reperfusion. The combination of peroxide generation and myeloperoxidase release is likely to result in production of hypochlorite. Hypochlorite is a potent activator of procollagenase, although it may not be as effective on fibroblast procollagenase as it is on leukocyte procollagenase [13]. Nevertheless, this potential system for activation of interstitial collagenase seems compelling in the ischemia-reperfusion setting. Given the interstitial residency of mast cells and evidence for their degranulation during ischemia-reperfusion [12], other mast cell granule substances should be considered as potential contributors to ischemic degradation of matrix. Two neutral serine proteases, tryptase and chymase, are specific for mast cells. The presence of chymase in mast cells appears to vary significantly among species. However, mast cell tryptase has been found in many species, and is considered a specific marker, along with histamine, for mast cell activity. Tryptase is a trypsin-like serine protease which is active under neutral conditions. There is evidence that tryptase activates stromelysin which in turn activates latent collagenase [14].

Acknowledgments. Supported in part by National Institutes of Health grant HL27219-11 and a Grant-in-Aid from the American Heart Association, New York City Affiliate.

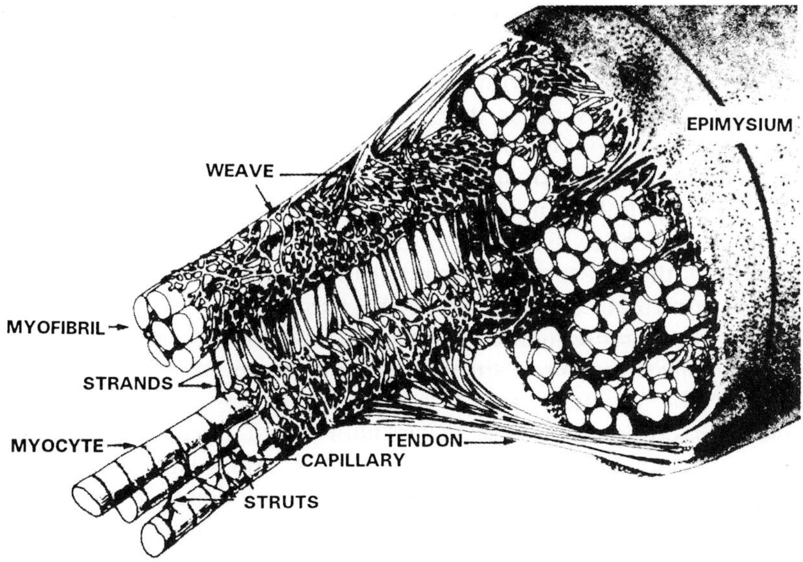

Fig. 1. Schematic depiction of the myocardial extracellular collagen matrix and its relation to myofibrils, myocytes, and capillaries. Shown are the epimysial, perimysial (i.e., tendon, weave, and strands) and endomysial (i.e., network surrounding myocyte and struts) components of the matrix. (From [52], with permission)

increases sixfold [12]. Based on this basal value and an assumed equilibrium, the half-life of myocardial collagen is estimated to be around 90 days.

Once deposited in fibrillar form and subsequently crosslinked, extracellular collagen is extremely stable and not easily degraded. Interstitial collagens consist of three peptide chains which intertwine to form a right-handed superhelix. This conformation makes interstitial collagens highly resistant to all proteinases except specific collagenases [13]. In the heart, the cellular source of collagenase is the fibroblast. Inflammatory cells, such as leukocytes and macrophages, add another dimension to collagenolytic activity in that they bring their proteolytic enzymes to the site of wound healing and inflammation. Because of the stability of fibrillar collagen, the rate limiting step in its degradation is the catalytic cleavage by interstitial collagenase. Once cleaved, collagen denatures and unwinds to form gelatin. Gelatinase then digests these products into smaller peptides that are further cleaved by nonspecific proteases [14]. A collagenase system has been identified within the myocardium by Montfort and Perez-Tamayo [15] using specific antibody and immunofluorescent staining. More recently, using immunofluorescence, we found collagenase to be concentrated in the endothelium and subendothelial space of the endocardium as well as throughout the interstitial space between groups of muscle fibers [16]. The amount of total collagenase in the rat myocardium was found to be 5 ± 2 pg/μg of tissue with 98% being latent [17].

Properties of Collagen that Affect Material Elasticity

Collagen is a stiff substance with low extensibility. Thus, small amounts of it in a composite material, such as the myocardium, could strongly influence the passive stress-strain relation of the material. Other characteristics besides the amount or concentration of fibrillar collagen may also be influential. These would include: spatial alignment of collagen, collagen fiber crimp properties, collagen fibril and fiber diameter, degree of crosslinking, and collagen types. Collagen fibers that are oriented parallel to the direction of locally generated stresses will contribute significantly to the elasticity of the composite material compared to an inconsequential influence from fibers which are aligned perpendicular to the direction of stress. The crimp property of fibrillar collagen is a measure of the amount to which a collagen fiber is corrugated. The greater the degree of crimping, the longer a fiber could be extended without the development of a significant stress. Thereafter, stress will increase exponentially. Coiled perimysial fibers oriented parallel or obliquely to the long axes of myocytes have been observed throughout the myocardium to undergo focal straightening as the myocardium is stretched [18]. Tissue that is subjected to a high tensile stress typically will have larger diameter collagen fibers that have a greater percentage of covalent crosslinks than tissue exposed to low stresses. Lastly, tissue with predominantly type I collagen (e.g., tendons) is stiffer than tissue with mostly type III collagen (e.g., uterus).

Functional Consequence of an Abnormal Increase in Myocardial Collagen

Interstitial fibrillar collagen is known to be increased from 40% to 150% in experimental [9,19–21] and genetic [20,22–24] hypertension. This remodeling of the collagen matrix consists of the following: an abnormal increase in collagen concentration related to fibroblast proliferation [25,26] and a sustained elevation in the collagen synthesis rate [12]; thickening of peri- and endomysial fibrils, fibers, and tendons; an increase in the density of the perimysial collagen weaves and myocyte collagen networks; newly formed collagen fibers; an expansion of perivascular collagen area; and microscopic scars. As a consequence of a rise in the concentration of this relatively inelastic material, both the myocardium and ventricle become stiffer. Bing and coworkers [19] noted hypertrophied papillary muscles with increased hydroxyproline concentration to be stiffer several days following the constriction of the aortic arch in rats. Holubarsch and colleagues [20] have argued that the increase in myocardial collagen which occurs in various forms of experimental hypertension in the rat was responsible for the greater diastolic stiffness found in the hypertrophied papillary muscle. Borg et al. [27] have hypothesized that the more extensive collagen weave separating myocyte groups in the hamster heart compared to that of the rat heart resulted in the twofold difference in ventricular stiffness between these two species. Subsequent studies have positively established a relation between myocardial and ventricular stiffness and collagen concentration in: the nonhuman primate with experimental hypertension [9]; in rats with renovascular [21], perinephritic [28], or genetic [22,23] hypertension; and in rats with myocardial fibrosis secondary to perinephritis and/or isoproterenol [28], or coronary embolization [29].

In addition to elevated collagen concentration in these models, a significant myocyte hypertrophy was noted. Several studies, however, have discounted the possibility that myocyte enlargement, not fibrosis, is responsible for the observed diastolic dysfunction. Bing et al. [30] prevented the increase in collagen content associated with chronic aortic constriction with β-amino proprionitrile and concluded that elevations in resting tension depend upon an increase in collagen content but not hypertrophy. Narayan and associates [22] were able to prevent myocyte hypertrophy in spontaneously hypertensive rats (SHR) with hydralazine but not the abnormal accumulation of collagen. The consequence of this fibrosis was an abnormally elevated passive myocardial stiffness which was similar to that measured in the untreated SHR with fibrosis and hypertrophy. Finally, Gelpi and colleagues [31] found left ventricular (LV) diastolic chamber compliance to be normal in dogs with normal collagen concentration and significant hypertrophy secondary to perinephritic hypertension.

From these experimental observations, it can be concluded that hypertrophy accompanied by a disproportionate increase in myocardial collagen represents a pathologic remodeling process. This also appears to be the case clinically. In the athlete with a significant increase in LV mass (i.e., physiologic hypertrophy), diastolic function is normal at rest and even enhanced during exercise [32,33], while in hypertensive patients with lesser amounts of hypertrophy, significant diastolic dysfunction is present [34] which is not related to the increase in LV mass [35,36]. Combining these clinical observations with experimental results and the postmortem finding that collagen concentration is increased in humans with systemic hypertension [24], it is reasonable to conclude that diastolic dysfunction in hypertensive patients is the result of abnormal accumulations of myocardial fibrillar collagen.

Functional Consequence of an Abnormal Decrease in Myocardial Collagen

As stated earlier, the rate limiting step in the degradation of fibrillar collagen is the catalytic cleavage by collagenase, which is normally present throughout the myocardium in its latent form. Evidence exists to indicate that with exposure to activated collagenase, myocardial collagen is rapidly degraded and as a result the ventricle dilates and becomes more compliant. For example, O'Brien and Moore [37] observed the LV pressure–volume curve in a nonliving rabbit heart with rigor to shift significantly to the right following a 90-min incubation in a solution of collagenase. This exogenous collagenase-induced increase in ven-

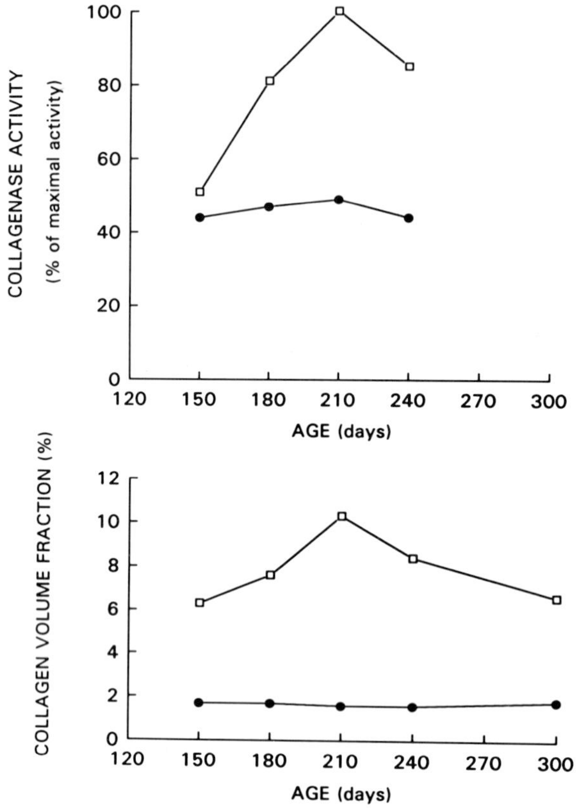

Fig. 2. Myocardial collagenase activity and collagen volume fraction at several ages in the cardiomyopathic hamster (*squares*) compared to age-matched golden Syrian hamsters (*circles*). At each age, both quantities are greater in the cardiomyopathic than in the control hamsters and both reached a maximum at an age of 210 days. It is around 240 days of age that the left ventricle of the cardiomyopathic hamster begins to dilate with thinning of its wall

tricular size and distensibility was not obtained after similar incubation times in saline, elastase, or trypsin. Studies in rats have indicated rapid collagen degradation within 24 h after experimental myocardial infarction. In addition, collagen breakdown was significantly greater in infarcted hearts of rats with normal leukocyte response than in rats with experimental leukopenia [38]. In infarcted regions, Takahashi et al. [39] reported decreases of up to 50% in myocardial collagen after 3 h of infarction. The loss was associated with a 2- to 3-fold increase in activities of tissue collagenase and lysosomal serine proteases. As a result of extensive collagen degradation, the infarcted region was noted to thin and expand outward during systole. Before healing, this area devoid of collagen is prone to rupture, particularly if the infarct is transmural [4,40].

Table 1. Structural and functional consequences of collagen degradation.

Group	%H_2O	CVF	Ultrastructural	V_0	Diastolic stiffness
3 h saline	↑ 2%*	↓ 12%*	↓	↑ 44%	↔
3 h glutathione	↑ 3%*	↓ 8%*	↓	↑ 58%	↔
3 weeks saline	↔	↓ 40%*	↔	↔	↔
3 weeks glutathione	↔	↓ 44%*	↓	↑ 69%*	↓ 35%*
5 weeks saline	↔	↓ 40%*	↔	↔	↔
5 weeks glutathione	↔	↓ 56%*	↔	↔	↔

* $P < 0.05$; ↑, increase; ↓, decrease; ↔, no change *vs* nonperfused, control group.

While these results suggest a major role of inflammatory cell collagenase in collagen breakdown during myocardial infarction, another consideration is that the increase in the sulfhydryl-active compound oxidized glutathione (GSSG), which is known to occur in the ischemic zone [41], activates latent collagenase in this area. GSSG has recently been shown to activate myocardial collagenases by Tyagi et al. [17]. This would explain the rapid disruption of collagen struts and loss of collagen weaves in stunned myocardium, where inflammatory infiltrate is not yet present [42,43]. Similar observations were made by Sato et al. [44] in the infarcted area within 2 to 3 h after coronary artery occlusion and prior to any appreciable influx of leukocytes.

We [45] and others [3] investigated the structural and functional consequences of collagen degradation using an assumed in vivo model of global collagenase activation (Table 1). Rats were infused either with ($n = 12$) or without ($n = 12$) 2 m*M* oxidized glutathione in 20 ml of 0.9% saline over 3 h on two occasions separated by a week. Total plasma protein concentration (TPC) was measured pre- and postinfusion. Three hours, 3 weeks, and 5 weeks after the second infusion, rats were killed and LV unstressed volume (V_0) and diastolic stiffness assessed. LV tissue was used to determine myocardial H_2O content (%H_2O) and amounts of microscopic—i.e., collagen volume fraction (CVF)—and ultrastructural fibrillar collagen. The results indicated: (a) hemodilution (22% decrease in TPC); (b) myocardial edema in the 3-h groups (c) degradation of myocardial ultrastructural and microscopic fibrillar collagen in the 3-h saline, 3-h glutathione and 3-week glutathione groups; (d) LV dilatation and increased diastolic compliance in groups with ultrastructural collagen degradation; and (e) a return to normal collagen ultrastructure and ventricular size and stiffness in the 3-week saline and 5-week glutathione groups. Thus the increase in ventricular size and compliance best correlated with the degradation of the ultrastructural components of the collagen matrix [45].

Evidence is accumulating to indicate that collagenase activation and fibrillar collagen breakdown are responsible for the dilatation, the change in shape, and the increase in distensibility of the cardiomyopathic left ventricle. We found that, in the cardiomyopathic hamster, left ventricular dilatation and wall thinning were associated with increased collagenase activity and degradation of collagen in the myocardium [46]. As can be seen in Fig. 2, collagenase activity was significantly increased in cardiomyopathic hamsters compared to that in age-matched golden Syrian hamsters. In golden Syrian hamsters, the collagen volume fraction was invariant with age, while in cardiomyopathic hamsters there was significant reparative fibrosis which reached a peak value at 210 days and subsequently declined. The age at which collagen began to decline corresponded to the age when maximum collagenase activation occurred. In the cardiomyopathic hamster, left ventricular dilatation and wall thinning become apparent around 240 days of age [47]. An inadequate myocardial collagen matrix has also been found in postmortem hearts of patients with dilated cardiomyopathy [48]. Thick coiled perimysial fibers were rare. Numerous widened interstitial spaces were present with conspicuous reduction or disruption of lateral connections of collagen between muscle fibers. A recently documented increase in collagenase activity in endomyocardial biopsies obtained from patients with dilated cardiomyopathy (i.e., 65% ± 34% *vs* 8% ± 5% measured in biopsies from post-transplant patients with assumed normal myocardium) [49] would account for the fibrillar collagen degradation seen in these patients.

Finally, in end-stage heart failure one would predict that an inadequate collagen matrix is responsible for the progressive left ventricular dilatation, together with wall thinning and sphericalization. Experimentally, chronic supraventricular tachycardia is widely used to create a model of heart failure. Within three weeks of rapid pacing, both ventricles are significantly dilated and wall thickness reduced. Histologic changes characteristic of collagen degradation including reduced collagen concentration, significant myocardial edema, and disrupted fibrillar collagen tethers have been reported to occur within 6 h of rapid ventricular pacing [50]. With continued rapid pacing, these changes were persistent for weeks [50,51]. After 3 weeks of rapid pacing Spinale et al. [51] found hydroxyproline concentration to be significantly reduced and associated with a large (8%) increase in myocardial water content. Thus, breakdown of myocardial fibrillar collagen appears to play a major role in the pathophysiology of heart failure.

References

1. Janicki JS, Matsubara BB (1993) Myocardial collagen and left ventricular diastolic function. In: Gaasch WH, LeWinter MM (eds) Left ventricular diastolic dysfunction. Lea and Febiger, Philadelphia, pp 125–140
2. Matsubara BB, Henegar JR, Janicki JS (1992) Functional and morphological consequences of induced myocardial collagen damage. Circulation 86:I-171
3. Caulfield JB, Norton P, Weaver RD (1992) Cardiac dilatation associated with collagen alterations. Mol Cell Biochem 118:171–179
4. Factor SM, Robinson TF, Dominitz R, Cho S (1986) Alterations of the myocardial skeletal framework in acute myocardial infarction with and without ventricular rupture. Am J Cardiovasc Pathol 1:91–97

5. Robinson TF, Factor SM, Sonnenblick EH (1986) The heart as a suction pump. Sci Am 254:84–91
6. Robinson TF, Cohen-Gould L, Factor SM (1983) The skeletal framework of mammalian heart muscle: arrangement of inter- and pericellular connective tissue structures. Lab Invest 49:482–487
7. Ahumada GG, Saffitz JE (1984) Fibronectin in rat heart: a link between cardiac myocytes and collagen. J Histochem Cytochem 32:383–388
8. Contard F, Koteliansky V, Marotte F, Dubus I, Rappaport L, Samuel J (1991) Specific alterations in the distribution of extracellular matrix components within rat myocardium during the development of pressure overload. Lab Invest 64:65–75
9. Weber KT, Janicki JS, Shroff SG, Pick R, Chen RM, Bashey RI (1988) Collagen remodeling of the pressure-overloaded, hypertrophied nonhuman primate myocardium. Circ Res 62:757–765
10. Eghbali M, Czaja MJ, Zeydel M, Weiner FR, Seifter S, Blumenfeld OO (1988) Collagen mRNAs in isolated adult heart cells. J Mol Cell Cardiol 20:267–276
11. Eghbali M, Blumenfeld OO, Seifter S, Buttrick PM, Leinwand LA, Robinson TF, Zern MA, Giambrone MA (1989) Localization of types I, III, IV collagen mRNAs in rat heart cells by in situ hybridization. J Mol Cell Cardiol 21:103–113
12. Bonnim CM, Sparrow MP, Taylor RR (1981) Collagen synthesis and content in right ventricular hypertrophy in the dog. Am J Physiol 241:H708–H713
13. Woolley DE (1984) Mammalian collagenases. In: Piez K, Reddi AH (eds) Extracellular matrix biochemistry. Elsevier, New York, pp 119–158
14. Woessner JF Jr (1991) Matrix metalloproteinases and their inhibitors in connective tissue remodeling. FASEB J 131:2145–2154
15. Montfort I, Perez-Tamayo R (1975) The distribution of collagenase in normal rat tissues. J Histochem Cytochem 23:910–920
16. Tyagi SC, Ratajska A, Weber KT (1994) Myocardial matrix metalloproteinase(s): localization and activation. Mol Cell Biochem 126:49–59
17. Tyagi SC, Matsubara L, Weber KT (1993) Direct activation and estimation of collagenase(s) activity by zymography in microquantities of rat myocardium and uterus. Clin Biochem 26:191–198
18. Robinson TF, Cohen-Gould L, Factor SM, Eghbali M, Blumenfeld OO (1988) Structure and function of connective tissue in cardiac muscle: Collagen types I and III in endomysial struts and pericellular fibers. Scanning Elect Microsc 2:1005–1015
19. Bing OHL, Matsushita S, Fanburg BL, Levine HJ (1971) Mechanical properties of rat cardiac muscle during experimental hypertrophy. Circ Res 28:234–245
20. Holubarsch CH, Holubarsch T, Jacob R, Medugorac I, Thiedemann K (1983) Passive elastic properties of myocardium in different models and stages of hypertrophy: A study comparing mechanical, chemical, and morphometric parameters. Perspect Cardiovasc Res 7:323–336
21. Doering CW, Jalil JE, Janicki JS, Pick R, Aghili S, Abrahams C, Weber KT (1988) Collagen network remodeling and diastolic stiffness of the rat left ventricle with pressure overload hypertrophy. Cardiovasc Res 22:686–695
22. Narayan S, Janicki JS, Shroff SG, Pick R, Weber KT (1989) Myocardial collagen and mechanics after preventing hypertrophy in hypertensive rats. Am J Hypertens 2:675–682
23. Brilla CG, Janicki JS, Weber KT (1991) Cardioprotective effects of lisinopril in rats with genetic hypertension and left ventricular hypertrophy. Circulation 83:1771–1779

24. Pearlman ES, Weber KT, Janicki JS, Pietra GG, Fishman AP (1982) Muscle fiber orientation and connective tissue content in the hypertrophied human heart. Lab Invest 46:158–164
25. Morkin E, Ashford TP (1968) Myocardial DNA synthesis in experimental cardiac hypertrophy. Am J Physiol 215:1409–1413
26. Skosey JL, Zak R, Martin AF (1972) Biochemical correlates of cardiac hypertrophy. V. Labeling of collagen, myosin and nuclear DNA during experimental myocardial hypertrophy in the rat. Circ Res 31:145–157
27. Borg TK, Ranson WF, Moshlehy FA, Caulfield JB (1981) Structural basis of ventricular stiffness. Lab Invest 44:49–54
28. Jalil JE, Doering CW, Janicki JS, Pick R, Shroff S, Weber KT (1989) Fibrillar collagen and myocardial stiffness in the intact hypertrophied rat left ventricle. Circ Res 64:1041–1050
29. Carroll EP, Janicki JS, Pick R, Weber KT (1989) Myocardial stiffness and reparative fibrosis following coronary embolization in the rat. Cardiovasc Res 23:655–661
30. Bing OHL, Fanburg BL, Brooks WW, Matsushita S (1978) The effect of the lathyrogen β-amino proprionitrile (BAPN) on the mechanical properties of experimentally hypertrophied rat cardiac muscle. Circ Res 43:632–637
31. Gelpi RJ, Pasipoularides A, Lader AS, Patrick TA, Chase N, Hittinger L, Shannon RP, Bishop SP, Vatner SF (1991) Changes in diastolic cardiac function in developing and stable perinephritic hypertension in conscious dogs. Circ Res 68:555–567
32. MacFarlane N, Northridge DB, Wright AR, Grant S, Dargie HJ (1991) A comparative study of left ventricular structure and function in elite athletes. Br J Sports Med 25:45–48
33. Nixon JV, Wright AR, Porter TR, Roy V, Arrowood JA (1991) Effects of exercise on left ventricular diastolic performance in trained athletes. Am J Cardiol 68:945–949
34. Shapiro LM, McKenna WJ (1984) Left ventricular hypertrophy: relation of structure to diastolic function in hypertension. Br Heart J 51:637–642
35. Shahi M, Thom S, Poulter N, Sever PS, Foale RA (1990) Regression of hypertensive left ventricular hypertrophy and left ventricular diastolic function. Lancet 336:458–461
36. Szlachcic J, Tubau JF, O'Kelly B, Massie BM (1990) Correlates of diastolic filling abnormalities in hypertension: A Doppler echocardiographic study. Am Heart J 120:386–391
37. O'Brien LJ, Moore CM (1966) Connective tissue degradation and distensibility characteristics of the non-living heart. Experientia 22:845–847
38. Cannon RO, Butany JW, McManus BM, Speir E, Kravitz AB, Bolli R, Serranus VJ (1983) Early degradation of collagen after myocardial infarction in the heart. Am J Cardiol 52:390–395
39. Takahashi S, Barry AC, Factor SM (1990) Collagen degradation in ischemic rat hearts. Biochem J 265:233–241
40. Campbell SE, Diaz-Arias A, Weber KT (1991) Ventricular rupture and fibrillar collagen degradation. Circulation 84:II-558
41. Romero FJ, Montoro A, Saez GT, Alberola A, Gil F, Vina J, Such L (1987) Myocardial glutathione alterations in acute coronary occlusion in the dog. Free Radic Res Commun 4:27–30
42. Zhao M, Zhang H, Robinson TF, Factor SM, Sonnenblick EH, Eng C (1987) Profound structural alterations of the extracellular collagen matrix in postischemic dysfunctional ("stunned") but viable myocardium. J Am Col Cardiol 10:1322–1334

43. Charney RH, Takahashi S, Zhao M, Sonnenblick EH, Eng C (1992) Collagen loss in the stunned myocardium. Circulation 85:1483–1490
44. Sato S, Ashroy M, Millard RW, Fujiwara H, Schwartz A (1983) Connective tissue changes in early ischemia of porcine myocardium: an ultrastructural study. J Mol Cell Cardiol 15:261–267
45. Janicki JS, Henegar JR, Matsubara BB (1993) Myocardial fibrillar collagen degradation induced by hemodilution (abstract). J Mol Cell Cardiol 25:S26
46. Janicki JS, Tyagi SC, Henegar JR, Campbell SE (1993) Myocardial collagenase activity and ventricular dilatation in cardiomyopathic hamsters (abstract). Circulation [Suppl]:I-381
47. Gertz EW (1972) Cardiomyopathic Syrian hamster: a possible model of human disease. Prog Exp Tumor Res 16:242–260
48. Weber KT, Pick R, Janicki JS, Gadodia G, Lakier JB (1988) Inadequate collagen tethers in dilated cardiopathy. Am Heart J 116:1641–1646
49. Reddy HK, Tyagi SC, Tjahja IE, Voelker DJ, Campbell SE, Weber KT (1993) Enhanced endomyocardial collagenase activity in dilated cardiomyopathy: a marker of dilatation and architectural remodeling (abstract). Circulation [Suppl]:I-407
50. Weber KT, Pick R, Silver MA, Moe GW, Janicki JS, Zucker IH, Armstrong PW (1990) Fibrillar collagen and the remodeling of the dilated canine left ventricle. Circulation 82:1387–1401
51. Spinale FG, Tomita M, Zellner JL, Cook JC, Crawford FA (1991) Collagen remodeling and changes in LV function during development and recovery from supraventricular tachycardia. Am J Physiol 261:H308–H318
52. Weber KT, Clark WA, Janicki JS, Shroff SG (1987) Physiologic versus pathologic hypertrophy and the pressure-overloaded myocardium. J Cardiovasc Pharmacol 10:S37–S50

Part 3

Pathophysiology and Treatment of Heart Failure

Causes of Heart Failing

3.1 Alterations of the Sympathetic Nervous System in Heart Failure

Ron M. Oren[1,2] and Edward M. Gilbert[1]

Summary. Recent concepts regarding the pathophysiology of heart failure have focused on neurohumoral abnormalities. The heart failure state is characterized by many abnormalities of the autonomic nervous system including activation of the sympathetic neural system and reduced activity of the parasympathetic nervous system. Many abnormalities of autonomic reflex circulatory control have been demonstrated in heart failure as well. These impaired reflexes include the cardiopulmonary baroreflex, arterial baroreflex, muscle metaboreflex, and chemoreflex. On a cellular level, abnormalities of the receptor-G protein-adenylate cyclase complex are present in heart failure as well. Medications which comprise standard heart failure therapy probably have significant effects on these abnormalities of the autonomic nervous system. These interactions probably have an impact on the therapeutic efficacy of these agents.

Key words: Heart failure—Autonomic nervous system—Cardiomyopathy—Beta receptor

Introduction

Concepts regarding the pathophysiology of heart failure have undergone dramatic change in recent years. Although long thought of exclusively as a hemodynamic disease, current evidence from both experimental and clinical studies has demonstrated that neurohormonal abnormalities are of significant pathophysiologic importance in the development and progression of the heart failure

[1] Heart Failure Treatment Program, The Division of Cardiology, 4A-100, University of Utah School of Medicine, Salt Lake City, UT 84132, USA
[2] Current Address: Assistant Professor of Medicine, Division of Cardiology, University of Iowa Hospitals, Iowa City, IA 52246, USA

syndrome. Abnormalities of the sympathetic nervous system play a large role in the neurohormonal derangements that are seen in heart failure patients. These alterations include an increased activation of sympathetic neural activity, abnormalities of reflex circulatory control mechanisms, and alterations in β-adrenergic receptor pathways. This review will outline the normal autonomic neural reflex control mechanisms and the normal β-adrenergic receptor pathways, and review the abnormalities of the sympathetic nervous system that characterize the heart failure state.

Autonomic Cardiovascular Control Mechanisms

The autonomic control of the heart and peripheral vasculature is closely regulated by homeostatic reflex mechanisms [1,2]. Changing environmental factors, such as exercise or orthostatic stress, are detected via the afferent receptors of these reflexes and the activity of the reflex is then altered to adjust the cardiovascular system to the changing environmental circumstances. These reflex pathways include the arterial and cardiopulmonary baroreflexes, arterial and ventricular chemoreceptors, and skeletal muscle metaboreceptors. In normal humans, the baroreflexes exert a tonic inhibitory afferent input to the brainstem cardiovascular control centers, while the chemoreflex and muscle metaboreflex give rise to excitatory afferent influences. In the brainstem these afferent inputs are then integrated with input from higher central centers and the sympathetic and parasysmpathetic neural outflow is modulated.

Autonomic adjustments to changes in hemodynamics are mediated via the baroreflexes. The afferent limb of the baroreflexes comprises mechanoreceptors which are activated by stretch of the structures in which they are located [1,2]. The cardiopulmonary baroreceptors are located diffusely throughout the cardiopulmonary tree. The arterial baroreflexes are located in the aortic arch and carotid sinus [3]. The activity of the cardiopulmonary baroreceptors is determined by cardiac filling pressures and inotropic state [4–6], while the arterial baroreceptor activity is principally determined by static (systolic, diastolic, mean) and dynamic (pulse frequency and dP/dt) arterial pulse parameters [7,8]. When deactivated by a decrease in cardiac filling pressure (cardiopulmonary receptors) or by a fall in arterial pressures (arterial receptors) the tonic inhibitory restraint of the baroreflexes is lessened and efferent sympathetic neural activation is produced. Alternatively, when pressures are increased and baroreceptors are activated, the inhibitory afferent influence is augmented which results in efferent sympathoinhibition. Arterial baroreflexes are felt to be the major regulators of short-term beat-to-beat autonomic tone and the cardiopulmonary baroreflexes probably modulate the cardiovascular system over a longer period such as seconds to hours.

Excitatory influences to the brainstem vasomotor centers arise from arterial or ventricular chemoreceptors [1,9] and from metaboreceptors located in exercising muscle [10,11]. The muscle metaboreflex is responsible for regulating systemic arterial pressure and perfusion to exercising skeletal muscle in the presence of metabolic vasodilation. This reflex, which provides excitatory afferent inputs to the brainstem, is primarily responsible for the sympathoexcitation seen during exercise [10]. The receptors of the metaboreflex are located in the interstitium of skeletal muscle [11]. Although the exact stimulus to the metaboreceptor during exercise is unclear, studies utilizing phosphorus-31 nuclear magnetic resonance have suggested that the metaboreceptors are activated by intracellular acidosis [12]. The arterial chemoreceptors are located in the carotid sinus region and are activated during hypoxia, acidemia, or hypercarbia. When activated, the excitatory afferent influences from the muscle metaboreflex or the arterial chemoreflex result in an increase in efferent sympathetic neural activity. Chemically sensitive receptors are also located in the left ventricular myocardium. These receptors are activated following the intracardiac injection of contrast agents and prostaglandins, and produce reflex bradycardia and hypotension [1,2,13].

The efferent autonomic neural outflow consists of the sympathetic and parasympathetic nervous systems. Preganglionic parasympathetic neurons exit the medulla and travel with the vagus to innervate end-organs including the cardiovascular system. Sympathetic efferent neurons course with the spinal cord where they synapse in the intermediallateral cell column. Neurons from these cells then exit the cord to synapse in the sympathetic ganglia. Postganglionic fibers then travel to end-organs including the heart and renal, splanchnic, and skeletal muscle vasculature.

Neuroeffector responses are mediated at the cellular level by the binding of agonist "first messengers" to receptors which are located on the cell membrane of the effector organs. The interaction of agonists with their receptors results in receptor coupling to a family of guanine nucleotide regulatory (G) proteins including both stimulatory (Gs) and inhibitory (Gi) protein subtypes [14,15]. The G proteins serve to transduce and amplify (up to 100-fold) the signal from the membrane receptor to adenylate cyclase which then produces changes in the intracellular cAMP concentrations. The G proteins may either activate (Gs) or inhibit (Gi) the adenylate cyclase system. The particular G protein activated during the receptor couping is dependent upon the receptor type involved. The β-1, β-2, histamine, and vasoactive intestinal peptide (VIP) receptors are coupled to the Gs protein [14]. Binding of agonists to these receptor types results in coupling with Gs proteins and activation of adenylate cyclase. The adenosine, somatostatin, and muscarinic receptors couple with the Gi protein, and binding to these receptors reduces adenylate cyclase activity. Activation of adenylate cyclase results in an increase in intracellular cAMP levels and activation of intracellular protein kinases [15]. These protein kinases then phosphorylate proteins of the sarcolemma and sarcoplasmic reticulum which allow increased intracellular calcium flux and thereby improve cardiac contractility and relaxation.

The function of the nonfailing human heart is predominantly influenced by the binding of catecholamines (either circulating or from synaptic release) to the β-adrenergic receptor. In normal myocardium the approximate ratio of β-1 to β-2 receptors is 80/20 [16]. Also, the affinity of norepinephrine (the primary in-vivo cardiac neurotransmitter) is much greater for the β-1 receptor than it is for the β-2 receptor [17]. Thus, because of the increased receptor numbers and agonist affinity, the β-1 receptor is the primary influence on regulation of cardiac contractility in normal humans.

Other receptor subtypes are felt to be of lesser importance than are the β-receptors. For example, the normal human myocardium contains small quantities of VIP [18]. In addition, in in-vitro studies, activation of the VIP receptor produces less than one-half of the contractile response noted following β-agonist administration [19]. Similarly, only a minimal increase in contractility is seen following stimulation of the H2 histamine receptor [20]. The effect of alpha receptor stimulation on human myocardial contractility is unclear. Although these receptors have been demonstrated in human myocardium [21], in-vitro studies on the inotropic effects of alpha stimulation in humans have been conflicting [22,23]. Recent studies have examined the effect of intracoronary injection of the alpha adrenergic receptor antagonist phentolamine and agonist phenylephrine in normal humans [24]. These data suggested that while alpha receptors do not contribute to the resting the cardiac inotropic state, when stimulated they do result in increases in myocardial contractility.

Abnormalities of the Autonomic Nervous System in Heart Failure

The heart failure state in associated with significant alterations in the normal autonomic control of the cardiovascular system. In patients with established heart failure the tone of the sympathetic nervous system is heightened while parasympathetic tone is blunted. In addition, significant disturbances in autonomic reflex circulatory control are seen. Finally, the intracellular events following β-adrenergic receptor activation are abnormal.

Activation of the Sympathetic Nervous System in Heart Failure

Heart failure is characterized by sympathetic neural activation which has been demonstrated by a variety of techniques. Concentrations of circulating catecholamines have been frequently utilized to assess the sympathetic nervous system in heart failure patients. Studies have shown that venous plasma norepinephrine levels are markedly elevated in the heart failure state [25,26] and are inversely related to prognosis [27,28]. Catecholamine measurements from arterial and coronary sinus samples have been used to assess myocardial catecholamine balance in heart failure patients [29,30]. These studies suggest that the net myocardial release of norepinephrine is increased in heart failure. Also, similar to many other parameters of clinical heart failure, coronary sinus norepinephrine levels have been shown to correlate with cardiac filling pressures but not resting cardiac index or left ventricular ejection fraction [37].

Measurements of plasma norepinephrine have been used to help delineate the pathophysiology of the heart failure state. Although neurohormonal activation has been thought to be a consequence of heart failure, recent data from the Studies of Left Ventricular Dysfunction (SOLVD) trial indicate that neurohormone levels are elevated in patients with depressed ventricular function before the onset of clinical symptoms [32]. This suggests that sympathoexcitation may contribute to the pathophysiology of heart failure.

Although commonly used to assess the sympathetic nervous system, plasma norepinephrine measurements are indirect assessments of sympathetic neural activity. For example, studies suggest that plasma norepinephrine levels account for less than 1% of norepinephrine present in the synaptic cleft, indicating that only small amounts of released norepinephrine reach the circulation [33,34]. The norepinephrine released from nerve terminals can be either locally metabolized or sequestered by neuronal reuptake. Thus, increased plasma norepinephrine levels do not necessarily indicate increased efferent sympathetic outflow and may be related to other mechanisms, including augmented norepinephrine release from peripheral neurons and altered local norepinephrine metabolism or reuptake. However, recent studies, utilizing techniques to define plasma norepinephrine kinetics and techniques to directly assess efferent sympathetic neural activity, have been performed to determine the contribution of these potential mechanisms to the increased plasma norepinephrine levels seen in heart failure patients.

Measurements of norepinephrine turnover with the use of a continuous infusion of radiolabeled norepinephrine have been employed by Hasking et al. [35] to evaluate the sympathoexcitation in heart failure patients. In these studies the elevated plasma norepinephrine levels were noted to reflect both an increased release and reduced clearance of norepinephrine. In addition, these studies demonstrated that a marked regional variation in sympathetic neural activation is seen in heart failure with a pronounced increase in cardiac sympathetic neural activity. A lesser degree of sympathoexcitation is seen in the renal bed and no increase is seen in either the pulmonary or the hepatomesenteric sympathetic tone. Rose et al. [36] employed a technique for assessing both neuronal uptake and release of norepinephrine which utilized an injection of radiolabeled norepinephrine and reference tracers for measurement of intravascular and interstitial spaces. These parameters, in combination with measurements of endogenous norepinephrine concentrations and mathematical modeling, yielded steady state assessments of cardiac neuronal uptake and release. These studies, in contrast to those of Hasking et al., demonstrated a reduction in cardiac norepinephrine release and uptake in patients with heart failure. Further preliminary studies utilizing the methods of Rose et al. demonstrate that norepinephrine uptake is reduced to a greater degree than is release [37] and therefore coronary sinus, interstitial, and synaptic cleft norepinephrine levels are likely increased. Additional insight into myocardial catecholamine balance may be obtained from studies of myocardial catecholamine content. These studies show that myocardial norepinephrine [38,39] and its cotransmitter neuropeptide Y [40] are depleted in heart failure. The observation that dopamine [40] is similarly depressed indicates that an abnormal conversion of dopamine to norepinephrine is not present in the heart failure state.

The techniques utilizing catecholamine determinations are indirect measures of sympathetic neural outflow. Recent studies using the technique of microneurography have provided direct evidence for an increased central sympathetic neural outflow in patients with heart failure. In this technique a small microelectrode is placed within a peripheral nerve and directly records efferent postganglionic sympathetic neural activity directed to muscle vasculature [41]. Microneurography is not influenced by the uptake, release, or metabolism of norepinephrine [41]. Leimbach et al. [42] first utilized microneurography in clinical heart failure and demonstrated a significantly increased resting efferent sympathetic neural activity to muscle in these patients. These observations were confirmed and expanded upon by further studies by Ferguson and coworkers [43] who noted that heart failure patients have levels of muscle sympathetic neural activity 2–3 times that seen in age-matched normal subjects. In addition, the magnitude of sympathoexcitation correlated with the hemodynamic severity of clinical heart failure. Furthermore, as has been shown with other clinical parameters, the resting level of muscle sympathetic nerve activity has been shown to correlate moderately with the ejection fraction of the right but not the left ventricle [44]. Finally, an inverse relationship has been demonstrated between exercise capacity and resting sympathetic nerve activity to muscle in heart failure patients [45].

Insight into abnormalities of the parasympathetic nervous system in heart failure patients has been gained with the use of the power spectral analysis of heart rate variability. This technique utilizes observations by Akselrod et al. [46] and others who demonstrated that frequency-specific variations in heart rate can be attributed to activity of either sympathetic or parasympathetic neural systems. For example, high frequency (>0.1 Hz) variations in heart rate are exclusively under parasympathetic control. Therefore, by quantifying the frequency content of the variation of the heart rate over time, an assessment of parasympathetic activity can be obtained. Binkley et al. [47] examined the spectral analysis of heart rate variability in the heart failure state. They demonstrated that both experimental and clinical heart failure were associated with a reduction in the parasympathetically mediated high-frequency area of the power density spectrum that was similar to that seen in normal subjects following the administration of atropine. Studies by Kienzle et al. [48] have suggested that the impairment in parasympathetic mechanisms is inversely related to the sympathoexcitation seen in heart failure patients. Thus, parasympathetic withdrawal, in addition to sympathoexcitation, is an important aspect of the dysautonomia seen in the heart failure state.

Alterations in Autonomic Reflex Circulatory Control in Heart Failure

The autonomic reflexes are critically important in maintaining cardiovascular homeostasis during environmental stress. Abnormalities in these reflexes may compromise the ability of the cardiovascular system to adjust to physiologic changes such as exercise or orthostatic stress and would probably contribute to clinical symptoms. A variety of clinical and experimental studies have focused on evaluating autonomic reflex circulatory control mechanisms in feart tailure. These studies have demonstrated that patients with heart failure exhibit abnormalities of both the cardiopulmonary baroreflex and the arterial baroreflex as well as abnormalities of the muscle metaboreflex.

Cardiopulmonary Baroreflex Abnormalities

Reflex sympathetic control mediated by cardiopulmonary baroreflex afferents has been evaluated in two dog models of heart failure including the high-output arteriovenous fistula model and the rapid ventricular pacing model. Zucker et al. employed the former model and observed the sympathetic neural responses following occlusion of the mitral valve orifice [49]. This intervention increases the pressures in the atria and pulmonary vasculature and therefore activates cardiopulmonary baroreceptors. In contrast to the sympathoinhibition noted in control animals, the heart failure dogs demonstrated paradoxical sympathoexcitation. More recently, Dibner-Dunlap and Thames noted a blunted increase in renal sympathetic nerve activity in dogs with the rapidly paced model of heart failure following the inflation of a balloon located at the atrial–pulmonary vein junction [50].

Clinical studies of the cardiopulmonary baroreflex in patients with heart failure have examined either neurohumoral or vasoconstrictor responses to mechanical unloading of the cardiopulmonary baroreceptors with either lower body negative pressure [51,52] or upright tilt [53,54]. These perturbations of the cardiopulmonary baroreflex resulted in blunted vasoconstrictor or paradoxical vasodilatory responses in the patients with heart failure. Other reports demonstrated attenuated neurohormone increases (including plasma norepinephrine and renin activity) in response to cardiopulmonary baroreflex activation with these techniques [52,54]. These baroreflex impairments appear to be related to the severity of heart failure. Finally, Goldsmith has demonstrated that the reflex response to baroreflex loading is also abnormal as suggested by impaired baroreflex suppression of arginine vasopressin in response to head down tilt [55]. These experimental and clinical studies offer substantial evidence for an impairment in cardiopulmonary baroreflex function in the heart failure state.

Arterial Baroreflex Abnormalities

Abnormalities of arterial baroreflex cardiovascular control have also been demonstrated in experimental heart failure models and in heart failure patients. These studies have included those which examine the arterial baroreflex mediated control of heart rate and others which evaluate the arterial baroreflex control of efferent sympathetic nerve activity.

The predominant influence on the control of heart rate in humans is mediated by the arterial baroreflex [1]. Clinical studies have suggested that, in heart failure, there is an attenuated arterial baroreflex control of heart rate in response to changes in systemic blood pressures [56–59]. In these studies, pharmacologic elevations in blood pressure are accompanied by blunted heart rate decreases when patients are compared with normal subjects. Similarly, diminished increases in heart rate are noted following the pharmacologic lowering of blood pressure. Impairments in the baroreflex control of heart rate have also been demonstrated in canine models of heart failure induced by tricuspid avulsion [60] or rapid ventricular pacing [61].

Recent clinical studies have suggested that the heart failure state is also associated with alteration of arterial baroreflex control of peripheral sympathetic tone. Patients with heart failure have been shown to exhibit blunted plasma norepinephrine [55,62] and muscle sympathetic neural responses [63] to arterial baroreceptor deactivation via systemic blood pressure lowering with vasodilator administration. In contrast, arterial baroreceptor activation with vasoconstrictor agents does not seem to be associated with an abnormal decrease in sympathetic tone [63]. The abnormalities of arterial baroreflexes have prognostic significance as patients with the most severe baroreflex impairment have poorer survival than do patients with intact baroreflex mechanisms [55].

Mechanisms Responsible for Baroreflex Abnormalities

Although the presence of baroreflex abnormalities in patients with heart failure has been clearly demonstrated, the mechanisms responsible for these abnormalities have not been precisely defined. Because of the constraints of performing experiments in intact humans, studies evaluating these potential mechanisms in patients with heart failure are limited. However, studies in animal models of heart failure have yielded significant insight into several factors which may contribute to the baroreflex abnormalities noted in the heart failure state.

Structural abnormality of the baroreceptors is one factor which may decrease baroreflex responsiveness. Such alterations have been noted in the microscopic examination of baroreceptor endings from dogs with high-output heart failure [64]. These studies demonstrated baroreceptors with loss of end arborizations and in various stages of degeneration. These structural changes were associated with a decreased discharge sensitivity which returned towards normal following reversal of the heart failure state [65].

Baroreceptors are stretch receptors whose activity is determined by deformity of the cardiovascular structures in which the baroreceptors are located. A second potential mechanism which may decrease baroreceptor activity in heart failure is an altered compliance of baroreceptor regions. Recent studies in heart failure patients have reported decreased compliance of large arteries [66]. Other reports demonstrated a smaller change in cardiac chamber volumes for a given degree of orthostatic stress in heart failure patients compared to normal subjects [52]. Such a decrease in compliance of either the aortic arch and carotid sinus or of the cardiopulmonary tree may result in impaired stretch of mechanically sensitive baroreceptors and blunted sympathetic neural response to pressure perturbations.

Biochemical abnormalities of baroreceptor cell membranes have been proposed as a mechanism of blunted baroreflex activity in heart failure. Baroreceptors from an animal model of heart failure exhibit an augemented activity of the membrane Na-K-ATPase [67]. This results in membrane hyperpolarization and decreased activation threshold. The mechanism of this abnormality of baroreceptor membrane function is unknown but can be reversed with the application of rapidly acting digitalis glycosides which reduce the activity of the membrane Na-K-ATPase pump [68].

Another potential mechanism of suppression of baroreceptor function in heart failure would be via the effect of circulating substances on baroreflex activity. While this mechanism has not been extensively investigated, recent reports indicate that baroreflex circulatory control is normalized within two to four weeks following cardiac transplantation [57]. Such a rapid improvement in reflex function suggests that the removal of the "circulating neurohormonal milieu" of the heart failure state contributes to normalization of baroreflex function [57].

Alteration in the central processing of afferent baroreflex inputs to the medullary cardiovascular control centers has been proposed to be at least partially responsibile for baroreflex abnormalities in heart failure. Dibner-Dunlap and Thames [69] have speculated that central control is abnormal since the sensitivity of baroreflex circulatory control is relatively preserved in experimental heart failure even though the operating range of baroreflexes is reduced. However, other lines of experimental evidence suggest that central factors are of lesser importance. For example, heart failure patients exhibit preserved responses to nonbaroreflex stimuli such as the cold pressor test [70]. In addition, studies utilizing single-fiber recordings from the carotid sinus dogs with induced heart failure show preserved renal sympathetic neural responses during electrical stimulation of the afferent nerve fiber [71]. There data can be interpreted to suggest that central neural processing of baroreflex afferent input is maintained in heart failure. Thus, the data evaluating the role of this potential mechanism of baroreflex abnormalities remains inconclusive.

A final potential means by which the baroreflex amy be abnormal is through diminished end-organ responsiveness. Collluci et al. [72] have shown that the chronotropic response to isoproterenol is blunted in heart failure patients when compared to controls. In addition, vascular responses to a variety of stimuli are blunted in the heart failure state [73–75]. These data become important when interpreting studies where end-organ responses are utilized as indirect indices of baroreflex responsiveness. While blunted end-organ responses play some role in altered baroreflex circulatory control, the studies which utilize direct assessments of sympathetic neural activity indicate other mechanisms are operating. These studies include data from experimental models and from human studies utilizing the technique of microneurography.

Abnormalities of Baroflex Control in Early Heart Failure

It has been suggested that abnormalities of the baroreflexes may occur early in the development of heart failure and may contribute to pathophysiology of the sympathoexcitation that characterizes the heart failure state via a diminished tonic afferent inhibitory influence. Experimental evidence in support of this hypothesis is limited. Few studies have evaluated the function of the baroreflexes in early heart failure. In experimental heart failure, the arterial baroreflex control of heart rate during increases in systemic pressure induced pharmacologically is maintained until overt heart failure develops [76]. In contrast, preliminary studies suggest that, in an animal model of heart failure, cardiopulmonary baroreflexes become abnormal when the cardiac filing pressures are only minimally elevated [77]. In addition, the heart rate response to nitroprusside-induced hypotension is abnormal as early as one week after onset of rapid ventricular pacing [78]. Studies of the reflex circulatory control in early heart failure in humans have not been performed to date.

Abnormalities in Metaboreceptor Function

The muscle metaboreflex serves the important role of maintaining blood flow to skeletal muscle during exercise [1,11]. Unlike the baroreflexes, the function of the metaboreflex in patients with heart failure has not been extensively investigated. Sterns et al. [79] have reported studies in which microneurographic sympathetic neural activity was recorded during period of post-handgrip regional circulatory arrest. This experimental technique isolates the sympathoexcitatory response to the metaboreflex. They found that heart failure patients exhibited a significantly reduced increase in the sympathetic neural response to this metaboreflex stimulus when compared to normal control subjects. Since the development of intracellular acidosis (the metaboreflex stimulus) was similar between patients and controls, these studies suggest that a significant attenuation of the metaboreflex is present in the heart failure state. Additional studies are needed to confirm these findings.

Abnormalities in Chemoreceptor Function

Like the metaboreflex, the function of the chemoreflexes in patients with heart failure has not been extensively examined. No studies to date have evaluated the function of the chemoreceptors located in the carotid sinus in heart failure. Mukharji et al. [80] examined the function of chemosensitive receptors in the left ventricle of heart failure patients. In normal subjects, reflex-mediated bradycardia and hypotension occurs following receptor stimulation with intra coronary injection of a contrast agent. In this study, heart failure patients showed only minimal heart rate effects following this stimulus, suggesting diminished chemoreceptor function. This is in contrast to preliminary observations in experimental heart failure which indicate that an augmented reflex response occurs following chemoreceptor stimulation with prostaglandin [81].

Abnormalities of the Receptor–G Protein–Adenylate Cyclase Complex in Heart Failure

The receptor–G protein–adenylate cyclase (RGC) complex in patients with established heart failure differs in several important ways from the normal nonfailing heart. These alterations have been most extensively evaluated in the β-receptors. The total population of β-1 receptors is decreased or "down regulated" such that the ratio of β-1 receptors to β-receptors is 60/40 rather than the 80/20 which is observed in the normal heart [15,82–85]. The degree of down regulation is related to the severity of the underlying heart failure [83]. In addition, while the density of the β-2 receptors is similar to that of the nonfailing heart, the β-2 agonist responsiveness is reduced [82,84]. This suggests an uncoupling of the β-2 receptors from adenylate cyclase is present in heart failure. These abnormalities of the β-1 and β-2 receptors in heart failure have functional consequences as demonstrated by a 50% reduction in the inotropic response to β agonists administered either in vivo or in vitro [83,85].

Abnormalities have been observed in other receptors as well. The density of the VIP receptor is decreased [18]. However, the affinity for agonist binding is increased and therefore the effects of the receptor down-regulation are somewhat blunted. Studies performed thus far suggest that the function of the α-1 receptor [21], M-2 muscarinic receptor, and H-2 histamine receptor [20] are not significantly effected by the heart failure state.

Other components of the RGC system are also altered in heart failure patients. A significant increase in the activity of the Gi protein has been demonstrated, which has been suggested to account for the uncoupling of the β-2 receptor [85]. Further experiments utilizing immunochemistry techniques suggest that levels of Gi are unchanged in heart failure and therefore indicate that the increase in Gi activity is not explainable by an increased level of Gi protein [86]. The function of the Gs protein has been suggested to be decreased in some studies and unchanged in others [87,88]. The existing studies which have evaluated the molecular and biochemical mechanisms responsible for these abnormalities in the G proteins are conflicting. Eschenhagen et al. [89] found an increase in the mRNA for a subunit of the Gi protein in heart failure patients. However, in recent experiments Feldman et al. [90,93] found no difference in the mRNA levels between failing and nonfailing human hearts.

Mechanisms of RCG Abnormalities

Despite the likely importance of the RCG abnormalities to the pathophysiology of heart failure, the precise mechanisms responsible for the changes are unknown. A growing body of evidence suggests that the chronic exposure of the heart to elevated norepinephrine levels plays an important role in the genesis of the RCG alterations seen in the heart failure state. These data include: (1) chronic exposure to norepinephrine is a powerful stimulus to β-receptor down-regulation [91]; (2) β-receptor density is inversely correlated with coronary sinus norepinephrine levels [37]; (3) β-1 receptors (which are down regulated) have greater affinity for norepinephrine than do either the β-2 or the α-1 receptor, whose densities are normal [17]; (4) treatment of heart failure patients with competitive β-blocking agents, which decrease agonist binding to the receptor, results in increasing β-receptor density [86]. However, it is likely that exposure to catecholamines is not the sole factor responsible for the RCG abnormalities that occur in heart failure. For example, only a moderate correlation exists between coronary sinus norepinephrine and β-receptor density and at least some β-1 receptors are resistant to down-regulation despite chronic norepinephrine exposure.

Although these abnormalities of the RCG system are present in most forms of cardiomyopathy, recent data suggest that the abnormalities may be affected by the underlying etiology of the heart failure state. For example, the degree of β-1 receptor down-regulation is greater in nonischemic compared to ischemic cardiomyopathy [88]. Similarly, the increases in Gi protein are comparatively greater in the nonischemic patient [92]. The clinical consequences and underlying causes of the differences in the RCG system in patients with varying etiologies of heart failure are unclear.

One potential mechanism underlying these observed differences is that cardiac adrenergic activity (and therefore possibly the down-regulation stimulus) may be somewhat greater in nonischemic heart failure patients when compared to those patients with an ischemic etiology.

Therapeutic Modulation of the Sympathetic Nervous System in Heart Failure

It is likely that the alterations in the sympathetic nervous system in patients with heart failure are related to both the symptoms of heart failure and progression of the disease process. Recent attention has focused on the ability of pharmacologic agents to modulate these abnormalities in heart failure patients. Medications which constitute standard heart failure therapy have been demonstrated to exert significant interactions with the sympathetic nervous system that likely impact on the therapeutic efficacy of these agents.

Calcium Channel Blocking Agents

Patients with heart failure commonly receive therapy with calcium channel blocking agents. Recent clinical reports have indicated that calcium channel blockers (especially nifedipine and other dihydropyridines) are detrimental in some patients with heart failure [96,97]. Although this is probably related in part to the negative inotropic properties of these agents, evidence indicates that nifedipine is a potent stimulus to the sympathetic and renin-angiotensin systems [96,97]. Newer, second-generation dihydropyridines have less myocardial depressor activity and commonly lead to acute hemodynamic improvements. However, their effect on the neurohormonal axis is not well defined and reports of their chronic efficacy in clinical heart failure are conflicting [98]. Amlodipine, a third-generation dihydropyridine has been shown, in preliminary reports, to improve the clinical course of heart failure [99]. Studies of the effect of amlodipine on the neurohormonal activity in heart failure are ongoing.

Angiotensin Converting Enzyme Inhibitors

Recent studies have indicated that angiotensin converting enzyme (ACE) inhibitors produce beneficial effects on the survival of patients with heart failure when compared to direct vasodilator combinations [100]. These effects are seen even though the direct acting agents result in greater improvements in exercise capacity and hemodynamics. This suggests that at least a portion of the benefit of ACE inhibitors is related to their effect of lowering neurohumoral activation. ACE inhibitors have significant interactions with the sympathetic nervous system in heart failure patients. Experimental evidence indicates that angiotensin II enhances sympathetic neural influence on the cardiovascular system. For example, sympathetic nerve discharge and norepinephrine release are augmented by angiotensin II [101–103]. These actions are likely blunted by ACE inhibitor therapy. Recent studies have also indicated that ACE inhibitors interact significantly with baroreflex mechanisms in heart failure patients. Arterial baroreflex sensitivity is improved by these agents [104]. Similarly, the acute and chronic administration of ACE inhibitors improves the hemodynamic and neurohumoral responses to orthostatic stress [105,106]. These studies suggest that ACE inhibitors produce a central modulation of the sympathetic nervous system as the response to nonspecific stimuli such as the cold pressor test is normalized [105].

Digitalis Glycosides

The digitalis glycosides have been employed in the therapy of heart disease for many years. Skepticism regarding the efficacy of digitalis has recently diminished as clinical trials have indicated that it is beneficial in patients with moderate or severe heart failure and sinus rhythm. Digitalis is most commonly considered a inotropic agent; however, several lines of experimental evidence now suggests that it also exhibits important "neurotropic" effects in heart failure as well. In animal models of heart failure, digitalis preparations have resulted in sympathoinhibition that appears to be related to the known actions of digitalis on the membrane Na-K ATPase. Digitalis results in inhibition of the Na-K ATPase which increases baroreceptor sensitivity [67,68].

In human heart failure studies, Ferguson et al. utilized the technique of microneurography to demonstrate that digitalis acutely decreases efferent sympathetic neural outflow [107]. These effects occurred immediately following drug administration and before any observed hemodynamic effects. Dobutamine, given in eqi-inotropic doses, had no measurable effect on sympathetic nerve activity. This suggested that factors other than the inotropic actions of digitalis were responsible for the observed sympathoinhibition. Schobel et al. [108] have demonstrated that digitalis results in an augmentation of the sympathoexcitatory response to baroreceptor unloading with lower body negative pressure in studies performed in normal human subjects. These clinical studies support the concept that digitalis acutely sensitizes the baroreceptors. However, other human studies have been unable to detect an effect of digitalis on baroreceptor function. In contrast, Goldsmith et al. [109], found that digitalis did not alter either resting sympathetic neural activity or the response to baroreceptor loading, using a method which measured the "spillover" kinetics of infused radiolabeled norepinephrine. The reasons for these apparently conflicting findings are unclear but may relate to differences in the patients studied or the experimental techniques used to assess sympathetic neural activity.

β-Adrenergic Receptor Blocking Agents

Contrary to what one would expect, β-adrenergic receptor blockage has been demonstrated to result in improvements in several clinical parameters in heart failure patients. Waagstein et al. first reported beneficial effects of these agents [110]. Since this initial report, studies have demonstrated that β blockade, if continued for several months, will produce improvements in hemodynamics and reductions in symptoms in the majority of patients with idiopathic dilated cardiomyopathy [111].

The mechanisms of improvements in myocardial function following β blockade are unclear. Several possible mechanisms exist. Waagstein first postulated in his initial report that β-blockers result in reduction in the resting tachycardia seen in heart failure. In this manner, myocardial function may be improved by decreasing the myocardial oxygen demand. Second, cardiac improvement may be produced in heart failure by reducing the degree of sympathoexcitation, and by reducing renin and vasopressin release. Third, a reduction in catecholamine cardiotoxicity may be produced by lowering sympathetic tone and by competitive β-receptor antagonism. Studies on the effects of β-blockade on circulating catecholamine concentrations have been conflicting. For example, plasma venous norepinephrine levels following therapy with the β-blocker bucindolol have been reported to be decreased in our placebo-controlled study [112] but unchanged in an uncontrolled trial [113].

An additional mechanism whereby long-term β-receptor blockade may result in improvements in cardiac function is by reducing the degree of β-receptor down-regulation. As just outlined, heart failure is accompanied by a reduced density of myocardial β-adrenergic receptors that in turn limits the inotropic responsiveness to β-agonists. Heilbrunn and co-workers [86] evaluated the ability of long-term therapy with metoprolol to reverse this abnormality. They reported that, following six months of treatment, the density of β receptors was increased more than 100%. The improved β-receptor density with metoprolol had functional consequences as the inotropic response to the β-agonist dobutamine increased significantly following treatment. However, recent studies suggest that the improved myocardial β-receptor density does not seem necessary for the improvements in ventricular function to be demonstrated. We recently evaluated this concept by observing the improvements in clinical course and β-receptor density in response to β blockade with either metoprolol or carvedilol [114]. These β-blocking agents differ in several respects. Carvedilol is a mildly β1-selective β-blocker with vasodilator activity via alpha-1 blockade and without intrinsic sympathomimetic activity. Carvedilol, but not metoprolol, exhibits the properties of guanine nucleotide modulated binding and results in the down-regulation of β-receptors in cultured cells. In placebo-controlled trials, both carvedilol and metoprolol improved left ventricular function and symptoms of heart failure. Myocardial β-receptor density increased in subjects treated with metoprolol. In contrast, myocardial β-receptor changes were not observed in subjects treated with carvedilol. Thus, improvements can occur in left ventricular function with β-blocker therapy in the absence of β-receptor up-regulation.

Conclusion

Heart failure is characterized by both sympathetic neural activation and a withdrawal of parasympathetic activity. These alterations have been demonstrated by many independent techniques. Autonomic reflex circulatory control mechanisms are noted to be abnormal in experimental as well as clinical heart failure. In addition, the β-adrenergic receptor pathways of the patients with heart failure have been shown to differ significantly from those seen in the normal heart. Therapeutic modulation of these abnormalities in autonomic neural function is likely to benefit the clinical outcome of patients with heart failure.

References

1. Abboud FM, Heistad DD, Mark AL, Schmid PG (1976) Reflex control to the peripheral circulation. Prog Cardiovasc Dis 18:371
2. Shepherd JT (1982) Reflex control of arterial blood pressure. Cardiovasc Res 16:357

3. Coleridge H, Coleridge J, Dangel A, Kidd C, Luck J, Sleight P (1973) Impulses in slowly conducting vagal fibers from afferent endings in the veins, atria, and arteries of dogs and cats. Circ Res 33:87–97
4. Thoren P (1977) Characteristics of left ventricular receptors with nonmedullated vagal afferents in cats. Circ Res 40:415–421
5. Ferguson DW, Thames MD, Mark Al (1983) Effects of propranolol ion reflex vascular responses to orthostatic stress in humans. Role of ventricular baroreceptors. Circulation 67:802–807
6. Karim F, Kidd C, Malpus CM (1972) The effects of stimulation of left atrial receptors on sympathetic efferent nerve activity. J Physiol (Lond) 227:243–260
7. Sanders JS, Mark AL, Ferguson DW (1989) Importance of aortic baroreflex in regulation of sympathetic responses during hypotension: Evidence from direct sympathetic nerve recordings in man. Circulation 79:83
8. Niebaurer MJ, Zucker IH (1985) Static and dynamic responses of carotid sinus baroreceptors in dogs with chronic volume overload. J Physiol (Lond) 369: 295–319
9. Sommers VK, Mark AL, Abboud FM (1988) Potentiation of sympathetic nervous responses to hypoxia in borderline hypertensive subjects. Hypertension 11:608
10. Mark AL, Victor RG, Nerhed C, Wallin BG (1985) Microneurographic studies of the mechanisms of sympathetic nervous responses to static exercise in humans. Circ Res 57:461
11. McCloskey DI, Mitchell JH (1972) Reflex cardiovascular and respiratory responses originating in exercising muscle. J Physiol (Lond) 224:173–186
12. Victor RG, Bertocci LA, Pryor SL, Nunally RL (1988) Sympathetic nerve discharge is coupled to muscle cell pH during exercise in humans. J Clin Invest 82:1301–1305
13. Arrowood JA, Mohanty PK, Hodgson J McB, Dibner-Dunlap ME, Thames MD (1989) Ventricular sensory endings mediate reflex bradycardia during coronary arteriography in humans. Circulation 80:1293–1300
14. Kessler PD, VanDop C, Feldman AM (1988) G proteins: transmembrane signal processors in the heart. Heart Failure 3:239–247
15. Bristow MR, Laser JA, Ginsburg R, Minobe W (1985) β-1 and β-2 receptors are coupled to adenylate cyclase in human ventricular myocardium. Clin Res 33:171A
16. Bristow MR (1988) The β-adrenergic receptor: configuration, regulation, mechanism of action. Postgrad Med Feb 28:19–26
17. Kaumann AJ, Lemoine H (1987) β-2 adrenoceptor mediated positive inotropic effect of adrenaline in human ventricular myocardium. Naunyn-Schmiedeberg Arch Pharmacol 225:403–411
18. Hershberger RE, Anderson FL, Bristow MR (1989) Vasoactive intestinal peptide receptor in failing human ventricular myocardium exhibits increased affinity and decreased density. Circ Res 66:283–294
19. Hershberger RE, Anderson FL, Bristow MR (1989) Vasoactive intestinal peptide receptor pharmacology in nonfailing and failing human heart. Heart Failure 5: 51–61
20. Bristow MR, Cubicciotti R, Ginsburg R, Stinson EB, Johnson C (1982) Histamine-mediated adenylate cyclase stimulation in human myocardium. Mol Pharmacol 21:671–679
21. Bristow MR, Minobe W, Rasmussen R, Hershberger RE, Hoffmann BB (1988) Alpha-1-adrenergic receptors in the nonfailing and failing human heart. J Pharmacol Exp Ther 247:1039–1045

22. Bruckner R, Meyer W, Mugge A, Schmitz W, Scholz H (1984) Alpha-adrenoceptor-mediated positive inotropic effect of phenylephrine in isolated human ventricular myocardium. Eur J Pharmacol 99:345–347
23. Jakob H, Nawrath H, Rupp J (1988) Adrenoceptor-mediated changes of action potential and force of contraction in human isolaed ventricular heart muscle. Br J Pharmacol 94:584–590
24. Landzberg JS, Parker JD, Gauthier DF, Colucci WS (1991) Effects of myocardial alpha-1-adrenergic receptor stimulation and blockade on contractility in humans. Circulation 84:1608–1614
25. Thomas LA, Marks BH (1978) Plasma norepinephrine in congestive heart failure. Am J Cardiol 41:233
26. Levine TB, Francis GS, Goldsmith SR, et al. (1982) Activity of the sympathetic nervous system and renin-angiotensinogen system assessed by plasma hormone levels and their relationship to hemodynamic abnormalities in congestive heart failure. Am J Cardiol 49:1659
27. Cohn JN, Levine TB, Olivari MT, et al. (1984) Plasma norepinephrine as a guide to prognosis in patients with chronic congestive heart failure. N Engl J Med 311:819
28. Rector TS, Olivari MT, Levine TB, et al. (1987) Predicting survival for an individual with congestive heart failure using the plasma norepinephrine levels. Am Heart J 114:148
29. Swedberg K, Viquerat C, Rouleau J-L, Roizen M, Atherton B, Parmley WW, Chatterjee K (1984) Comparison of myocardial catecholamine balance in chronic congestive heart failure and in angina pectoris without failure. Am J Cardiol 54:783–786
30. Swedberg K, Hjalmarson A, Holmberg S (1979) Effects of work and acute betareceptor blockade on myocardial noradrenaline release in congestive cardiomyopathy. Clin Cardiol 2:424–430
31. Petch MC, Mayler WG (1979) Uptake of catecholamines by human cardiac muscle in vitro. Br Heart J 41:336–339
32. Francis GS, Benedict C, Johnstone DE, et al. (1990) Comparison of neuroendocrine activation in patients with left ventricular dysfunction with and without congestive heart failure. A substudy of the studies of left ventricular dysfunction (SOLVD). Circulation 82:1724
33. Goldstein DS, Zimlichman R, Stull R, Keiser HR, Kopin IJ (1986) Estimation of intrasynaptic norepinephrine concentrations in humans. Hypertension 8:471
34. Hoeldtke RD, Cilmi KM, Reichard GA Jr, Boden G, Owen OE (1983) Assessment of norepinephrine secretion and production. J Clin Lab Med 101:772
35. Hasking GJ, Esler MD, Jennings GL, Burton D, Korner PI (1986) Norepinephrine spillover to plasma in patients with congestive heart failure: evidence of increased overall and cardiorenal sympathetic nervous activity. Circulation 73:615
36. Rose CP, Burgess JH, Cousineau D (1985) Tracer norepinephrine kinetics in coronary circulation in patients with heart failure secondary to chronic pressure and volume overload. J Clin Invest 76:1740–1747
37. Sandoval A, Gilbert EM, Ginsburg R, et al. (1988) Is β-1 receptor down-regulation in the failing human heart the result of exposure to cardiac-derived norepinephrine? (abstract) J Am Coll Cardiol 11:117A
38. Chidsey CA, Braunwald E, Morrow AG, Mason DT (1963) Myocardial norepinephrine concentrations in man: effects of reserpine and congestive heart failure. N Engl J Med 269:653–658

39. Pierpont GL, Francis GS, DeMaster EG, Olivari MT, Ring WS, Goldenberg IF, Reynolds S, Cohn JN (1987) Heterogeneous myocardial catecholamine concentrations in patients with congestive heart failure. Am J Cardiol 60:316–321
40. Anderson FL, Port JD, Reid BB, Larrabee P, Hanson G, Bristow MR (1992) Myocardial catecholamine and neuropeptide Y depletion in failing ventricles of patients with idiopathic dilated cardiomyopathy. Circulation 85:46–53
41. Anderson E, Mark A (1989) Microneurographic measurement of sympathetic nerve activity in humans. In: Schneidermann, Weiss S, Kaufmann P, eds Handbook of research methods in cardiovascular behavioral medicine. Plenum, p 107
42. Leimbach WN, Wallin BG, Victor RG, Aylward PE, Sundlof G, Mark AL (1986) Direct evidence from intraneural recordings for increased central sympathetic outflow in patients with heart failure. Circulation 73:913
43. Ferguson DW, Berg WJ, Sanders JS (1990) Clinical and hemodynamic correlates of sympathetic neural activity in normal humans and patients with heart failure. J Am Coll Cardiol 16:1125–1134
44. Oren RM, Roach PJ, Berg WJ, Schobel HP, Ferguson DW (1990) Resting muscle sympathetic nerve activity correlates with right rather than left venticular ejection fraction in human heart failure. Clin Res 38(3):883A
45. Oren RM, Zavala DC, Berg WJ Schobel HP, Roach PJ, Ferguson DW (1990) Resting muscle sympathetic nerve activity predicts exercise capacity in human heart failure. Circulation 82(4):2750A
46. Akselrod S, Gordon D, Madwed JB, et al. (1985) Hemodynamic regulation: investigation by spectral analysis. Am J Physiol 294:H867
47. Binkley PF, Nunziata E, Hass GJ, et al. (1991) Parasympathetic withdrawal is an integral component of autonomic imbalance in congestive heart failure: demonstration in human subjects and verification in a paced canine model of ventricular failure. J Am Coll Cardiol 18:464
48. Kienzle MG, Ferguson DW, Burkett CL, Berg WJ, Mariano DJ (1992) Clinical, hemodynamic, and microneurographic correlates of respiratory heart rate variability in heart failure. Am J Cardiol 69:761–767
49. Zucker IH, Gorman AJ, Cornish KG, Lang M (1985) Impaired atrial receptor modulation of renal nerve activity in dogs with chronic volume overload. Cardiovasc Res 19:411–418
50. Dibner-Dunlap ME, Thames MD (1989) Atrial mechanoreflex control of renal sympathetic nerve activity is blunted in heart failure (abstract). Circulation 80(Suppl II): II–393
51. Ferguson D, Abboud F, Mark A (1984) Selective impairment of baroreflex mediated vasoconstrictor responses in patients with ventricular dysfunction. Circulation 69:451
52. Mohanty PK, Arrowood JA, Ellenbogen KA, Thames MD (1989) The neurohumoral and hemodynamic effects of lower body negative pressure in patients with congestive heart failure. Am Heart J 118:78
53. Levine TB, Francis GS, Goldsmith SR, Cohn JN (1983) The neurohumoral and hemodynamic responses to orthostatic tilt in patients with congestive heart failure. Circulation 67:1070
54. Goldsmith SR, Francis GS, Levine TB, Cohn JN (1983) Regional blood flow response to orthostasis in patients with congestive heart failure. J Am Coll Cardiol 1:1391–1395
55. Olivari MT, Levine TB, Cohn JN (1983) Abnormal neurohumoral response to nitroprusside infusion in congestive heart failure. J Am Coll Cardiol 2:411–417

56. Eckberg DL, Drabinsky M, Braunwald E (1971) Defective cardiac parasympathetic control in patients with heart disease. N Engl J Med 285:877–883
57. Ellenbogan KA, Mohanty PK, Szentpetery S, Thames MD (1989) Arterial baroreflex abnormalities in heart failure. Reversal after orthotopic cardiac transplantation. Circulation 79:51
58. Binkley PF, Nunziata E, Haas GJ, Cody RJ (1991) Autonomic response to baroreceptor loading vs unloading in congestive heart failure: definition by analysis of heart rate variability. Clin Res 39(2):231A
59. Goldstein RE, Beiser GD, Stampfer M, Epstein SE (1975) Impairment of autonomically mediated heart rate control in patients with cardiac dysfunction. Circ Res 36:571–578
60. White CW (1981) Abnormalities in baroreflex control of heart rate in canine heart failure. Am J Physiol 240:H793–H799
61. Chen J-S, Wang W, Bartholet T, Zucker IH (1991) Analysis of baroreflex control of heart rate in conscious dogs with pacing-induced heart failure. Circulation 83:260–267
62. Goldsmith SR (1992) Baroreflex loading maneuvers do not suppress increased plasma arginine vasopressin in patients with congestive heart failure. J Am Coll Cardiol 19:1180
63. Ferguson DW, Berg WJ, Roach PJ, Oren RM, Mark AL (1992) Effects of heart failure on baroreflex control of sympathetic neural activity. Am J Cardiol 69: 523–531
64. Zucker IH, Earle AM, Gilmore JP (1977) The mechanism of adaptation of left atrial stretch receptors in dogs with chronic congestive heart failure. J Clin Invest 60:323
65. Zucker IH, Earle AM, Gilmore JP (1979) Changes in the sensitivity of left atrial receptors following the reversal of heart failure. Am J Physiol 237:H556–H622
66. Arnold JMO, Marchiori GE, Imrie JR, Burton GL, Pflugfelder PW, Kostuk WJ (1991) Large artery function in patients with chronic heart failure. Studies of brachial artery diameter and hemodynamics. Circulation 84:2418
67. Wang W, Chen J-S, Zucker IH (1990) Carotid sinus baroreceptor sensitivity in experimental heart failure. Circulation 81:1959
68. Wang W, Chen J-S, Zucker IH (1991) Postexcitatory depression of baroreceptors in dogs with experimental heart failure. Am J Physiol 260:H1160
69. Dibner-Dunlap ME, Thames MD (1989) Baroreflex control of renal sympathetic nerve activity is preserved in heart failure despite reduced arterial baroreceptor sensitivity. Circ Res 65:1526–1535
70. Oren RM, Schobel HP, Berg WJ, Kempf JS, Ferguson DW (1991) Sympathetic responses of heart failure patients to the cold pressor stimulus. Am J Cardiol 67:993–1001
71. Wang W, Chen J-S, Zucker IH (1991) Carotid sinus baroreceptor reflex in experimental heart failure. Circ Res 68:1294–3004
72. Colucci WS, Ribeiro JP, Creager MA, Hartley H (1989) Impaired chronotropic response to exercise in patients with congestive heart failure. Circ 80:314
73. LeJemtel TH, Maskin CS, Lucido D, Chadwick BJ (1986) Failure to augment maximal limb blood flow in response to one-leg versus two-leg exercise in patients with severe heart failure. Circ 74:245
74. Sinoway LI, Minotti JR, Davis D, Pennock JL, Burg JE, Musch TI, Zelis R (1988) Delayed reversal of impaired vasodilation in congestive heart failure after heart transplantation. Am J Cardiol 61:1076

75. Kaiser L, Spickard RC, Olivier NB (1989) Heart failure depresses endothelium-dependent responses in canine femoral artery. Am J Physiol 256:H962
76. Dibner-Dunlap ME, Thames MD (1989) Arterial baroreflexes are preserved until late in the course of developing heart failure. FASEB J 3:A858
77. Kinugawa T, Dibner-Dunlap ME, Thames MD (1992) Cardiopulmonary baroreflex control of renal sympathetic nerve activity is blunted in left ventricular dysfunction without heart failure. Circulation 86:I-781
78. Angus C, Moe GW, Howard RJ, Armstrong PW (1988) Alteration of cardiac size modulates baroreflex sensitivity in experimental heart failure. Circulation 78:II-106
79. Sterns DA, Ettinger SM, Gray KS, Whisler SK, Mosher TJ, Smith MB, Sinoway LI (1991) Skeletal muscle metaboreceptor exercise responses are attenuated in heart failure. Circulation 84:2034–2039
80. Mukharji J, Thames MD, Newton M, Hirsh PD, Lewis SA, Rehr RB, Cowley MJ, Hess ML, Hastillo A, Lower RR, Vetrovec GW (1987) Contrast injection bradycardia curing coronary angiography: Effects in the denervated heart. J Heart Transplant 6:44–48
81. Hintze TH, Xu X, Wang J (1991) Enhanced ventricular reflex prostaglandin mediated bradycardia during pacing induced heart failure in conscious dogs. Circulation 84:II-100
82. Bristow MR, Ginsburg R, Fowler M, Minobe W, Rasmussen R, Zera P, Menlove R, Shah P, Stinson E (1986) β-1 and β-2 adrenergic receptor subpopulations in normal and failing human ventricular myocardium: coupling of both receptor subtypes to muscle contraction and selective β-1 receptor down-regulation in heart failure. Circ Res 59:297–309
83. Fowler MB, Laser JA, Hopkins GL, Minobe W, Bristow MR (1986) Assessment of the β-adrenergic receptor pathway in the intact failing human heart: progressive receptor down-regulation and subsensitivity to agonist response. Circulation 74: 1290–1302
84. Bristow MR, Hershberger RE, Port JD, Rasmussen R (1989) β-1 and β-2 adrenergic receptor mediated adenylate cyclase stimulation in nonfailing and failing human ventricular myocardium. Mol Pharmacol 35:293–303
85. Feldman AM, Cates AE, Veazey WB, Hershberger RE, Bristow MR, Baughman KI, Baumgartner WA, Van Dop C (1988) Increase of the 40 ,000 mol wt pertussis toxin substrate (G protein) in te failing human heart. J Clin Invest 82:189–197
86. Heilbrunn SM, Shah P, Bristow MR, Valantine HA, Ginsburg R, Fowler MB (1989) Increased β-receptor density and improved hemodynamic response to catecholamine stimulation during chronic metoprolol therapy. Circulation 79:483–490
87. Neumann J, Schmitz W, Scholz H, Meyerinck LV, Doring V, Kalmar P (1988) Increase in myocardial Gi proteins in heart failue. Lancet 78:1373–1379
88. Ransnas LA, Hjalmarson A, Insel PA (1988) Dilated cardiomyopathy is associated with an impaired activation of the stimulatory G-protein, Gs, by GTP in heart membranes. Circulation 78:II-178
89. Eschenhagen T, Mende U, Nose M, Schmitz W, Scholz H, Haverich A, Hirt S, Doring V, Kalmar P, Hoppner W, Seitz H-J (1992) Increased messenger RNA level of the inhibitory G protein subunit in human end-stage heart failure. Circ Res 70:688–696
90. Feldman AM, Cates AE, Bristow MR, Van Dop C (1989) Altered expression of alpha-subunits of G proteins in failing human hearts. J Mol Cell Cardiol 21: 359–365

91. Port JD, DeBellis C, Wiederin J, et al. (1989) Long-term β-adrenergic receptor desensitization in cultured chick myocardial cells. FASEB J 3:47–56
92. Bohm M, Gierschik P, Jakobs KH, Pieske B, Schnabel P, Ungerer M, Erdmann E (1990) Increase of G in human hearts with dilated but not ischemic cardiomyopathy. Circulation 82:1249–1265
93. Feldman AM, Ray PE, Bristow MR (1991) Expression of alpha-subunits of G proteins in failing human heart: a reappraisal utilizing quantitative polymerase chain reaction. J Mol Cell Cardiol 23(12):1355–1358
94. Francis GS (1991) Calcium channel blockers and congestive heart failure. Circulation 83:336–337
95. Packer M (1989) Pathophysiological mechanisms underlying the adverse effects of calcium channel blockers in patients with chronic heart failure. Circulation 80:IV-59–IV-6767
96. Fifer MA, Colucci WS, Lorell BH, Jaski BE, Barry WH (1985) Inotropic, vascular and neuroendocrine effects of nifidipine in heart failure: comparison with nitroprusside. J Am Coll Cardiol 5:731–737
97. Fray JCS, Lush DJ, Valentine AMD (1983) Cellular mechanisms of renin secretion. Fed Proc 42:3150–3154
98. Packer M (1989) Second generation calcium channel blockers in the treatment of chronic heart failure: are they any better than their predecessors? J Am Coll Cardiol 14:1339–1440
99. The Amlodipine Investigators (1991) Randomized, multicenter, double-blind placebo-controlled evaluation of amlodipine in patients with mild to moderate heart failure. J Am Coll Cardiol 15:274A
100. Cohn JN, Johnson G, Ziesche S, et al. (1991) A comparison of enalipril with hydralizine-isosorbide dinitrate in the treatment of chronic heart failure. N Eng J Med 325:303–311
101. Zimmerman BG, Sybertz EJ, Wong PC (1984) Interaction between sympathetic and renin-angiotensin systems. J Hypertens 2:581–587
102. Zimmerman BG, Gomer SK, Liao JC (1972) Action of angiotensin on vascular nerve endings: facilitation of norepinephrine release. Fed Proc 31:1344–1350
103. Hatton R, Clough DP, Adigun Conway J (1982) Functional interaction between angiotensin and sympathetic reflexes in cats. Clin Sci 62:51–56
104. Osterziel KJ, Dietz R, Schmid, Milkulaschek K, Manthey J, Kubler W (1990) ACE inhibition improves vagal reactivity in patients with heart failure. Am Heart J 120:1120–1128
105. Cody RJ (1982) The effect of captopril on postural hemodymanics and autonomic responses in chronic heart failure. Am Heart J 104:1190–1196
106. Cody RJ, Franklin KW, Kluger J, Laragh JH (1982) Mechanisms governing the postural response and baroreceptor abnormalities in chronic heart failure: Effects of acute and chronic converting enzyme inhibition. Circulation 66:135–142
107. Ferguson DW, Berg WJ, Sanders JS, Roach PJ, Kempf JS, Kienzle MG (1989) Sympathoinhibitory responses to digitalis glycosides in heart failure patients. Circulation 80:65–77
108. Schobel HP, Oren RM, Roach PJ, Mark AL, Ferguson DW (1991) Contrasting effects of digitalis and dobutamine on baroreflex sympathetic control in normal humans. Circulation 84:1118–1129
109. Goldsmith SR, Simon AB, Miller E (1992) Effect of digitalis on norepinephrine kinetics in congestive heart failure. J Am Coll Cardiol 20:858–863

110. Waagstein F, Hjalmmarson A, Varnauskas E, Wallentin I (1975) Effect of β Adrenergic receptor blockade in congestive cardiomyopathy. Br Heart J 37: 1022–1036
111. Gilbert EM, O'Connell, Bristow MR (1991) Therapy of dilated cardiomyopathy with chronic β-adrenergic blockade. Heart Vessels 6:S29–S39
112. Gilberts EM, Anderson JL, Deitchman, et al. (1990) Long term β-blocker vasodilator therapy improves cardiac function in idiopathic dilated cardiomyopathy: a double blind, randomized study of bucindolol vs placebo. Am J Med 88:223–229
113. Eichorn EJ, McGhie AI, Bedotto JB (1991) Effects of bucindolol on neurohumoral activation in congestive heart failure. Am J Cardiol 67:67–73
114. Gilbert EM, Olsen SL, Renlund DG, Bristow MR (1993) Beta-adrenergic receptor regulation and left ventricular function in idiopathic dilated cardiomyopathy. Am J Cardiol 71:23C–29C

3.2 Calcium Overload as a Cause of Heart Failure

Yukihiro Koretsune, Hiroshi Sato, and Masatsugu Hori[1]

Summary. Although sympathetic activation is a compensatory mechanism to augment the contractile function of the heart, the excessive activation may be harmful for the failing heart since it may induce down-regulation of β-adrenoceptors and cause calcium overload. Recent reports demonstrate that calcium handling is abnormal in the severely failing heart in which calcium overload further deteriorates the cardiac function. Morgan and his colleagues reported that intracellular Ca^{2+} handling is abnormal in the human failing cardiac muscle. It is not clear whether this abnormality is the cause or the result of the failing myocardium; however, the excessive Ca may induce a number of adverse effects in cardiomyocytes, including activation of Ca^{2+}-sensitive proteases which may disrupt the membranous organellas and cytoskeletons. Recently, we observed that the microtubules of cardiomyocytes are disrupted when extracellular Ca^{2+} concentration is raised to 5 mM and when the cells are treated with calcium ionophores. Moreover, in the preliminary study, we observed the various extents of microtubular injuries in the biopsied myocardial samples obtained from the patients with cardiomyopathy. We also indicate that transient exposure to high $[Ca]_o$ without ischemia leaves behind distinctive contractile, metabolic, and histological sequelae in the isolated heart preparation. Therefore, calcium overload may play an important role in the deterioration of cardiac function.

Key words: Heart failure—Stunned myocardium—Microtubules—Adrenergic stimulation

Calcium ions play a key role as intermediaries of cell function in cardiac muscle. Such physiological actions are made possible by the low Ca^{2+} concentration normally present within the cells of the myocardium. The cytoplasmic

[1]The First Department of Medicine, Osaka University Medical School, 1-1-50 Fukushima, Fukushima-ku, Osaka, 553 Japan

Ca^{2+} concentration ($[Ca^{2+}]_i$) of unstimulated cells is approximately $10^{-7} M$, whereas extracellular Ca^{2+} concentration ranges around $10^{-3} M$ [1]. This chemical gradient for Ca^{2+} is magnified by the normal electronegativity of the interior of the resting cell. It is well known that the influx of Ca^{2+} into the myocardial cell occurs during the plateau phase of the action potential through a set of membrane proteins which are permeable primarily to Ca^{2+}, termed "slow channels" or voltage-dependent calcium channels [2]. The absolute quantity of Ca^{2+} that crosses the sarcolemma during each beat is relatively small and incapable by itself of bringing about full activation of the contractile apparatus in mammalian heart cells [3,4]. Instead, the major portion of the Ca^{2+} used to activate contraction is stored within the cell, largely in the sarcoplasmic reticulum from which Ca^{2+} is released by the Ca^{2+} which enters the cell through the slow channels (calcium-induced calcium release) [5]. The released Ca^{2+} then diffuses toward the myofibrils and triggers the contractile process by binding to troponin C and enabling the interaction of actin and myosin. The number of activated contractile elements and the resultant force generated are directly related to the quantity of Ca^{2+} present in the vicinity of the myofibrils, which ultimately depends on the influx of Ca^{2+} through the slow channels. Relaxation of cardiac muscle results from a cessation of the inward slow Ca^{2+} current coupled with the uptake of Ca^{2+} by sarcoplasmic reticulum and the extrusion of Ca^{2+} by the sarcolemmal Na^+–Ca^{2+} exchange. Therefore, the abnormal handling of Ca^{2+} in cardiac muscle may lead to dysfunction of contraction and relaxation of the heart. The role of abnormal Ca handling in myocardial dysfunction is discussed in this chapter.

Calcium Overload in Failing Heart

Direct measurements of $[Ca^{2+}]_i$ in human heart muscle are very limited. Recently, Morgan and his colleagues [6] reported that intracellular Ca^{2+} handling is abnormal in the human failing cardiac muscle. They measured $[Ca^{2+}]_i$ using aequorin during isometric contraction of myocardium from patients with end-stage heart failure undergoing heart transplantation. Contractions and Ca^{2+} transients of the failing muscle were markedly prolonged and the Ca^{2+} transient was biphasic [Fig. 1, early peak (L_1) and late plateau phase (L_2)]. In contrast to the control muscle, the failing muscle demonstrated a raised residual component L_2 which probably reflects Ca^{2+} entry through voltage-dependent sarcolemmal channels. Thus, their observations are not incompatible with previous findings that the Ca^{2+} uptake by sarcoplasmic reticulum is depressed in the failing heart [7,8]. It should be noted that the early peak of the Ca^{2+} transient, L_1, is minimally depressed in the failing heart, suggesting that the release of Ca^{2+} from sarcoplasmic reticulum is not significantly affected. Thus, these results may imply that the dysfunction of Ca uptake by sarcoplasmic reticulum, and/or the augmented Ca^{2+} entry through voltage-dependent Ca^{2+} channels, mainly cause the Ca overload in the failing cardiac

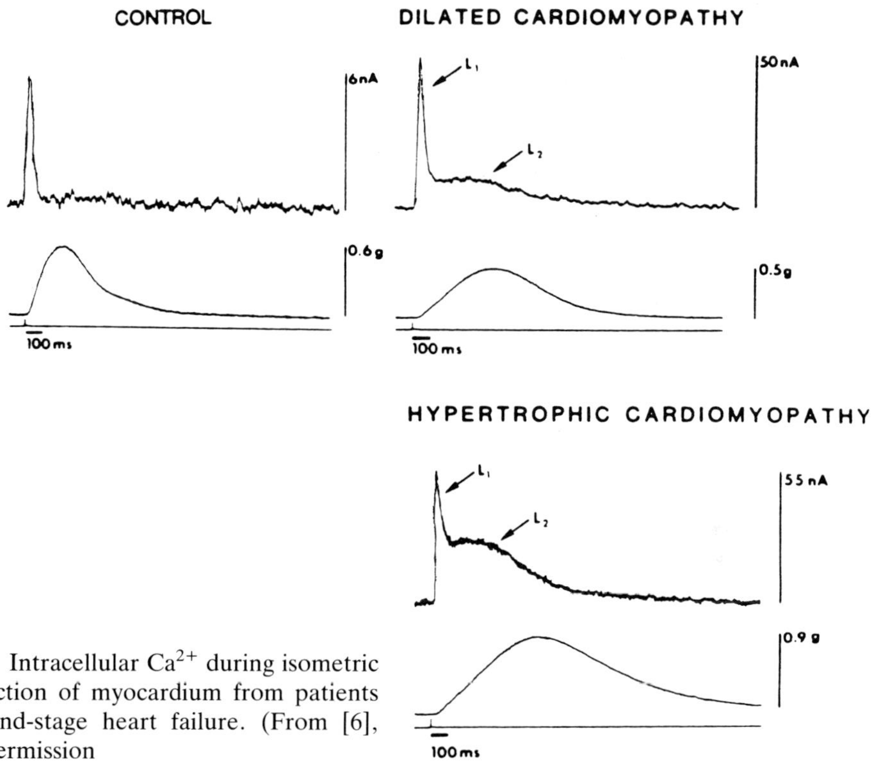

Fig. 1. Intracellular Ca^{2+} during isometric contraction of myocardium from patients with end-stage heart failure. (From [6], with permission

muscle. Ca overload in turn may impair relaxation of the heart, thus decreasing rapid ventricular filling and leading to the low cardiac output during tachycardia. Ca overload also would increase diastolic myocardial stiffness, raising the left ventricular (LV) end-diastolic pressure which causes the pulmonary congestion. The important results of Morgan et al. may be subject to technical limitations related to the chemical loading method for aequorin; confirmation by other methods is eagerly awaited.

The excessive Ca may induce a number of adverse effects in cardiomyocytes, including activation of Ca^{2+}-sensitive proteases which may disrupt the membranous organelles and cytoskeletons. Recently, we observed that the microtubules of cardiomyocytes are disrupted when the extracellular Ca^{2+} concentration is raised to 5 m*M* and when the cells are treated with calcium ionophores [9].

Given the Ca overload hypothesis, one may raise the possibility that long-term treatment with Ca^{2+} antagonists may be beneficial for patients with chronic heart failure. In a prospective clinical trial, the calcium channel antagonist, diltiazem, was given to 22 patients with dilated cardiomyopathy in addition to conventional therapy of digitalis, diuretics, and vasodilators [10]. The mean survival time was 29 months in the control group, whereas no patient in the diltiazem group died over a mean follow-up period of 15.4 months, and the mean LV ejection fraction increased from 0.34 to 0.44 with an improvement of clinical symptoms. Nifedipine is a primarily arteriolar vasodilator and produces an increase in cardiac output due to a decrease in systemic vascular resistance. However, in some patients with severe low cardiac output failure, it worsened ventricular performance through its negative inotropic effect [11]. Although some acute and chronic clinical trials have demonstrated hemodynamic improvement both at rest and during exercise [12–14], favorable results have not been obtained in other studies [11,15,16]. Since large-scale placebo-controlled studies have not been reported, the clinical efficacy of Ca antagonists in heart failure is still controversial. To clarify the role of Ca antagonists in treatment of chronic heart failure, well-designed, large-scale clinical trials are necessary. The underlying mechanism of Ca overload in the failing heart also merits further scrutiny.

Does Transient Ca Overload even in the Absence of Ischemia Induce Myocardial Dysfunction?

To evaluate the role of calcium as a mediator of injury during myocardial dysfunction, it is important to determine whether calcium overload per se is sufficient to produce myocardial injury. To determine the contractile, histological, and metabolic sequelae of transient Ca overload, developed pressures in perfused ferret hearts were measured before and 20 min after three 5-min periods of perfusion with a 10 m*M* $[Ca]_o$, 1 m*M* $[Mg]_o$ solution (high-Ca group) without ischemia, and in control hearts exposed transiently to the same total divalent cation concentration without a change in $[Ca]_o$ (9 m*M* $[Mg]_o$, 2 m*M* $[Ca]_o$) [17]. Developed pressures (DP), measured at various $[Ca]_o$ (0.5–5 m*M*), were depressed in the high-Ca group relative to control (Fig. 2a). The hearts in the control group were histologically normal, whereas foci of "reversible" injury (mitochondrial swelling, glycogen deposition, and clumping of nuclear chromatin) were infrequently observed in hearts from the high-Ca group. Maximum calcium-activated pressure (MCAP) was also decreased in the high-Ca group (Fig. 2b). $[Ca]_o$ sensitivity, determined by normalization of the DP–$[Ca]_o$ relationship to the corresponding MCAP, was shifted to higher $[Ca]_o$ in the high-Ca group (Fig. 2c). Phosphorus nuclear magnetic resonance (NMR) spectra were also obtained in high-Ca hearts. [ATP] declined by 30%–40% after exposure to high $[Ca]_o$, but inorganic phosphate, phosphocreatine, and pH remained unchanged. These results of Kitakaze et al. [17] indicate that transient exposure to high $[Ca]_o$ without ischemia leaves behind distinctive contractile, metabolic, and histological sequelae.

There is another analogy of myocardial failure in the postarrhythmic contractile dysfunction described by Koretsune and Marban [18]. During ventricular fibrillation induced by burst pacing, $[Ca^{2+}]_i$ rose rapidly and dramatically, exceeding by four times the control value within 5 min. $[Ca^{2+}]_i$ remained

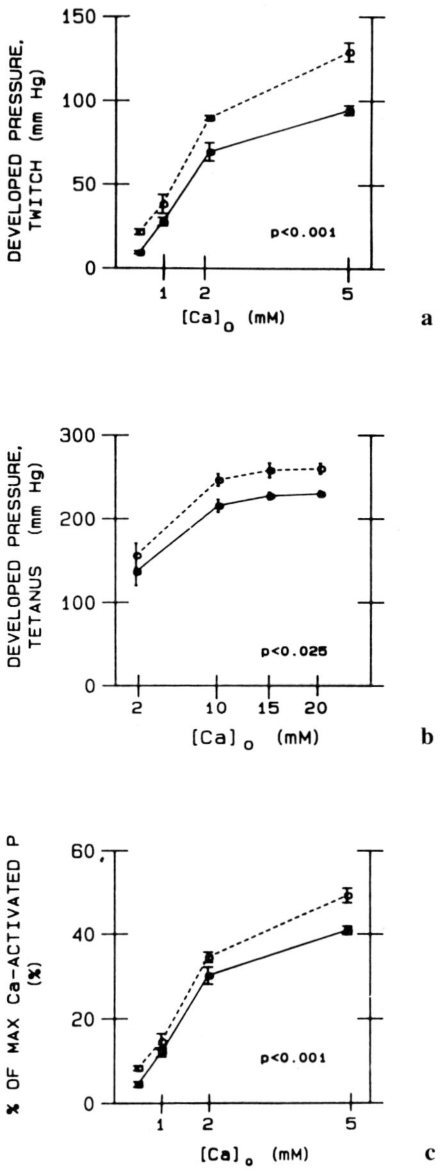

Fig. 2a–c. Characterization of contractile dysfunction in transiently Ca-overloaded hearts. Results from control groups (n = 5) are shown as *open circles*, whereas these from high-Ca hearts (n = 8) are presented as *filled circles*. **a** $[Ca]_o$ responsiveness. **b** Developed pressure during tetani maximum calcium-activated pressure (MCAP) in various $[Ca]_o$. **c** Ca_o sensitivity, i.e., Ca_o responsiveness normalized by the corresponding MCAP. *P*, pressure. (From [62], with permission)

markedly elevated throughout 20 min of fibrillation, but it returned to control values shortly after defibrillation. In hearts which contract isovolumically with a balloon in the left ventricle, acidosis and high-energy phosphate depletion developed despite the maintenance of normal coronary pressure. Even when the left ventricular volume was decreased during fibrillation to reduce the wall stress to avoid this adverse effect, $[Ca^{2+}]_i$ still increased remarkably and the developed pressure did not recover to the control level after defibrillation. Thus, the increase in $[Ca^{2+}]_i$ in postarrhythmic hearts may cause the contractile dysfunction. It should be noted that adriamycin-induced heart failure is associated with an increase in $[Ca^{2+}]_i$ even with the perfusion maintained [19]. These lines of evidence strongly suggest that Ca overload per se is sufficient to induce reversible myocardial injury.

Cytoskeletal Changes of Myocardium with Ca Overload

It is well recognized that the sympathetic nervous system is activated during heart failure [20,21]. Although the sympathetic activation supports the cardiovascular regulation, a number of studies have shown that excessive sympathetic activity deteriorates the cardiac contractile and metabolic functions [22–24], and β-adrenoceptor blocker therapy improves cardiac function and prevents functional deterioration in ischemic heart disease and chronic heart failure [25–27]. Previous studies suggest that intracellular calcium overload through β-adrenoceptor stimulation plays a key role in catecholamine-induced myocardial necrosis [28,29]. However, abnormal calcium handling in the failing hearts could not fully explain the progression of cardiac dysfunction and the histological changes in calcium-overloaded cells.

Recently, we observed that the cytoskeletal structures, microtubules, which support the integrity of the plasma membrane, myofibrils, and other membranous organelles, were disassembled and their structural integrity lost prior to irreversible injury in ischemic myocardium [30]. The microtubules were also disrupted in stunned myocardium due to intracellular calcium overload [31]. There have been several reports that microtubules are sensitive to intracellular Ca^{2+} [32,33]. Recently, we observed microtubular disruption in the rat heart when it was stimulated with continuous norepinephrine infusion [34]. In view of these findings, we hypothesized that microtubules are also injured by catecholamine stimulation through an excessive calcium influx.

Figure 3a shows a representative anti-β-tubulin immunofluorescent staining of cultured neonatal rat cardiomyocytes. Microtubules were observed as tortuous filaments distributed throughout the cytoplasm and encircling the nucleus.

Treatment with $10\,\mu M$ norepinephrine partially disrupted microtubules as shown in Fig. 3b. Loss of microtubular staining and fragmentation of microtubular filaments into small dotted spots were often observed. Actin filaments labeled with rhodamine-phalloidin showed fine cross-striations of the sarcomeres, even in the cells with microtubular disruption, indicating that the contractile apparatus remained intact (Fig. 3c).

Pretreatment with phentolamine (100 μ*M*) minimally attenuated the norepinephrine (10 μ*M*) induced microtubular disruption. In contrast, propranolol (100 μ*M*) significantly inhibited the norepinephrine effect. Pretreatment with a combination of propranolol (100 μ*M*) and phentolamine (100 μ*M*) completely inhibited the effect of norepinephrine. These results indicate that the role of norepinephrine in microtubular disruption is mostly mediated by β-adrenoceptor stimulation.

This conclusion was further confirmed by the observation that α-adrenergic stimulation by phenylephrine minimally affected the microtubules. In contrast, β-adrenoceptor stimulation with isoproterenol caused a marked decrease (Fig. 3d) in the incidence of normally stained myocytes. Pretreatment with propranolol (100 μ*M*) almost inhibited the microtubular disruption induced by 10 μ*M* isoproterenol. Furthermore, treatment with denopamine, a β_1-selective adrenergic agonist, disrupted the microtubular structures in a dose-dependent manner, indicating that the role of norepinephrine in microtubular disruption is mediated by β_1-adrenoceptor stimulation.

Both forskolin and dibutyryl cAMP increased the microtubule disruption score in a dose-dependent manner, indicating that the effect of β_1-adrenoceptor stimulation on microtubular disruption is cAMP-mediated. Furthermore, we observed that the microtubular disruption during β-adrenoceptor stimulation is directly dependent on Ca^{2+} influx; a decrease in $CaCl_2$ concentration in the medium from 2 m*M* to 0.5 m*M* during the treatment with 10 μ*M* isoproterenol significantly attenuated both the spontaneous contracting rate and the microtubule disruption score. Pretreatment with diltiazem also attenuated the effect of isoproterenol on the spontaneous contraction rate and microtubular disruption, suggesting that Ca^{2+} influx during β-adrenergic stimulation is responsible for microtubular disruption. In contrast, increases in extracellular $CaCl_2$ concentration disrupted microtubules in a dose-dependent manner even without β-adrenergic stimulation. Furthermore, treatment with the calcium ionophore A23187 severely disrupted the microtubules. These results indicate that intracellular calcium overload could disrupt the microtubules. It should be noted that treatment with calcium ionophore completely inhibited spontaneous contraction, suggesting that mechanical stress by spontaneous contraction is not necessary for calcium-induced microtubular disruption.

The role of microtubules in cardiac cells has not been extensively studied, and their physiological importance is still unclear. Although it is conceivable that the microtubular filamentous network throughout the cytoplasm may contribute to the structural support of cellular components, e.g., plasma membrane, myofibrils, and membranous organelles [35], a direct relation between the microtubules and cardiac contractile function has not been demonstrated. Indeed, the neonatal cardiomyocytes were contracting even with markedly disrupted microtubules. Treatment with colchicine depolymerizes the microtubular filaments; however, the contraction rate is even increased [36]. These

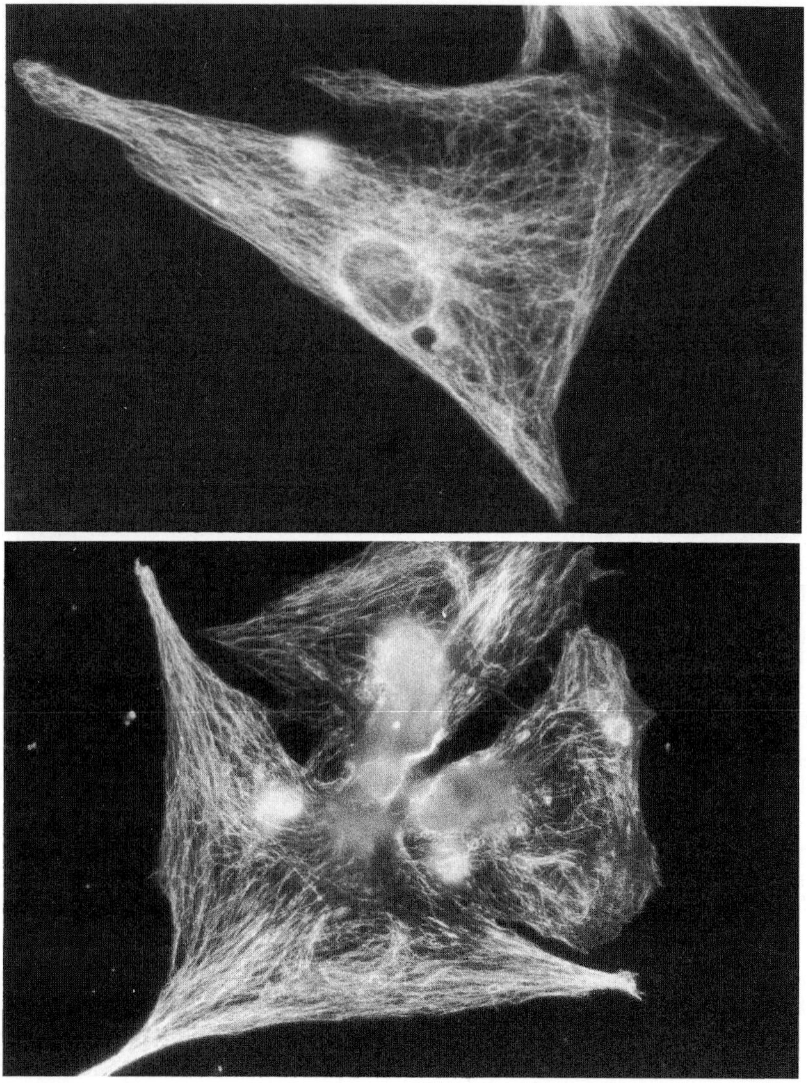

a

b

Fig. 3. Photomicrographs showing double staining of cultured neonatal rat cardiomyocytes with a mouse monoclonal antibody against β-tubulin (**a**, **b**, and **d**) and rhodamine–phalloidin (**c**). **a** A representative anti-β-tubulin immunofluorescent staining. Note that microtubular structures are observed as tortuous filaments throughout the cytoplasm and around the nucleus. **b** Microtubular staining after 60-min exposure to 10 μ*M* norepinephrine. Partial loss of microtubular staining and fragmentation of microtubular filaments (dotted spots staining) were observed. Microtubular structures around the nucleus almost disappeared whereas those in the peripheral region were minimally affected. **c** Cross-striations of actin filaments were well preserved (the same cell as **b**). **d** Microtubular structures after 60-min exposure to 10 μ*M* isoproterenol. Characteristic filamentous patterns of microtubular stains were substantially lost

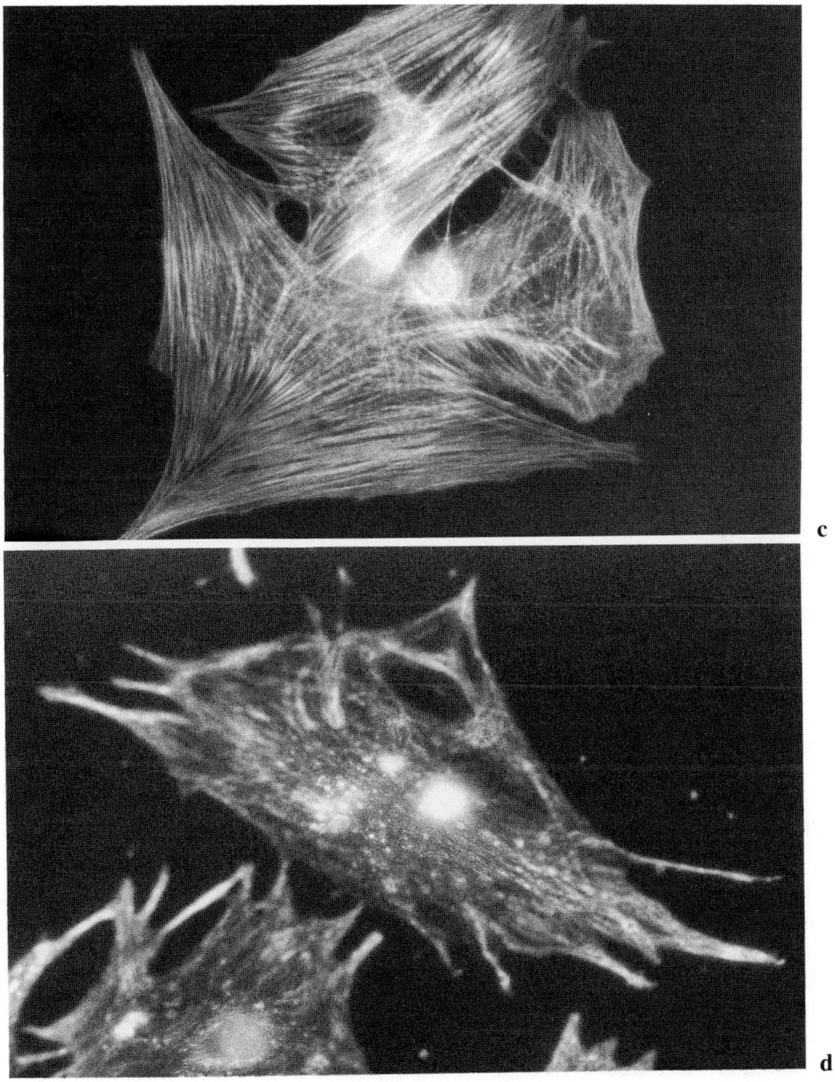

Fig. 3. *Continued*

lines of evidence may lead us to consider that the microtubules do not contribute to the cellular function. A recent report, however, indicates that an increase in microtubular filaments is responsible for contractile dysfunction in the hypertrophied heart induced by pressure overload [37]. Furthermore, a recent review indicates that the cytoskeleton plays a role in protein degradation and myofibrillogenesis in the heart [38]. In view of this hypothesis, it is of interest that disruption of microtubules by β-adrenoceptor stimulation is reversible. This may imply that the newly assembled microtubules contribute to the myofibrillogenesis, since catecholamine stimulation is known to be a potent trigger of protein synthesis. Thus, the disassembly of microtubules observed with β-adrenoceptor stimulation may contribute to the remodeling of cellular organization which in turn may affect cellular function.

It is well recognized that sympathetic nerves are activated in patients with severe heart failure. Although sympathetic activation is a compensatory mechanism to augment the contractile function of the heart, excessive activation may be harmful for the failing heart since it may induce down-regulation of β-adrenoceptors and cause calcium overload. Recent reports demonstrate that calcium handling is abnormal in the severely failing heart in which calcium overload further deteriorates the cardiac function [39]. These lines of evidence raise the hypothesis that microtubules may be injured in the failing heart. Indeed, we observed that sustained infusion of norepinephrine to rats exerted the disruption of microtubules in the heart; and furthermore, cardiac microtubules are disrupted in ischemic failing canine hearts [30]. Moreover, in preliminary study, we observed various extents of microtubular injury in biopsied myocardial samples obtained from patients with cardiomyopathy [40]. These findings suggest that microtubules may be injured in the human heart when stimulated by enhanced sympathetic activity. Although further studies are necessary to clarify the cause–effect relationship in the clinical setting, the present study indicates that β-adrenoceptor stimulation could cause reversible cytoskeletal injury in cardiomyocytes.

References

1. Blinks JR, Prendergast FG, Allen DG (1976) Proteins as biological calcium indicators. Pharmacol Rev 28:1–93
2. Beeler GW, Reuter H (1970) Membrane calcium current in ventricular myocardial fibers. J Physiol 207:191–209
3. New N, Trautwein W (1975) The ionic nature of the slow inward current and its relation to contraction. Pflugers Arch 354:55–74
4. Gibbons WR, Fozzard HA (1975) Slow inward current and contraction in sheep cardiac Purkinje fibers. J Gen Physiol 65:367–383
5. Katz AM (1977) Physiology of the heart. Raven, New York
6. Gwathmey JK, Copelas L, MacKinnon R, Schon FJ, Feldman MD, Grossman W, Morgan JP (1987) Abnormal intracellular calcium handling in myocardium from patients with end-stage heart failure. Circ Res 61:70–76
7. Lentz RW, Harrison CE Jr, Dewey DA, Barnhorst GK, Danielson GK, Pluth JR (1978) Functional evaluation of sarcoplasmic reticulum and mitochondria in human pathologic states. J Mol Cell Cardiol 10:3–30
8. Lindenmayer GE, Sordahl LA, Harigaya S, Allen JC, Besch HR Jr, Schwartz A (1971) Some biochemical studies on subcellular systems isolated from fresh recipient human cardiac tissue obtained during transplantation. Am J Cardiol 27: 277–283

9. Sato H, Hori M, Iwai K, Kagiya T, Takashima S, Tada M (1990) Ca^{2+} overload disrupts microtubules in cultured rat cardiomyocytes. Circulation 82[Suppl III]:III-297
10. Figulla HR, Rechenberg JV, Wiegand V, Soballa R, Kreuzer H (1989) Beneficial effects of long-term diltiazem treatment in dilated cardiomyopathy. J Am Coll Cardiol 13:653–658
11. Agostoni PG, Cesare ND, Doria E, Polese A, Tamborini G, Guazzi MD (1986) Afterload reduction: a comparison of captoril and nifedipine in dilated cardiomyopathy. Br Heart J 55:391–399
12. Bellocci F, Ansalone G, Santarelli P, Loperfido F, Scabbia E, Zecchi P, Manzoli U (1982) Oral nifedipine in the long-term management of severe chronic heart failure. J Cardiovasc Pharmacol 4:847–855
13. Zeng X, Du C, Zhang T, Luo D (1987) Low dose nifedipine therapy for dilated congestive heart failure. Circulation 76[Suppl IV]:IV-70
14. Thomas P, Sheridan DJ (1988) Acute and chronic hemodynamic effects of nicardipine in patients with congestive heart failure. Br J Clin Pharmacol 26:243
15. Metra M, Bonandi L, Canna GL, Nordio G, Nodari S, Raddino R, Guaini T, Danesi R, Cas LD (1988) Acute and chronic hemodynamic effects of nisoldipine in chronic heart failure. Eur Heart J 9[Suppl I]:184
16. Tan LB, Murray RG, Litter WA (1987) Felodipine in patients with chronic heart failure: discrepant hemodynamic and clinical effects. Br Heart J 58:122–128
17. Kitakaze M, Weisman HF, Marban E (1987) Contractile dysfunction and ATP depletion after transient calcium overload in perfused ferret hearts. Circulation 77:685–695
18. Koretsune Y, Marban E (1989) Cell calcium in the pathophysiology of ventricular fibrillation and in the pathogenesis of post-arrhythmic contractile dysfunction. Circulation 80:369–379
19. Kusuoka H, Futaki S, Koretsune Y, Kitabatake A, Suga H, Kamada T, Inoue M (1991) Alterations of intracellular calcium homeostasis and myocardial energetics in acute adriamycin induced heart failure. J Cardiovasc Pharmacol 18:437–444
20. Levine TB, Francis GS, Goldsmith SR, Simon AB, Cohn JN (1982) Activity of the sympathetic nervous system and renin–angiotensin system assessed by plasma hormone levels and their relation to hemodynamic abnormalities in congestive heart failure. Am J Cardiol 49:1659
21. Francis GS, Goldsmith SR, Levine TB, Olivia MT, Cohn JN (1984) The neurohumoral axis in congestive heart failure. Ann Intern Med 101:370–377
22. Bhagat B, Sullivan JM, Fischer VW, Nadel EM, Dhalla NS (1978) cAMP activity and isoproterenol-induced myocardial injury in rats. In: Kobayashi Y, Ito Y, Rona G (eds) Recent advances in studies on cardiac structure and metabolism. University Park Press, Baltimore, MD, pp 465–470
23. Wheatley AM, Thandroyen FT, Opie LH (1985) Catecholamine induced myocardial cell damage: Catecholamines or adrenochrome. J Mol Cell Cardiol 17:349–359
24. Rona G (1985) Catecholamine cardiotoxicity. J Mol Cell Cardiol 17:291–306
25. Waagstein F, Hjalmarson A, Varnauskas E, Wallentin I (1975) Effects of chronic beta-adrenergic receptor blockade in congestive cardiomyopathy. Br Heart J 37: 1022–1036
26. Swedberg K, Hjalmarson A, Waagstein F, Wallentin I (1979) Prolongation of survival in congestive cardiomyopathy by beta-receptor blockade. Lancet i:1374–1376

27. Swedberg K, Hjalamarson A, Waagstein F, Wallentin I (1980) Adverse effects of beta-blockade withdrawal in patients with congestive cardiomyopathy. Br Heart J 44:134–142
28. Bloom S, Davis DL (1972) Calcium as mediator of isoproterenol induced myocardial necrosis. Am J Pathol 69:459–470
29. Mann DL, Kent RL, Persons B, Cooper G IV (1992) Adrenergic effects on the biology of the adult mammalian cardiocyte. Circulation 85:790–804
30. Iwai K, Hori M, Kitabatake A, Kurihara H, Uchida K, Inoue M, Kamada T (1990) Disruption of microtubules as an early sign of irreversible ischemic injury. Immunohistochemical study of in situ canine hearts. Circ Res 67:694–706
31. Sato H, Hori M, Kitakaze M, Iwai K, Takashima S, Kurihara H, Inoue M, Kamada T (1993) Reperfusion after brief ischemia disrupts the microtubule network in canine hearts. Circ Res 72:361–375
32. Kieth C, Dipaola M, Maxfield FR, Shelanski ML (1983) Microinjection of Ca^{2+}-calmodulin causes a localized depolymerization of microtubules. J Cell Biol 97: 1918–1924
33. Schliwa M, Euteneuer U, Bulinski JC, Izant JG (1981) Calcium lability of cytoplasmic microtubules and its modulation by microtubule-associated proteins. Proc Natl Acad Sci USA 78:1037–1041
34. Sato H, Hori M, Iwai K, Kagiya T, Takashima S, Tada M (1990) Ca^{2+} overload disrupts microtubules in cultured rat cardiomyocytes (abstract). Circulation 82:III-297
35. Goldstein MA, Entman ML (1979) Microtubules in mammalian heart muscle. J Cell Biol 80:183–195
36. Klein I (1983) Colchicine stimulates the rate of contraction of heart cells in culture. Cardiovasc Res 17:459–465
37. Tsutsui H, Ishihara K, Cooper G IV (1993) Cytoskeletal role in the contractile dysfunction of hypertrophied myocardium. Science 260:682–687
38. Samarel AM (1993) Hemodynamic overload and the regulation of myofibrillar protein degradation. Circulation 87:1418–1420
39. Gwathmey JK, Copelas L, MacKinnon R, Schoen FJ, Feldman MD, Grossman W, Morgan JP (1987) Abnormal intracellular calcium handling in myocardium from patients with end-stage heart failure. Circ Res 61:70–76
40. Iwai K, Hori M, Sato H, Takashima S, Hoki Y, Fukunami M, Naka M, Kurihara H, Uchida K, Kitabatake A (1991) Disruptions of microtubules in human cardiomyopathy (abstract). Circulation 84[Suppl II]:II-440
41. Schaper J, Froede R, Hein St, Buck A, Hashizume H, Speiser B, Fridl A, Bleese N (1991) Impairment of the myocardial ultrastructure and changes of the cytoskeleton in dilated cardiomyopathy. Circulation 83:504–514

3.3 Systolic and Diastolic Dysfunction in Heart Failure

KAZUO KOMAMURA, RICHARD P. SHANNON, and STEPHEN F. VATNER[1]

Summary. In this review, we summarize the effects of heart failure, induced by chronic rapid ventricular pacing, on the sequence of development of left ventricular (LV) systolic and diastolic dysfunction in conscious dogs. LV systolic and diastolic dysfunction were evident within 24 h after initiation of pacing, and progressed over a 3-week period. These alterations were associated with significant increases in LV end-diastolic and LV end-systolic volumes and wall stresses. When stresses and heart rate were matched at the same levels in the control and failure stages, the abnormalities in diastolic function were no longer observed, whereas LV systolic function remained depressed. There were no increases in connective tissue content in this model of heart failure at this advanced stage. Thus, pacing-induced heart failure in conscious dogs is characterized by major alterations in LV diastolic function under conditions of increased loading, which were correctable when loading conditions were normalized.

Key words: Collagen—Diastole—Heart failure—Pacing—Systole—Ventricular function

Congestive cardiomyopathies, both experimental and clinical, are associated with abnormalities in systolic and diastolic function [1–4]. Data derived principally from isolated heart or muscle preparations have suggested that these abnormalities can be attributed to alterations in excitation-contraction coupling. However, there are numerous other factors such as ventricular loading conditions [5], changes in ventricular geometry [1,3], or alterations in the extracellular matrix [6] which may contribute to both systolic and diastolic dysfunction in the intact state.

[1]Department of Cardiovascular Medicine, Harvard Medical School, New England Regional Primate Research Center, Southborough, MA 01772, USA

In the current review, we summarize the alterations in left ventricular (LV) systolic or diastolic function in the model of pacing-induced heart failure in conscious dogs [1]. This model shows numerous phenotype similarities to human congestive cardiomyopathy including the nature and extent of contractile dysfunction [1,3,7], ventricular remodelling [1,3,7], neurohumoral activation [8], alterations in beta-adrenergic signalling [9,10], and excitation-contraction coupling [11].

To accomplish these goals, mongrel dogs were instrumented with LV pressure transducers, aortic and left atrial catheters, and three sets of ultrasonic dimension crystals placed across the long and short axes of the left ventricle and across the left ventricular free wall [1,3,7]. A sutureless pacing lead was placed on the right ventricular (RV) free wall for initiation of the insult and on the left atrial appendage to control heart rate. The details of the surgical instrumentation and protocols have been described in detail previously [1,3,7].

All dogs were studied in the control state, 2–3 weeks after instrumentation, when they were healthy and had completely recovered from the effects of surgery, and at frequent intervals after the initiation of rapid RV pacing ($240\,min^{-1}$) including an early stage of contractile dysfunction (24 h), following ventricular dilatation in the absence of symptoms (14 days), and finally during symptomatic congestive heart failure (23 ± 2 days). All hemodynamic measurements were made with the RV pacer turned off, after which the dogs were allowed to stabilize for 30 min. To investigate the role of altered loading conditions as determinants of LV systolic and diastolic dysfunction, loading conditions were matched between the control and symptomatic congestive failure states in seven dogs by reducing the elevated LV wall stresses in the heart failure state through controlled hemorrhage and inferior vena caval occlusion, and increasing loading conditions by volume loading and aortic constriction in the control state. Heart rate was matched in the control and failure states using atrial pacing at 150 beats/min. In addition, pathological analyses were obtained from dogs with advanced heart failure and a group of sham-operated controls. Calculation and analyses of digitized LV dimension and pressure data were made to obtain systolic and diastolic functional parameters as described previously [1].

Serial Changes in LV and Systemic Hemodynamics

Serial changes in LV end-diastolic and end-systolic stresses and volumes are shown in Fig. 1. LV end-diastolic and end-systolic wall stresses increased early (within 1 day) after initiating rapid ventricular pacing and progressed further at 1, 2, and 3 weeks, peaking at $53 \pm 6\,g/cm^2$ and $87 \pm 9\,g/cm^2$, respectively. There were similar significant increases in LV end-diastolic volume from 56 ± 2 ml to 79 ± 3 ml and end-systolic volume from 28 ± 2 to 56 ± 2 ml. Both LV systolic pressure and mean arterial pressure fell significantly from 119 ± 3 mmHg to 102 ± 2 mmHg and from 96 ± 3 to 87 ± 3 mmHg, respectively, while LV end-diastolic pressure rose from 8 ± 1 mmHg to 28 ± 2 mmHg over

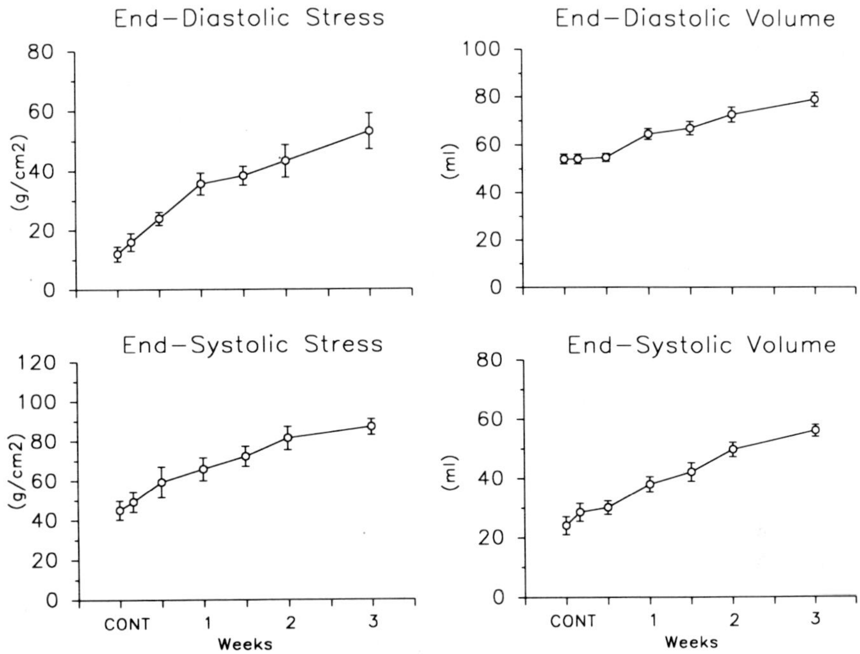

Fig. 1. Serial changes in systolic and diastolic left ventricular wall stresses and volumes are shown at control, at 1 day and at selected intervals after initiating rapid pacing. Both left ventricular (LV) end-diastolic and end-systolic wall stresses were increased at 1 day after initiation of rapid pacing and continued to increase progressively over the 3-week monitoring period, as did LV end-diastolic and end-systolic volumes. (From [1], with permission)

the 3-week period of observation. Stroke volume was maintained over the 1st week, but fell progressively thereafter.

Serial Changes in Indexes of LV Systolic Function

Figure 2 depicts serial changes in indexes of LV systolic function. Early systolic dysfunction was evident within 1 day and progressed over the 3-week period of study. The contractile dysfunction involved both isovolumic and ejection phase indices. These findings are in keeping with prior reports from this laboratory [3] using indices of ventricular elastance.

Serial Changes in Indexes of LV Diastolic Function

Figure 3 depicts serial changes in indexes of LV diastolic function. The isovolumic relaxation time constant (Tau) was increased significantly by 6.8 ± 1.7 ms ($P < 0.05$) at 1 day and was elevated by 14.0 ± 2.8 ms ($P < 0.001$) after

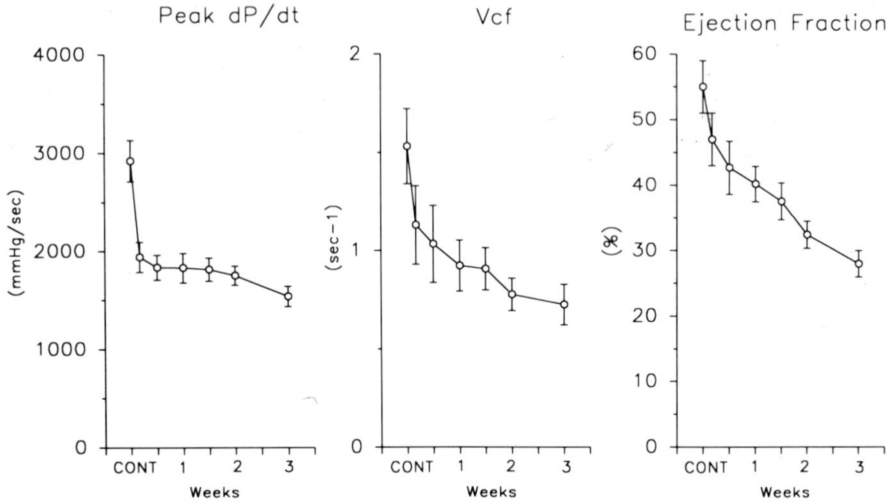

Fig. 2. Time course of the changes in LV dP/dt, mean velocity of circumferential fiber shortening (*Vcf*), and ejection fraction. LV dP/dt, Vcf, and ejection fraction were decreased within 1 day after initiation of rapid pacing and continued to decline gradually over the remainder of the 3-week monitoring period. *CONT*, control. (From [1], with permission)

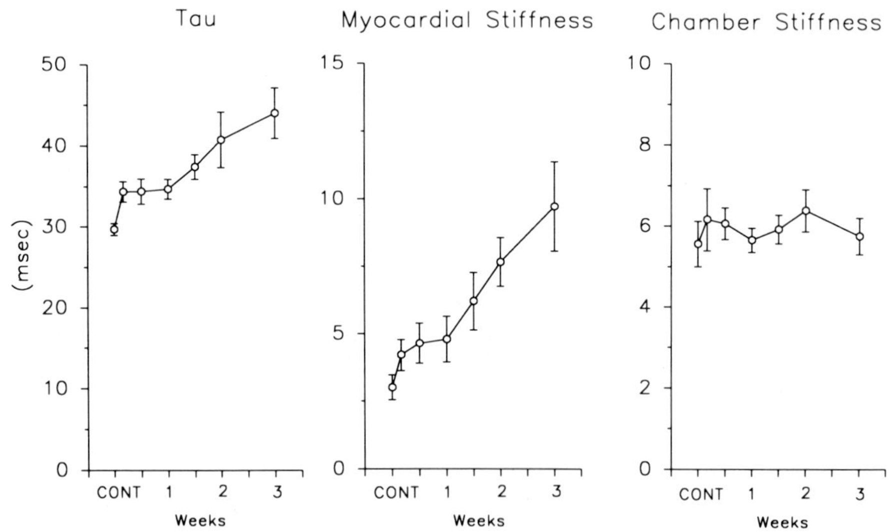

Fig. 3. Time course of the changes in the isovolumic relaxation time constant (*Tau*), myocardial stiffness, and the coefficient of chamber stiffness. The isovolumic relaxation time constant and myocardial stiffness were increased at 1 day after initiation of rapid pacing and continued to increase further over the 3-week monitoring period, whereas chamber stiffness remained unchanged over the study period. (From [1], with permission)

3 weeks of pacing. The myocardial stiffness constant was increased significantly by 1.2 ± 0.3 ($P < 0.05$) at 1 day and was elevated further to 9.5 ± 1.5 ($P < 0.002$) after 3 weeks of pacing. However, the chamber stiffness coefficient was not changed significantly over the 3-week period of study, despite the increase in myocardial stiffness, because the chamber stiffness constant was normalized for the increase in diastolic volume that occurred as heart failure evolved.

LV Systolic and Diastolic Function with Matched Loading Conditions

Figure 4 summarizes the effects of 3 weeks of pacing on heart rate, LV wall stresses, and LV systolic and diastolic function. After 3 weeks of pacing, heart rate was elevated by 21 ± 6 beats/min ($P < 0.001$). LV end-diastolic stress was elevated by 40 ± 5 g/cm^2 ($P < 0.001$); LV end-systolic stress was elevated by 29 ± 6 g/cm^2 ($P < 0.001$); LV dP/dt was significantly reduced by 1327 ± 105 mmHg/s ($P < 0.001$); ejection fraction was significantly reduced from 54 ± 5% to 28 ± 2% ($P < 0.001$); Tau was elevated by 14.0 ± 2.8 ms ($P < 0.001$); and the myocardial stiffness constant was elevated to 9.5 ± 1.5 ($P < 0.002$).

The effects of reducing LV preload and afterload in the heart failure state to matched levels observed in the control state are shown on indexes of LV systolic and diastolic function in Figs. 5 and 6, respectively. Normalizing the elevated loading conditions in heart failure to those observed in control

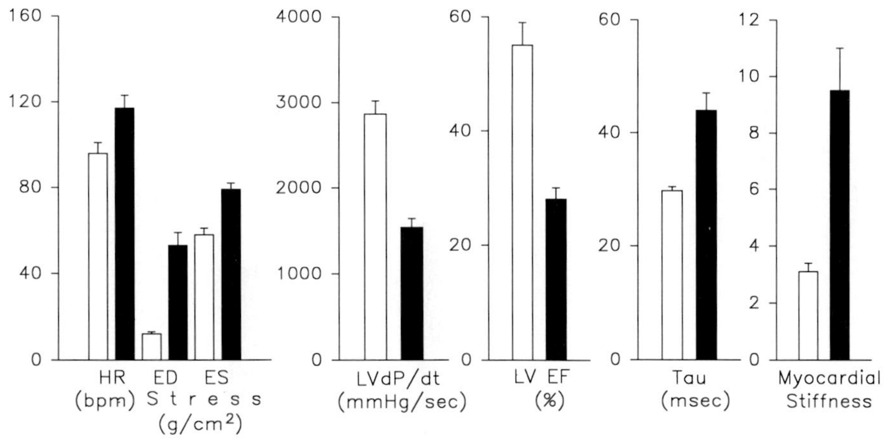

Fig. 4. LV systolic and diastolic function compared before (control, *open bars*) and 3 weeks after (CHF, *solid bars*) rapid pacing. Values in both states were obtained under baseline conditions of loading. Heart rate (*HR*) as well as LV end-systolic (*ES*) and end-diastolic (*ED*) stresses were elevated in heart failure. The indices of LV systolic function [*LV dP/dt* and *LV* ejection fraction (*EF*)] were reduced in the failure state. Concomitantly, the indices of LV diastolic function (Tau and myocardial stiffness) were elevated in heart failure. *bpm*, beats per minute. (Data redrawn from [1], with permission)

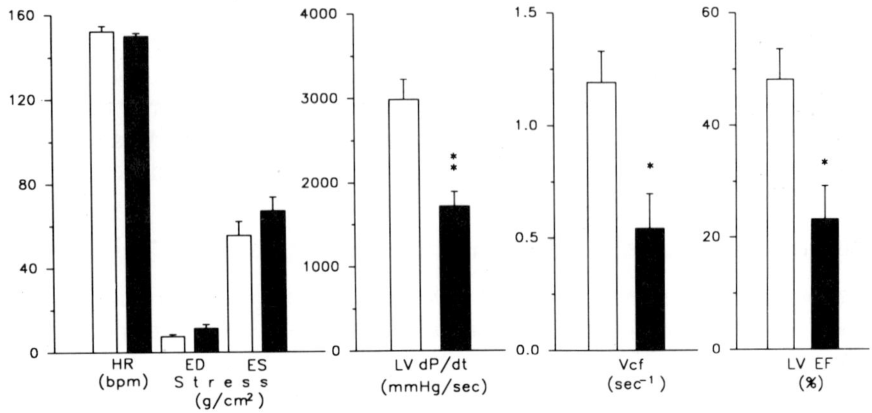

Fig. 5. LV systolic function compared before (control, *open bars*) and 3 weeks after (CHF, *solid bars*) rapid pacing. Values in the heart failure state were obtained with reduced loading conditions to match those attained in the control state. Heart rates for both the control and failure states were matched by left atrial pacing (150 beats/min). Even with matched LV end-diastolic and end-systolic stresses, LV systolic function was depressed significantly in failure. $^*P < 0.05$ *vs* control; $^{**}P < 0.01$ *vs* control). (From [1], with permission)

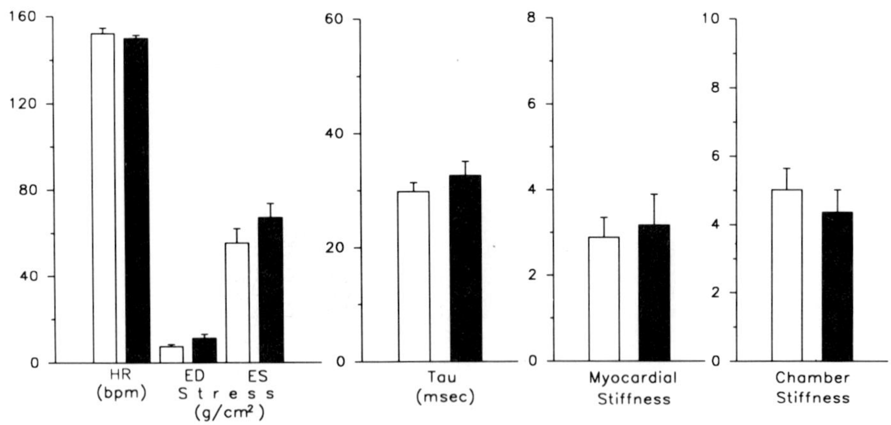

Fig. 6. LV diastolic function compared before (control, *open bars*) and 3 weeks after (CHF, *solid bars*) rapid pacing. Values in the heart failure state were obtained with reduced loading conditions to match those attained in the control state. Heart rates at both the control and failure states were matched by left atrial pacing (150 beats/min). There were no differences in the three indexes of diastolic function in the control and failure states at matched load, in contrast to the persistent depression in systolic function. (From [1], with permission)

resulted in return of diastolic indices to normal values (Fig. 6). Importantly, normalization of loading conditions did not correct the abnormalities in systolic function (Fig. 5).

Similarly, if we superimposed elevated loading conditions on the normal ventricle of these same dogs during control, we could recapitulate the abnormalities in isovolumic relaxation and myocardial stiffness (Figs. 7, 8).

Pathology

There were no significant differences in body weights between sham-operated controls and dogs with heart failure, nor in the LV plus septum weight/body weight in dogs with heart failure (5.2 ± 0.3 g/kg) compared with sham-operated controls (5.0 ± 0.1 g/kg). Quantitative analysis of connective tissue by measurement of hydroxyproline concentration revealed no differences in transmural, epi-, and endomyocardial layers between the dogs with heart failure and sham-operated controls.

Discussion

This review summarizes published findings from our laboratory with respect to the temporal development and determinants of systolic and diastolic

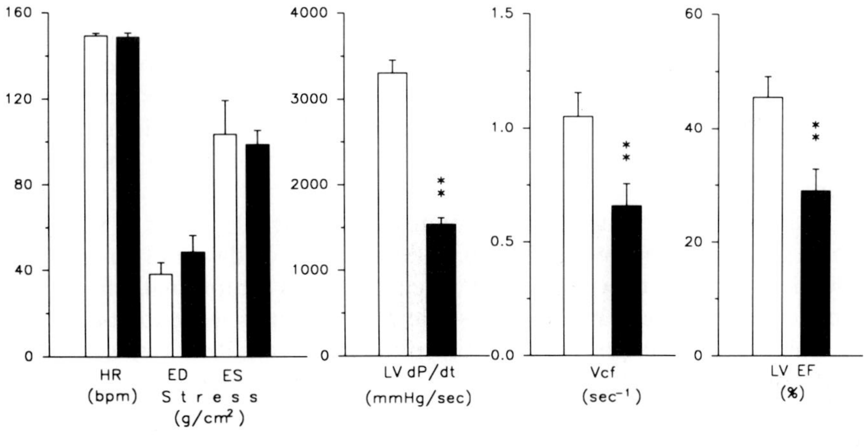

Fig. 7. LV systolic function compared before (control, *open bars*) and 3 weeks after (CHF, *solid bars*) rapid pacing. Values in the control state were obtained under elevated loading conditions to match those attained in heart failure. Heart rates for both the control and failure states were matched by left atrial pacing (150 beats/min). Even with matched LV end-diastolic and systolic stresses, LV systolic function was depressed significantly in failure. *Vcf*, mean velocity of circumferential fiber shortening. $^{**}P < 0.01$ *vs* control. (From [1], with permission)

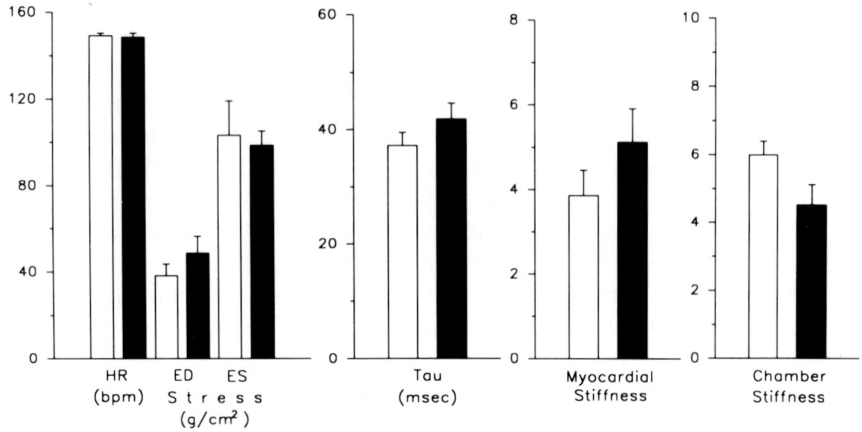

Fig. 8. LV diastolic function compared before (control, *open bars*) and 3 weeks after (CHF, *solid bars*) rapid pacing. Values in the control state were obtained under elevated loading conditions to match those attained in heart failure. Heart rates for both the control and failure states were matched by left atrial pacing (150 beats/min). There were no differences in the three indexes of diastolic function in the control and failure states at matched load, in contrast to the persistent depression in systolic function. (From [1], with permission)

abnormalities in conscious dogs with pacing-induced heart failure [1]. Importantly, the marked abnormalities in diastolic function were due to associated increases in loading conditions and were not due to structural changes in the extracellular matrix. Furthermore, while we [11] and others [4] have observed abnormalities in intracellular calcium handling in this model, which have been assumed to underlie the diastolic abnormalities, it appears that loading conditions were a more important determinant than these cellular abnormalities when studied in the intact state.

An additional finding involved the simultaneous development of systolic and diastolic abnormalities, which were evident within 1 day and progressed in parallel over the 3-week period over which advanced symptomatic heart failure was induced. Notably, while the diastolic abnormalities were load-dependent, the systolic abnormalities persisted despite load normalization, suggesting a distinctly different mechanism for the contractile dysfunction.

It is also important to note that while the extracellular matrix was not significantly altered at this stage of the heart failure process, there were significant ultrastructural changes including loss of collagen weave between myocytes and Z band disruption [7]. Despite these significant changes, load appeared to be potentially the most important factor in mediating diastolic abnormalities [1]. It is also possible that reducing load on the failing heart relieved resting myocardial ischemia. However, we noted an actual fall in transmural myocardial blood flow, measured by radioactive microspheres, arguing against significant ischemia as a mechanism of diastolic dysfunction. Rather, the fall in myocardial blood flow is in keeping with reduced oxygen requirements as load was normalized [12]. It should be kept in mind that with more advanced, end stage heart failure, there may be greater alterations in intracellular calcium homeostasis, extracellular matrix remodelling, or myocardium perfusion which render the diastolic abnormalities less sensitive to normalization of load. Nonetheless, these data suggest that during both early and advanced stages of symptomatic congestive heart failure, diastolic but not systolic dysfunction was load-dependent in conscious dogs with pacing-induced heart failure. Therefore, the clinical benefit attributed to drugs which alter ventricular load may be, in large measure, due to these improved diastolic abnormalities.

Acknowledgment. This study was supported in part by National Institutes of Health Grants HL-HL38070, HL33107 and RR00168 and NASA Grant NAG 2 451.

References

1. Komamura K, Shannon RP, Pasipoularides A, Ihara T, Lader AS, Patrick TA, Bishop SP, Vatner SF (1992) Alterations in left ventricular diastolic function in conscious dogs with pacing-induced heart failure. J Clin Invest 89:1825–1838
2. Grossman W, McLaurin LP, Rolett EL (1979) Alterations in left ventricular relaxation and diastolic compliance in congestive cardiomyopathy. Cardiovasc Res 13:514–522
3. Shannon RP, Komamura K, Stambler BS, Bigaud M, Manders WT, Vatner SF (1991) Alterations in myocardial contractility in conscious dogs with dilated cardiomyopathy. Am J Physiol 260 (Heart Circ Physiol 29):H1903–H1911
4. Tomita M, Spinale FG, Crawford FA, Zile MR (1991) Changes in left ventricular volume, mass, and function during the development and regression of supraventricular tachycardia-induced cardiomyopathy. Circulation 83:635–644
5. Gaasch WH, Blaustein AS, Andrias CW, Donahue RP, Avitall B (1980) Myocardial relaxation. II. Hemodynamic determinants of rate of left ventricular isovolumic pressure decline. Am J Physiol 239 (Heart Circ Physiol 8):H1–H6
6. Weber KT, Pick R, Silver MA, Moe GW, Janicki JS, Zucker IH, Armstrong PW (1990) Fibrillar collagen and remodeling of dilated canine left ventricle. Circulation 82:1387–1401
7. Komamura K, Shannon RP, Ihara T, Shen Y-T, Mirsky I, Bishop SP, Vatner SF (1993) Exhaustion of Frank-Starling mechanism in conscious dogs with heart failure. Am J Physiol 265 (Heart Circ Physiol 34):H1119–H1131
8. Kiuchi K, Shannon RP, Sato N, Bigaud M, Lajoie C, Morgan K, Vatner SF (1994) Factors involved in delaying the rise in peripheral resistance in developing heart failure. Am J Physiol 267 (Heart Circ Physiol 36):H211–H216
9. Kiuchi K, Shannon RP, Komamura K, Cohen DJ, Bianchi C, Homcy CJ, Vatner SF, Vatner DE (1993) Myocardial β-adrenergic receptor function during the development of pacing-induced heart failure. J Clin Invest 91:907–914

10. Kiuchi K, Sato N, Shannon RP, Vatner DE, Morgan K, Vatner SF (1993) Depressed β-adrenergic receptor- and endothelium-mediated vasodilation in conscious dogs with heart failure. Circ Res 73:1013–1023
11. Perreault CL, Shannon RP, Komamura K, Vatner SF, Morgan JP (1992) Abnormalities in intracellular calcium regulation and contractile function in myocardium from dogs with pacing-induced heart failure. J Clin Invest 89:932–938
12. Shannon RP, Komamura K, Shen Y-T, Bishop SP, Vatner SF (1993) Impaired regional subendocardial coronary flow reserve in conscious dogs with pacing-induced heart failure. Am J Physiol 265 (Heart Circ Physiol 34):H801–H809

3.4 Mechanisms of Exercise Intolerance in Patients with Chronic Heart Failure

HIDEYUKI SATO, HIROSHI YOKOYAMA, and MASATSUGU HORI[1]

Summary. In patients with chronic heart failure, aerobic exercise capacity is decreased as reflected by decreases in the maximal oxygen uptake and anaerobic threshold. This decrease in the maximal aerobic power is attributed primarily to a decrease in the blood flow to exercising muscles and consequent reduction in the oxygen availability in active tissues. An inadequate pressor response, due to impairments of inotropic and chronotropic responses of the failing heart to sympathetic activation during exercise, plays a central role in the reduced blood flow to exercising muscles. In normal subjects, the venous pressure drop by means of muscle venous pump has been demonstrated to play an important role in increasing the skeletal muscle blood flow through an increase in the arteriovenous pressure gradient and local venoarteriolar reflex-mediated vasodilation. In patients with chronic heart failure, muscle venous pump is attenuated due to an elevated central venous pressure, and this may also be a flow-limiting factor in chronic heart failure. Other mechanisms such as metabolic abnormalities in skeletal muscle may also account for exercise intolerance, by decreasing oxygen utilization. Thus, the exercise intolerance in patients with chronic heart failure may be induced by multifactorial abnormalities.

Key words: Exercise capacity—Exertional dyspnea—Chronic heart failure—Muscle venous pump—Sympathetic activity—Skeletal muscle abnormality

Introduction

During endurance exercise, resynthesis of adenosine triphosphate (ATP) in exercising muscles is indispensable. Under aerobic exercise conditions, ATP is produced mainly through aerobic metabolism and only partly by anaerobic

[1] First Department of Medicine, Osaka University School of Medicine, 2-2 Yamadaoka, Suita, Osaka 565, Japan

glycolysis. Under anaerobic conditions, however, anaerobic glycolysis predominates over aerobic metabolism and progressively accumulates lactate in working muscles, causing muscle fatigue. Therefore, the maximal oxygen availability in working muscles is a primary determinant of the maximal aerobic power and, thereby, of exercise capacity. The maximal aerobic power can be assessed from measurements of the maximal oxygen uptake or anaerobic threshold during exercise. The oxygen uptake increases at least tenfold from rest to maximal exercise. This increase in oxygen uptake is achieved with cooperation of the circulatory system, ventilatory system, and tissue metabolism, and any impairment in these systems results in a reduction of the maximal aerobic power.

In patients with chronic heart failure, the maximal aerobic power is decreased, as reflected by decreases in the maximal oxygen uptake and anaerobic threshold, and this abnormality is believed to be the most important mechanism of exercise intolerance. The decrease in the maximal aerobic power in heart failure is attributed primarily to decreased oxygen transport to working muscles [1–3]; however, abnormalities of skeletal muscle metabolism which cause a decrease in oxygen utilization may also play an important role [4–6]. Since blood-gas abnormalities are not usually observed during exercise in chronic heart failure, exercise-induced pulmonary congestion may not play an important role in reducing the maximal aerobic power [7]. However, pulmonary congestion may limit submaximal exercise performance by provoking exertional dyspnea.

Oxygen Supply to Working Muscles

Oxygen Extraction

During exercise, increased oxygen demand is fulfilled by increases in blood flow to working muscles and oxygen extraction by active tissues. During systemic circulation, the arterial oxygen content is extracted only by 30% at rest, whereas the extraction fraction increases up to 80% during peak exercise in normal subjects. This mechanism is not impaired in patients with chronic heart failure and therefore does not account for the reduced aerobic power [2].

Metabolic Vasodilation

The blood flow to exercising limbs is markedly decreased in patients with chronic heart failure; this abnormality primarily accounts for the reduced aerobic power [2,3]. The blood flow to active tissues is increased by both an increase in perfusion pressure and local metabolic vasodilation. The vascular resistance in exercising legs is decreased by 90% or more with tissue hypoxia or related metabolites such as H^+, K^+, inorganic phosphate, adenosine, and/or prostaglandins during maximal exercise in normal subjects [3]. The local

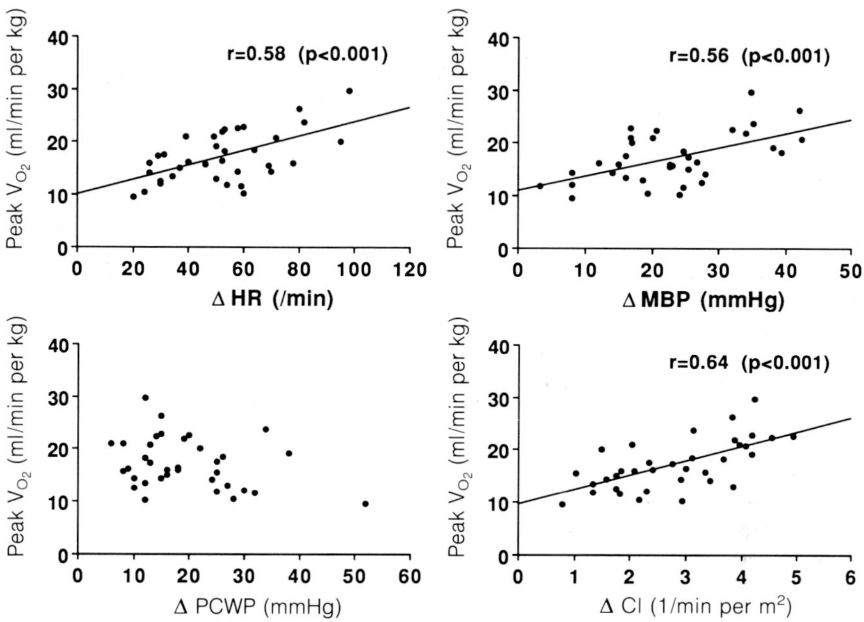

Fig. 1. Relationships between peak oxygen uptake (V_{O_2}) and changes (Δ) in hemodynamic parameters, i.e., heart rate (*HR*), mean blood pressure (*MBP*), pulmonary capillary wedge pressure (*PCWP*), and cardiac index (*CI*) during exercise in 35 patients with chronic heart failure

vasodilator response is reported to be quite well preserved in patients with nonedematous chronic heart failure [8]. Thus, the decreased blood flow to exercising limbs in chronic heart failure could be attributed mainly to an inadequate increase in arterial pressure during exercise. Indeed, we observed a significant correlation between the peak oxygen uptake and increase in mean arterial pressure during exercise (Fig. 1).

Pressor Response

Sympathetic activation plays a central role in the exercise pressor response, increasing cardiac output and constricting resistance vessels in nonworking areas. Cardiac output increases approximately fourfold during maximal exercise in normal subjects. Sympathetic-mediated vasoconstriction counteracts the effects of metabolic vasodilation so that total systemic vascular resistance decreases only by 50% even during maximal exercise. As a result, mean blood pressure increases approximately twofold during maximal exercise in normal subjects. Thus, two possible mechanisms can be raised for the attenuated pressor response in chronic heart failure: (1) inadequate sympathetic activation and (2) cardiovascular hyporesponses to sympathetic stimulation.

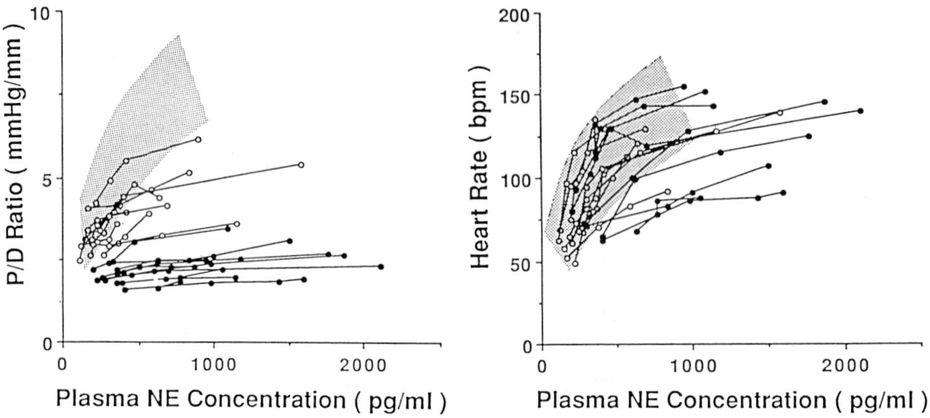

Fig. 2. The left ventricular contractile response (*P/D ratio*) and heart rate response to sympathetic activation indicated by plasma norepinephrine (*NE*) level during exercise in patients with dilated cardiomyopathy (*closed circles*) and aortic regurgitation without heart failure (*open circles*). P/D ratio indicates the ratio of systolic blood pressure to end-systolic left ventricular dimension. The *shaded areas* represent 95% confidence limits of the normal range. *bpm*, beats per minute

Sympathetic System

During exercise, sympathetic nerves are activated through central command mechanisms and somatic exercise reflexes originating from chemosensitive muscle afferents in active tissues. Chemosensitive muscle afferents respond to local hypoxic stimulus or related metabolites which cause metabolic vasodilation. Thus, the same chemical stimuli could initiate both reflex vasoconstriction and direct local vasodilation. The exercise reflex can be assessed from measurements of plasma norepinephrine responses to tissue hypoxia. Using this technique, we have demonstrated that the exercise reflex is not impaired in patients with chronic heart failure [9]. Therefore, the attenuated pressor response in patients with heart failure could be attributed to cardiovascular subsensitivities to sympathetic stimulation. However, the vasoconstriction response mediated by alpha-receptors is not impaired even in patients with chronic heart failure [10]. In contrast, we demonstrated that cardiac inotropic and chronotropic responses to exercise-induced sympathetic stimulation are markedly blunted in patients with chronic heart failure, probably because of down regulation of cardiac beta-receptors and/or cardiac norepinephrine depletion (Fig. 2) [11]. Thus, cardiac inotropic and chronotropic hyporesponses to exercise-induced sympathetic stimulation are primary mechanisms of the attenuated pressor response during exercise. Indeed, we observed that the peak oxygen uptake significantly correlates with increases in heart rate and cardiac output, as well as mean arterial pressure, during exercise in patients with chronic heart failure (Fig. 1).

3.5 Iodine-123 Metaiodobenzylguanidine Myocardial Imaging of Congestive Heart Failure

Tsunehiko Nishimura, Hidetoshi Yamagami, and Takakazu Morozumi[1]

Summary. To elucidate the sympathetic neural function in dilated cardiomyopathy, myocardial imaging with ^{123}I-metaiodobenzylguanidine (MIBG) was carried out in 20 patients. By simultaneous MIBG and thallium myocardial single photon emission computerized tomography (SPECT), ten had larger defects with MIBG than with thallium. MIBG defect sizes were correlated with left ventricular function. In nine patients, quantitative analysis of MIBG parameters (H/B ratio: heart to upper mediastinum uptake ratio and % WR: percent washout) were evaluated. We compared these two indices with the left ventricular ejection fraction (LVEF) and exercise capacity determined using a respiratory gas exchange analyzer during maximal bicycle exercise. H/B ratio correlated well with LVEF ($r = 0.77$) and anaerobic threshold ($r = 0.74$). % WR was significantly correlated with LVEF ($r = 0.79$), peak $\dot{V}_{O_2}$ ($r = -0.74$), and anaerobic threshold ($r = 0.81$). Thus, H/B ratio and % WR evaluated by ^{123}I-MIBG myocardial imaging were closely related to the depressed exercise capacity in patients with dilated cardiomyopathy. In conclusion, ^{123}I-MIBG myocardial imaging provides useful information concerning the severity of congestive heart failure.

Key words: ^{123}I-metaiodobenzylguanidine—Dilated cardiomyopathy—Myocardial SPECT—Left ventricular function—Exercise capacity

Introduction

Adrenergic nerves of the sympathetic nervous system play a major role in regulating cardiac function. These nerves have a stimulating effect on cardiac contraction and are a major support system for the heart. In dilated cardiomyopathy, beta blockade has resulted in improvement in signs and symptoms

[1] Department of Tracer Kinetics, Biomedical Research Center, Osaka University, Medical School, 2-2 Yamadaoka, Suita, Osaka, 565 Japan

of congestive heart failure, suggesting that sympathetic nerve overactivity may be causative or contributory to the manifestation of heart failure [1]. At present, means of studying the myocardial sympathetic nerve activity in vivo, however, are limited.

Metaiodobenzylguanidine (MIBG) is a norepinephrine (NE) analogue which was developed as an imaging agent for pheochromocytoma [2]. MIBG is taken up mainly by adrenergic tissues by a specific mechanism (uptake 1) as well as a nonspecific mechanism (uptake 2) which is probably due to diffusion [3,4]. Thus, the dense sympathetic innervation of the heart allows imaging of the myocardial sympathetic activity with ^{123}I-MIBG.

Animal and human studies using ^{123}I-MIBG have shown that the normal heart is easily visualized [5,6]. Cardiac MIBG uptake is decreased in conditions in which NE content and/or uptake is reduced, such as congestive heart failure [7,8]. In this study, ^{123}I-MIBG was used to evaluated the patients with dilated cardiomyopathy and the results were correlated with left ventricular function and exercise capacity to assess the severity of congestive heart failure.

Materials and Methods

Patient Population

Twenty patients with dilated cardiomyopathy were entered in this study. All patients were confirmed as having dilated cardiomyopathy by clinical symptoms, echocardiography, and cardiac catheterization. There were 15 men and 5 women. Their mean age was 49 years, ranging from 15 to 74 years. As for patient conditions, five had a functional class of NYHA I, 4 NYHA II, 9 NYHA III, and 2 NYHA IV.

^{123}I-MIBG Myocardial Imaging

The patients were intravenously administered 111 MBq (3 mCi) of ^{123}I-MIBG. Images were obtained at 15 min and 4 h later. Then, 111 MBq (3 mCi) of thallium was injected intravenously. Simultaneous ^{123}I-MIBG and thallium myocardial single photon emission computerized tomography (SPECT) was carried out. In nine patients, anterior planar images of ^{123}I-MIBG were obtained at 15 min and 4 h after ^{123}I-MIBG administration.

For all studies, a General Electric 400 AC/T camera (General Electric, Milwaukee, Wis., USA) equipped with an all-purpose, parallel-hole collimator interface to a STAR computer (Milwaukee, Wis., USA) was used. A total of 32 planar acquisitions were performed per 30 s, each over a 180° arc extending from the 45° left posterior oblique projection. Oblique, orthogonal tomographic slices, each 6 mm in thickness, were reconstructed parallel to the vertical and horizontal long axes and the short axis of the left ventricle.

The camera's energy discriminator was set on the 75 KeV photopeak of ^{201}Tl with a 20% window and the 159 KeV photopeak of ^{123}I with a 20% window.

Since two tracers were administered simultaneously, the effects of cross talk were evaluated. Standard samples of the two radionuclides containing the same radioactivity were placed without mixing in the center of the camera's field. The radioactive count was determined in each window, and the cross-talk values were estimated by simultaneous equations. The cross-talk values were 13% for ^{201}Tl to ^{123}I and 9% for ^{123}I to ^{201}Tl; however, the effect of cross talk on both images was not visually observed. Therefore, the cross-talk correction was not done quantitatively in this study [9].

Data Analysis

By using ^{123}I-MIBG and thallium short axial SPECT views, three representative tomographic slices were selected from the apical to the midventricular level. The defect sizes were visually assessed as (++), (+), or (−) by three nuclear medicine specialists unaware of the clinical status of the patients. By using anterior planar images, cardiac MIBG uptake was measured as follows. Left ventricular activity was recorded using a manually drawn region of interest (ROI). Another ROI was placed over the upper mediastinum area as background. The heart-to-background (H/B) ratio was then computed to quantify cardiac MIBG uptake. In this study, the H/B ratio in the delayed (4 h) planar images was adapted in the washout analysis. Furthermore, the percent MIBG washout (%WR) from 15 min to 4 h was calculated as follows (Fig. 1):

$$\text{MIBG washout (\%WR)} = \frac{(\text{H-B})_{\text{initial}} - (\text{H-B})_{\text{delayed}}}{(\text{H-B})_{\text{initial}}} \times 100$$

Cardiac Catheterization

All patients underwent cardiac catheterization. End-diastolic volume, end-systolic volume, and left ventricular ejection fraction were evaluated by contrast left ventriculography.

Exercise Testing

All patients underwent a symptom-limited multistage exercise test using a bicycle ergometer. Using a respiratory gas exchange analyzer (Minato RM-200, Tokyo, Japan), maximum $\dot{V}_{O_2}$ at anaerobic threshold (AT) was calculated [10]. Changes of heart rate to achieve AT and submaximal stress were also calculated as % ΔHR-AT and % ΔHR-maximum.

Statistical Analysis

Data were expressed as mean ± standard deviation. The nonparametric Wilcoxon statistics were used to test the significance of differences among groups. Statistical significance was determined by analysis of variance, linear

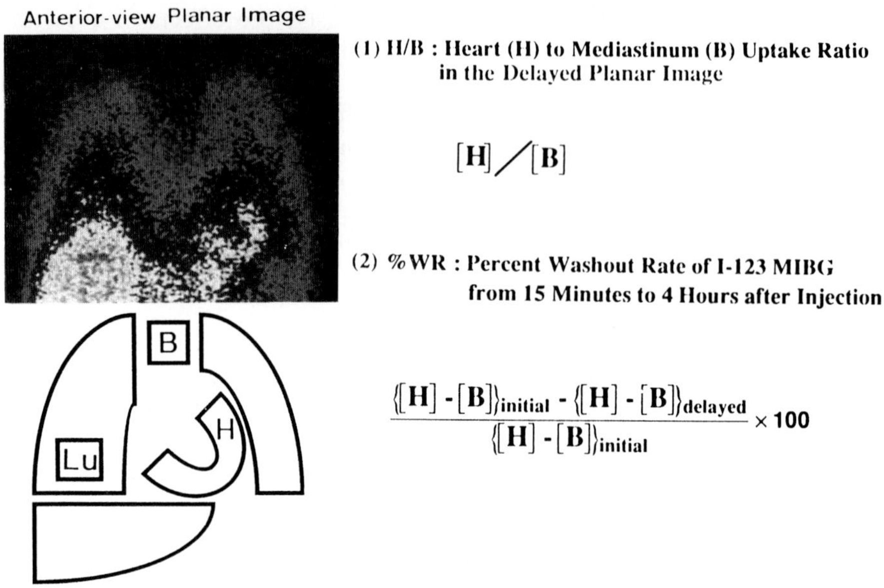

Fig. 1. Quantitative estimation of ^{123}I-MIBG cardiac uptake into the heart (*H*) compared with the upper mediastinum (*B*, background) (*H*/*B* ratio) and myocardial washout rate (% *WR*) from initial to delayed studies using the anterior-view planar scintigram image. *MIBG*, metaiodobenzylguanidine

regression, or Student's *t*-test. For all tests, a *P* value of less than 0.05 was considered as significant.

Results

Comparison of ^{123}I-MIBG and Thallium Myocardial SPECT

Figure 2 shows simultaneous ^{123}I-MIBG and thallium myocardial SPECT in a patient with dilated cardiomyopathy. The defect sizes measured by MIBG SPECT were larger than those from thallium SPECT. In MIBG myocardial SPECT, an extensive inferoposterior defect was observed. The functional class of this patient was NYHA III and the value of the left ventricular ejection fraction was 17%.

According to the comparison of the defect size between ^{123}I-MIBG and thallium myocardial SPECT, patients were divided into four groups as follows. There were 4 patients in group A: Tl (−) MIBG (+); 4 in group B: Tl (+) MIBG (+); 6 in group C: Tl (+) MIBG (++); and 6 in group D: Tl (++) MIBG (++). By visual assessment of simultaneous ^{123}I-MIBG and thallium myocardial SPECT, 10 of 20 patients showed larger defect size with MIBG than thallium. The defect sizes correlated well with the left ventricular end-

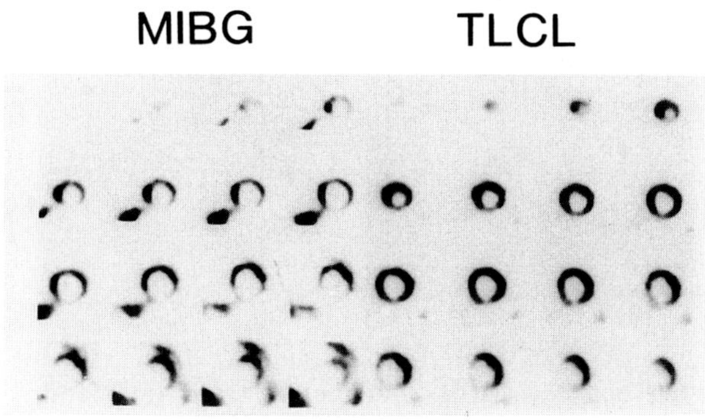

Fig. 2. Simultaneous ^{123}I-MIBG and thallium myocardial single photon emission computerized tomography (SPECT) in a 60-year-old female patient with dilated cardiomyopathy. The defect size measured with MIBG is larger than with thallium (*TLCL*) at the inferioposterior left ventricular wall. The patient was NYHA III, the end-diastolic volume index was 143 ml, and the ejection fraction was 17%

Table 1. Hemodynamic variables in relation to grades of scintigraphic defect.

	Tl/MTBC defect		*n*	EDVI (ml/m^2)	EF (%)	NYHA
A	Tl(−)	MIBG (+)	4	111 ± 11	55 ± 3	1.4 ± 0.5
B	Tl(+)	MIBG (+)	4	150 ± 29	41 ± 8*	2.1 ± 0.7
C	Tl(+)	MIBG (++)	6	179 ± 13**	26 ± 2**	3.1 ± 0.6**
D	Tl(++)	MIBG (++)	6	186 ± 33	17 ± 5***	3.2 ± 0.4

* $P < 0.05$ *vs* Grade I; ** $P < 0.05$ *vs* Grade 2; *** $P < 0.05$ *vs* Grade 3.
EDVI, left ventricular end-diastolic volume index; *EF*, left ventricular ejection fraction; *NYHA*, New York Heart Association functional class; *MIBG*, metaiodobenzylguanidine.

diastolic volume index and NYHA functional class, and inversely correlated with the left ventricular ejection fraction according to grades of defects (from group A to D) (Table 1).

MIBG Parameters in Relation to Ventricular Function

Intra- and interobserver differences for myocardial MIBG uptake (H/B ratio) were not different, when calculated repeatedly after setting the region of interest (ROI). H/B ratios were well correlated ($r = 0.90$). The mean myocardial MIBG uptake (H/B ratio) in nine patients with dilated cardiomyopathy was 0.62 ± 0.63, while that in normal patients was 2.20 ± 0.30 ($P < 0.01$). The H/B ratio correlated well with the left ventricular ejection fraction ($r = 0.77$, $P < 0.05$). On the other hand, the percentage washout of MIBG (%WR) in dilated cardiomyopathy was 58% ± 13%, while the normal value was 37% ± 5% ($P < 0.01$). MIBG washout was inversely correlated with the left ventricular ejection fraction ($r = -0.79$, $P < 0.05$). Therefore, in severely impaired

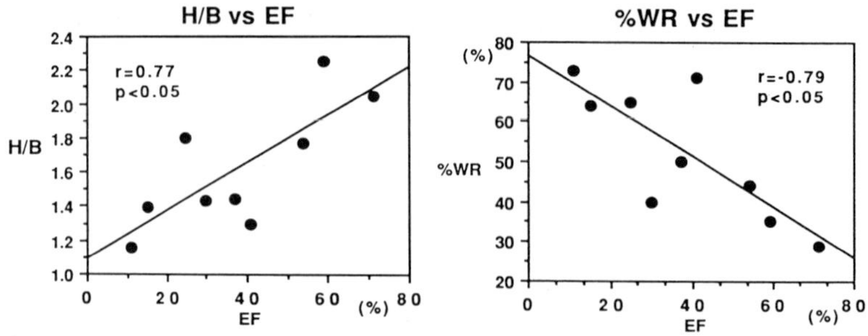

Fig. 3. Relationship between MIBG parameters (*H/B* ratio and % *WR*) and left ventricular ejection fraction (*EF*)

patients, decreased cardiac MIBG uptake and increased MIBG washout were demonstrated (Fig. 3).

MIBG Parameters in Relation to Exercise Testing

Figure 4 shows the relationship between MIBG parameters (H/B ratio and %WR) and the heart rate responce to exercise. The H/B ratio correlated with percent change in heart rate at the anaerobic threshold (AT) ($r = 0.81$, $P < 0.05$) and percent change in heart rate at peak exercise ($r = 0.69$, NS). Furthermore, MIBG washout inversely correlated with percent change in heart rate at AT ($r = -0.78$, $P < 0.05$), and percent change in heart rate at peak exercise ($r = -0.60$, NS). Patients with a decreased H/B ratio and increased %WR showed a poor heart rate response to exercise. Figure 5 shows the relationship between MIBG parameters and exercise capacity. The H/B ratio correlated with $\dot{V}_{O_2}$ at AT ($r = 0.74$, $P < 0.05$) and max $\dot{V}_{O_2}$ ($r = 0.53$, NS). Furthermore, MIBG washout inversely correlated with $\dot{V}_{O_2}$ at AT ($r = -0.74$, $P < 0.05$). Patients with a decreased H/B ratio and increased MIBG %WR also showed poor exercise capacity.

Discussion

By visual inspection, defect sizes measured using MIBG were larger than those using thallium, in 10 out of 20 patients with dilated cardiomyopathy. In the remaining ten patients, both defects showed similar sized defects. These results indicate that the sympathetic nerve abnormality precedes the perfusion abnormality in these patients. Therefore, ^{123}I-MIBG myocardial SPECT may be useful for the early detection of myocardial damage. In addition, patients could be divided into four groups based on the extent of perfusion defect measured using a combination of MIBG and thallium SPECT. The extents of MIBG defects correlated with the left ventricular end-diastolic volume index and

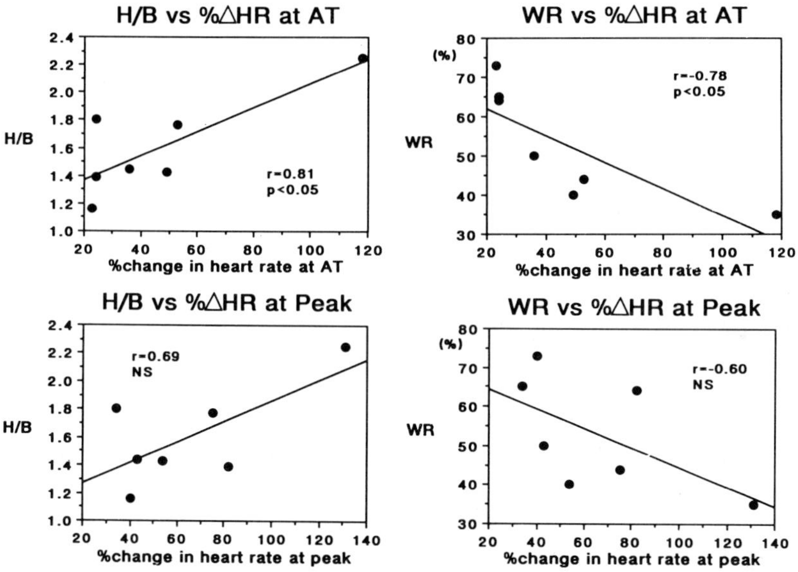

Fig. 4. Relationship between MIBG parameters (*H/B* ratio and % *WR*) and heart rate (*HR*) response to exercise. % *ΔHR at AT*, % change in HR at anaerobic threshold (*AT*); % *ΔHR at peak*, % change in HR at peak exercise

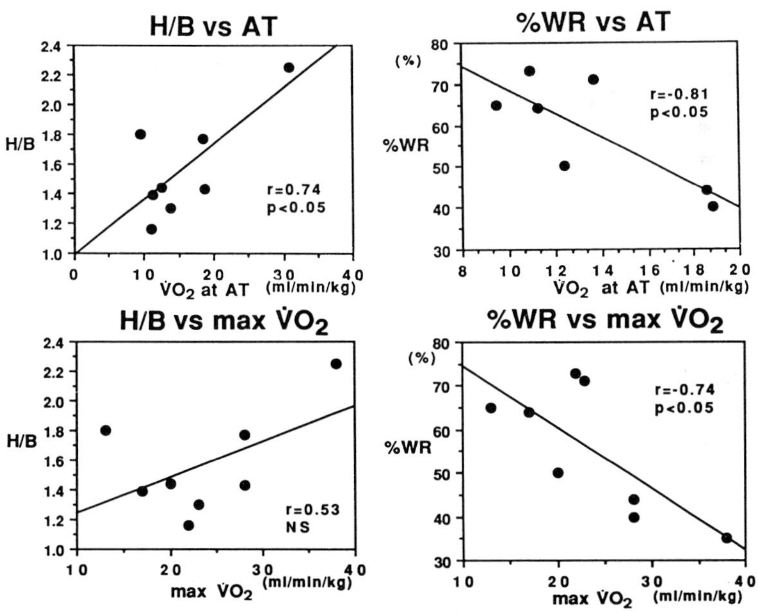

Fig. 5. Relationship between MIBG parameters (*H/B* ratio and % *WR*) and exercise capacity. $\dot{V}_{O_2}$ *at AT*, oxygen consumption at anaerobic threshold; *max* $\dot{V}_{O_2}$, maximum oxygen consumption

NYHA functional class, and inversely correlated with the left ventricular ejection fraction. Therefore, simultaneous MIBG and thallium myocardial SPECT is also useful for the global assessment of the severity of dilated cardiomyopathy.

Compared to normal controls, decreased cardiac MIBG and rapid washout of MIBG was demonstrated in dilated cardiomyopathy. These MIBG parameters correlated well with left ventricular funciton. The decreased MIBG uptake may reflect damage to the sympathetic neurons, while increased MIBG washout may reflect increased adrenergic sympathetic activity [8,9]. It was previously reported that cardiac stores of NE are decreased in heart failure. Plasma NE levels are elevated, suggesting increased sympathetic nerve activity [11,12]. However, myocardial sympathetic activity could not be evaluated by these methods; therefore, MIBG parameters may be useful for the evaluation of congestive heart failure.

In patients with congestive heart failure, impaired chronotropic and/or inotropic responses to exercise were reported [13,14]. In our study, MIBG parameters correlated with heart rate response to exercise. In addition, they correlated with exercise capacity. Thus, MIBG parameters were closely related to chronotropic and/or inotropic responses in these patients. Therefore, these results may be useful for the assessment of congestive heart failure from the viewpoint of quality of life.

In conclusion, we have shown that patients with dilated cardiomyopathy have decreased uptake and more rapid washout of MIBG from the heart than normal controls. The decreased uptake of MIBG suggests dysfunction of cardiac sympathetic neurons. The rapid washout of MIBG from the heart suggests increased cardiac sympathetic nerve activity in dilated cardiomyopathy. MIBG appears to be useful for studying the sympathetic nervous innervation of the heart noninvasively, which provides a unique means of investigating a relatively unexplored area of cardiac physiology.

References

1. Waagstein F, Hjalmarson A, Swedeberg K, et al. (1983) Beta-blockers in dilated cardiomyopathies: they work. Eur Heart J 4:173–178
2. Shapiro B, Copp JE, Sisson JC, et al. (1985) Iodine-131 metaiodobenzylguanidine for the locating of suspected pheochromocytoma: experience in 400 cases. J Nucl Med 26:576–585
3. Jaques S, Tobes MC, Sisson JC, et al. (1984) Comparison of the sodium dependency of uptake of meta-iodobenzylguanidine and norepinephrine into cultured bovine adrenomedullary cells. Mol Pharm 26:539–546
4. Tobes MC, Jaques S, Wieland DM, et al. (1985) Effect of uptake-one inhibitors on the uptake of norepinephrine and metaiodobenzylguanidine. J Nucl Med 26: 897–907
5. Kline RC, Swanson DP, Wieland DM, et al. (1981) Myocardial imaging in man with I-123 meta-iodobenzylguanidine. J Nucl Med 22:129–132

6. Sisson JC, Shapiro B, Myers L, et al. (1987) Metaiodobenzylguanidine to map the adrenergic nervous system in man. J Nucl Med 28:1625–1636
7. Glowniak TV, Turner FE, Gray LL, et al. (1989) Iodine-123 metaiodobenzylguanidine imaging of the heart in idiopathic congestive cardiomyopathy and cardiac transplants. J Nucl Med 30:1182–1191
8. Merlet P, Valette H, Syrota A, et al. (1992) Prognostic value of cardiac metaiodobenzylguanidine imaging in patients with heart failure. J Nucl Med 33:471–477
9. Nishimura T, Oka H, Sago M, et al. (1992) Serial assessment of denervated but viable myocardium following acute myocardial infarction in dogs using iodine-123 MIBG and tallium myocardial SPECT. Eur J Nucl Med 19:25–29
10. Beaver WL, Wasserman K, Whipp BJ (1986) A new method for detecting the anaerobic threshold by gas exchange. J Appl Physiol 60:2020–2027
11. Thomas JA, Marks BH (1978) Plasma norepinephrine in congestive heart failure. Am J Cardiol 41:233–243
12. Davis D, Zelis R (1986) The sympathetic nervous system in congestive heart failure. Heart Failure 2:21–32
13. Colucci WS, Ribeiro JP, Rocco MB, et al. (1989) Impaired chronic response to exercise in patients with congestive heart failure. Role of postsynaptic β-adrenergic desensitization. Circulation 80:314–323
14. Bristow MR, Ginsburg R, Minobe W, et al. (1982) Decreased catecholamine sensitivity and β-adrenergic-receptor density in failing human hearts. N Engl J Med 307:205–211

3.6 Long-Term β-Blocker Therapy in Patients with Dilated Cardiomyopathy

Masatake Fukunami and Noritake Hoki[1]

Summary. Evidence for the effectiveness of long-term β-blockade in the treatment of heart failure has been increasingly accumulated. We found that β-blocker was also effective in patients with dilated cardiomyopathy. In our 5-year follow-up study, Kaplan-Meier analysis revealed a significant improvement of mortality with β-blocker treatment, mainly due to the prevention of sudden death. Besides, although echocardiographical parameters also significantly improved, the extent of improvement largely depended on the severity of the intercellular type of fibrosis in endomyocardial biopsy samples. To search for the mechanism of this beneficial effect of β-blockade, the β-receptor density and efficacy in lymphocytes were examined serially at the time of administration, and before and after withdrawal, of β-blocker. In the case of β-blocker administration, an increase in β-receptor efficacy followed by an increase in density might play a role in β-blocker tolerance and effectiveness. Withdrawal exerted an adverse effect in terms of cardiac function and receptor modification. However, β-blocker acted as a negative inotropic agent, as in a normal heart, at a late stage when the cardiac function had already recovered to such an extent that β-blocker no longer seemed necessary. These results indicate that the beneficial effect of β-blockade therapy might derive from improvement in the response to sympathetic stimulation and prevention of catecholamine injury in the residual myocardial cells.

Key words: Dilated cardiomyopathy—Cardiac function—Catecholamine—β-receptor—β-blocker

Introduction

Intrinsic catecholamine is generally believed to have a dual action in the failing heart. One action appears to be compensatory to heart failure, and is based on

[1] Division of Cardiology, Osaka Prefectural Hospital, 3-1-56 Mandai-Higashi, Sumiyoshi-ku, Osaka, 558 Japan

a chronotropic and inotropic regulatory mechanism via β-adrenergic receptors. Another action, which could possibly be harmful to the myocardium [1], may be associated with Ca^{2+}-overloading in myocardial cells or various changes in the β-adrenergic pathway. Such a dual action possibly causes a vicious circle; that is, an increase in catecholamine level to compensate the failing heart will lead to further worsening of the condition of the failing heart. That might be one of the reasons why the level of plasma catecholamine can be used as a major predictor of mortality in patients with heart failure [2,3]. If the effect of catecholamine on the myocardium were adverse in dilated cardiomyopathy (DCM), some protective effects derived from chronic β-blockade might be expected.

Since 1975, a Swedish group [4–9] has reported that β-adrenergic blocking agents are useful in patients with severe DCM. However, controversy regarding their usefulness remains, from several controlled studies [10–14], although some investigators accumulated evidence of a favorable effect with chronic β-blockade [15,16]. We have also observed that long-term β-blocker therapy in patients with DCM improved cardiac function significantly compared with the control group [17]. The extent of improvement is likely to depend on the degree [17] and type [18] of fibrosis of the myocardium.

The present chapter aims to describe the beneficial effect of β-blocker for heart failure in patients with DCM, and to discuss the possible mechanisms for the improvement noted with long-term β-blockade, involving β-receptor density and efficacy (receptor-adenylate cyclase coupling).

Survival on β-Blockade in DCM

It is well known that DCM is a progressive disease with a poor prognosis. The 5-year survival rate in the natural course of the disease was initially reported to be less than 40%, with two-thirds of the deaths occurring within the first two years [19]. The effect of β-blocker on long-term survival remained to be elucidated. Therefore, to investigate the effect of β-blocker on survival, we followed up 105 DCM patients with (group G-1, $n = 40$) or without (group G-2, $n = 65$) β-blocker by annual interview and echocardiography for 9–104 months in G-1 and 6–122 months in G-2, although it was not a randomized control study. All the patients received the conventional therapy including digitalis and diuretics with or without vasodilators. The ratio of the patients who were administered angiotensin-converting-enzyme inhibitors, Ca^{2+}-antagonists, or antiarrhythmic agents were not significantly different between the two groups. As well, there were no significant differences in NYHA functional class, age, sex, or echocardiographical parameters (Dd, left ventricular end-diastolic dimension; Ds, left ventricular end-systolic dimension; EF, left ventricular ejection fraction) at entry.

Kaplan-Meier analysis revealed that the survival rate was significantly improved by the β-blocker therapy (Fig. 1). Incidentally, the survival rate at five

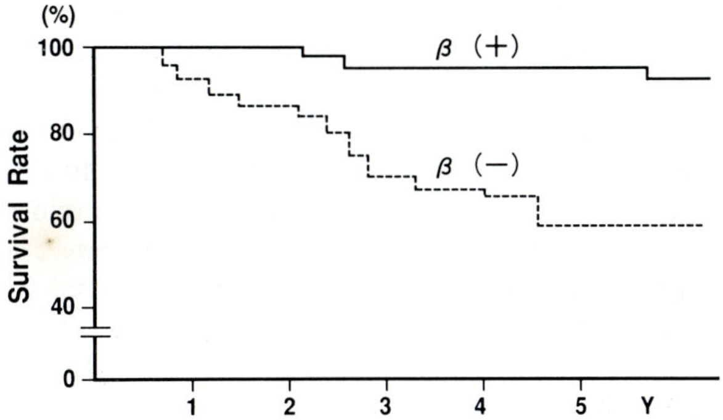

Fig. 1. Kaplan-Meier analysis of survival rate of dilated cardiomypathy patients. Note the marked improvement ($P < 0.001$) of prognosis with metoprolol administration. β (+), patients receiving metoprolol; β (−), patients receiving the conventional treatment without metoprolol; *Y*, years

Table 1. Transition of survival rate and left ventricular function in DCM patients with or without long-term beta-blocker therapy.

	Group	1 year	2 years	3 years	4 years	5 years
Survival rate	G-1	1.0	1.0*	0.96*	0.96*	0.89*
	G-2	0.95	0.91	0.82	0.78	0.59
DdR	G-1	0.95 ± 0.07	0.92 ± 0.09*	0.90 ± 0.10	0.90 ± 0.11	0.91 ± 0.11*
	G-2	0.95 ± 0.10	0.95 ± 0.11	0.93 ± 0.12	0.90 ± 0.12	1.13 ± 0.12
EFR	G-1	1.23 ± 0.36	1.31 ± 0.44	1.45 ± 0.43*	1.50 ± 0.56	1.46 ± 0.44*
	G-2	1.22 ± 0.36	1.18 ± 0.37	1.16 ± 0.35	1.25 ± 0.43	0.81 ± 0.44

DdR, left ventricular diastolic dimension at each follow-up/left ventricular diastolic dimension at entry; *EFR*, ejection fraction at each follow-up/ejection fraction at entry; *G-1*, patients with beta-blocker therapy; *G-2*, patients without beta-blocker therapy; *DCM*, dilated cardiomyopathy.
* $P < 0.05$ *vs* G-2.

years after entry improved from 0.59 to 0.89 (Table 1). As for the rate of sudden death, there was no sudden death case in G-1, whereas there were seven cases in G-2 ($P < 0.05$). On the other hand, the number of deaths from heart failure in both groups was similar (G-1/G-2 = 2/4 patients), although the changes in Dd at 2 and 5 years and EF at 3 and 5 years after entry showed a significant improvement (Table 1). In the analysis of only G-2 patients, followed up for more than one year, ten of 59 patients (G-2D) died during the study period and the remainder (G-2A) were still alive. Dd (71 ± 8 mm) at entry in G-2D was significantly greater than that (63 ± 6 mm) in G-2A, and EF (36% ± 6%) at entry in G-2D was significantly ($P < 0.05$) worse than that (42% ± 8%) for G-2A. The criteria of Dd > 68 mm or EF > 39% for death gave a sensitivity of 70% or 80% and a specificity of 86% or 63%, respectively.

Echocardiographical Follow-Up After Metoprolol Administration

To examine in further detail the effect of metoprolol on the hemodynamic parameters, we carried out a random-controlled study [17] on echocardiographical follow-up in 35 consecutive patients with DCM, who received no vasodilating agents. They were divided by the order at entry into this study into a β-blocker group and a control (conventional treatment) group, and were followed up echocardiographically without any changes of drug content. Metoprolol (final dose 60 mg/day) was administered in the β-blocker group only, in addition to the conventional treatment for heart failure. Ds and EF (6 months and more after) improved significantly earlier than Dd (12 months and more after) in the β-blocker group, compared with the control group, although there were no significant differences in the baseline data between the two groups. Interestingly, the extent of improvement of EF after administration of metoprolol inversely correlated ($r = -0.677$, $P < 0.01$) with percent fibrosis (%F) of the endomyocardial biopsy specimen estimated by the point counting method.

Our results are consistent with those of the Swedish group [4–9] or Engelmeier [13] with respect to the beneficial effect of chronic β-blockade in DCM. On the other hand, Ikram and Fitzpatrick [10] have demonstrated that β-blockers deteriorated the states of the patients, in the double-blind randomized crossover study. However, their use of β-blocker differed from ours in three ways. First, they started with a relatively high dose, while we started with a very low dose. Second, their observation period was as short as one month; ours was more than three months. Third, they used acebutolol which has intrinsic sympathetic activity (ISA), while metoprolol, which we used, has no ISA. An initial high dose might deteriorate the cardiac function even if it has ISA. Furthermore, Currie et al. [11] reported that their patients did not improve symptomatically or hemodynamically in a double-blind crossover trial, although metoprolol was administered gradually for one month. However, their starting dose was higher, and the dosage was increased in bigger steps, than was ours.

Selection of Good or Poor Candidates for β-Blocker Therapy

We also reported that not only percent fibrosis (%F) but also the fibrosis type in an endomyocardial biopsy specimen is a good predictor of the effectiveness of β-blocker therapy. Figure 2 shows the relationship between %F and the improvement of EF for 12 months, reevaluated in a total of 40 patients with DCM, taking the dominance of fibrosis type into consideration. The classification of the type of fibrosis was based on the histopathological report of Anderson et al. [20]. Interfascicular fibrosis (IF) was defined as that associated with collagenous tissue in the adventia of the vessels so as to encircle a fascicle or bundle of muscle fibers and to separate groups of fibers. On the other hand, intercellular fibrosis (IC) as defined as fibrosis located between individual muscle fibers.

The fibrosis type seems to be another independent factor. Therefore, we counted again separately two types of fibrosis points (%IC and %IF; total %F

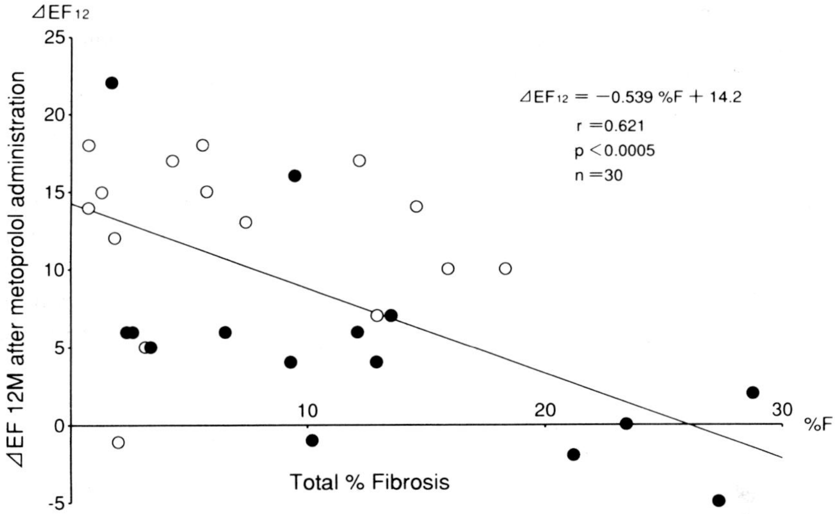

Fig. 2. Relationship between % fibrosis *(%F)* of endomyocardial biopsy specimens estimated by the point-counting method, and the extent of improvement of ejection fraction (ΔEF_{12}) 12 months (*M*) after the start of metoprolol administration. *Open circles* indicate cases with the interfascicular dominant type of fibrosis. *Closed circles* indicate cases with the intercellular dominant type of fibrosis. A close correlation between them is observed

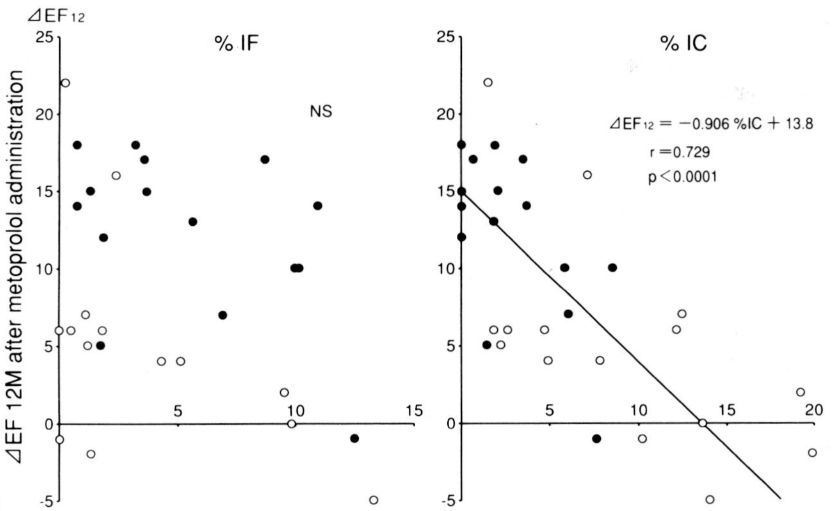

Fig. 3a,b. Relationships between percentages of each type of fibrosis and the extent of improvement of the ejection fraction ($\Delta\ EF_{12}$) for 12 months after metoprolol administration. **a** % fibrosis of interfascicular type (*open circles*)/total count (*%IF*); **b** % fibrosis of intercellular type (*closed circles*)/total count (*%IC*). Whereas %IF did not correlate, %IC closely correlated with $\Delta\ EF_{12}$

= %IC + %IF) with the point counting method of Weibel et al. [21] after Azan-Mallory staining. It should be noted that %IC correlated with the degree of EF improvement better than %F or %IF did (Figs. 2, 3). When a comparison was made between a group of 18 good responders showing improvement of at least one NYHA functional class or an increase in EF of 10% or more for 12 months, and a group comprising 12 poor responders to metoprolol without such an improvement, %F was significantly lower in good than in poor responders (7.6% ± 5.7% *vs* 14.2% ± 9.7%, $P < 0.05$). Moreover, when the type of fibrosis was classified into IF and IC types by the dominance of counted points, the majority (13 of 18 cases) of good responders showed IF dominance, while the majority (11 of 13 cases) of poor responders showed IC dominance ($P < 0.001$, sensitivity 72%, specificity 91%, predictive accuracy 80%) [18]. However, there were no significant differences between the two groups in age, gender, functional class, heart rate (HR), blood pressure (BP), pulmonary capillary wedge pressure (PCWP), cardiac index, Dd, and EF. In addition, the interval from the onset of symptoms to enrollment did not correlate with the extent of fibrosis and was not related to the dominance of fibrosis type. The relation between the extent of myocardial fibrosis and left ventricular dysfunction still remains controversial [22–25], although we found no significant difference between the groups.

Tolerance of β-Blocker in Heart Failure

It was considered a contraindication to administer β-blocker in heart failure because of the negative inotropic effect. Especially, it is natural to think that the acute administration of β-blocker deteriorates the failing heart, compensated by the sympathetic drive. Accordingly, to begin with, it is important to establish how the failing heart can tolerate β-blockade, in order to make the β-blocker treatment a success. The first point is the choice of β-blocking agent. We employed metoprolol, a cardioselective β-blocker without ISA. Metoprolol has been successfully used by many other investigators. Recently, third generation drugs such as labetalol [26,27], carvedilol [28], and bucindolol [29,30] were tried in expectation of a vasodilating effect and tolerability.

The second point is how to prescribe this drug. The initial dose should be very low to prevent the deterioration. Our protocol is as follows. The initial dose is 5–10 mg/day. The dose is stepwise increased by 5–20 mg/day every 2–8 weeks, guarding against deterioration or failure of the heart, up to the final therapeutic endpoint of 60 mg/day, unless severe hypotension (<80 mmHg), bradycardia (<40 beats/min) or any sign of clinical decompensation appears.

The third point is the status of the individual patient. Our study materials were limited to stable patients having NYHA functional class III or less, in whom intravenous administration of cardiotonic agents is not necessary. However, they had all experienced at least one episode of NYHA functional class IV. So far, there has been no dropout due to deterioration of cardiac function by β-blockade.

It has been reported that the tolerance of β-blockers in DCM might be at least partially predicted by the severity of structural abnormality, as qualitatively estimated from the extent of fibrosis, myocyte hypertrophy, and nuclear abnormality in endomyocardial biopsy samples. In that study, it was concluded that most patients with mild or moderate abnormalities could tolerate β-blocker therapy although there was a 50% chance of deterioration in the presence of the most severe histologic change [31].

Possible Mechanisms for the Beneficial Effect of β-Blocker

The possible mechanism for the beneficial effect of β-blocker in DCM has been explained from a variety of viewpoints [32–34]. The up-regulation of β-adrenoceptor is one explanation. Waagstein et al. [8] reported in their recent paper that a 60% increase in receptor density was observed after β-blockade. In our data, a similar result was obtained (Fig. 4), although the assay was performed with peripheral lymphocytes. However, it is needless to say that such a beneficial effect cannot be explained solely by an up-regulation mechanism.

In our preliminary study using a very low dose of metoprolol (less than 20 mg/day), NYHA functional class improved significantly (2.5 ± 0.2 to 1.6 ± 0.2, $P < 0.01$, follow-up period 8.8 ± 1.6 months) in the β-blockade group, compared with that in the control group (2.2 ± 0.2 to 1.8 ± 0.2, follow-up period 12.5 ± 2.5 months). Furthermore, only in the β-blockade group did cardiac output (CO) increase significantly (4.04 ± 0.40 to 5.60 ± 0.40 min,

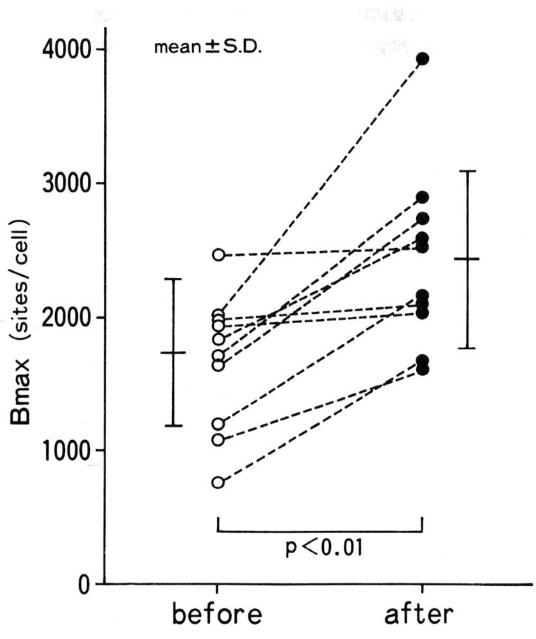

Fig. 4. Change in β-receptor density (B_{max}) one year after metoprolol. Note a significant increase in B_{max}

$P<0.01$) in spite of the tendency for PCWP to decrease (9.71 ± 2.12 to 5.71 ± 1.46 mmHg).

What is the mechanism for the beneficial effect of such a low dose of metoprolol? To elucidate the mechanism, we examined the behavior of the β-adrenoceptor of peripheral lymphocytes serially after the start of β-blocker administration, even though the majority of receptors on lymphocytes are β2. Twelve patients with DCM were entered for this study. Peripheral lymphocytes [35] were collected from them just before and 1, 2, and 3 months after the start of metoprolol administration. The density of β-adrenoceptor (B_{max}) on lymphocytes measured with radioligand ^{3}[H]-CGP12177 significantly increased throughout this three-month period, while the receptor affinity (kK_d) remained unchanged (Fig. 5). The cyclic AMP production of lymphocytes treated with 100 μ*M* isoproterenol (cAMP-ISP) or 100 μ*M* forskolin (cAMP-FSK) was also assayed by radioimmunoassay. It is of interest that, one month after metaprolol administration, cAMP-ISP had significantly increased, while cAMP-FSK remained unchanged throughout the three months (Fig. 6). The efficacy of receptor–adenylate cyclase coupling, designated as cAMP-ISP/B_{max}, was significantly improved only at one month (Fig. 7). These results indicate that β-blocker therapy not only increased the β-receptor density but also improved the efficacy of β-receptor–adenylate cyclase coupling especially during the early phase of treatment, which results in an increase of sensitivity to catecholamine and tolerance to the β-blocker.

As previously described, we found that patients with the interfascicular type of fibrosis (IF type) in the myocardium are good responders. The reason remains unknown. However, notable was the finding that down-regulation of the β-receptor was more severe for the IF type than for the intercellular fibrosis (IC) type. This finding was consistent with the observation that the plasma norepinephrine level at peak exercise (peak NE) was higher in the IF type than in the IC type. That is why the cardiac index at peak exercise, estimated by the Swan-Ganz catheter technique, in the IF type was less than that in the IC type without any difference in PCWP (Fig. 8). Consequently, it should be emphasized that although the hemodynamic response to catecholamine was impaired partly due to down-regulation of the β-receptor in the IF type, β-blocker therapy would be expected to be more effective than in the IC type.

To search for the cause of the difference in types of fibrosis, we counted leukocyte common antigen (LCA) positive cells in endomyocardial biopsy specimens. Interestingly, LCA-positive cells were denser in the IF type than in the IC type (3.3 ± 1.0 *vs* 1.0 ± 0.7 per high power field, $P < 0.01$), suggesting that interfascicular fibrosis might be attributed in part to some inflammatory process, although further studies will be needed to elucidate the possible mechanism in relation to fibrosis type.

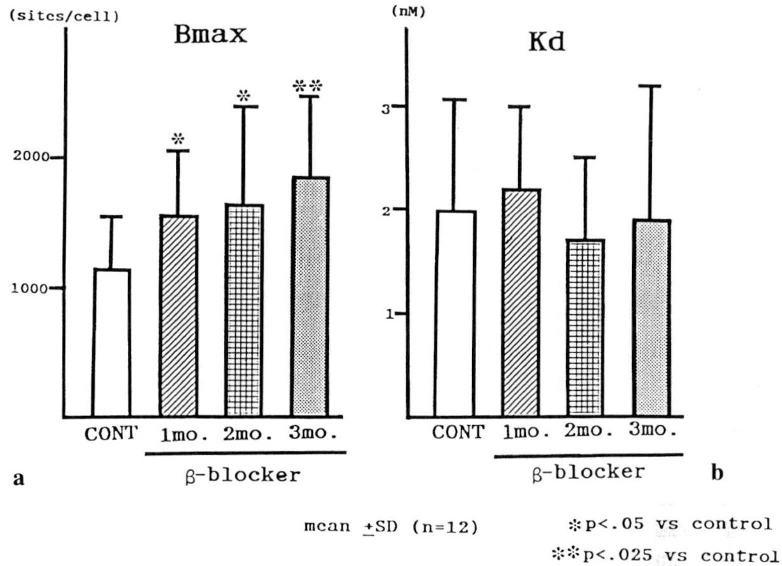

Fig. 5. Serial changes in B_{max}, β-receptor density (**a**) and K_d, the β-receptor affinity (**b**) after the start of metoprolol administration, indicating a significant increase in B_{max} even at one month, without any change in K_d. *CONT*, control; *mo.*, month

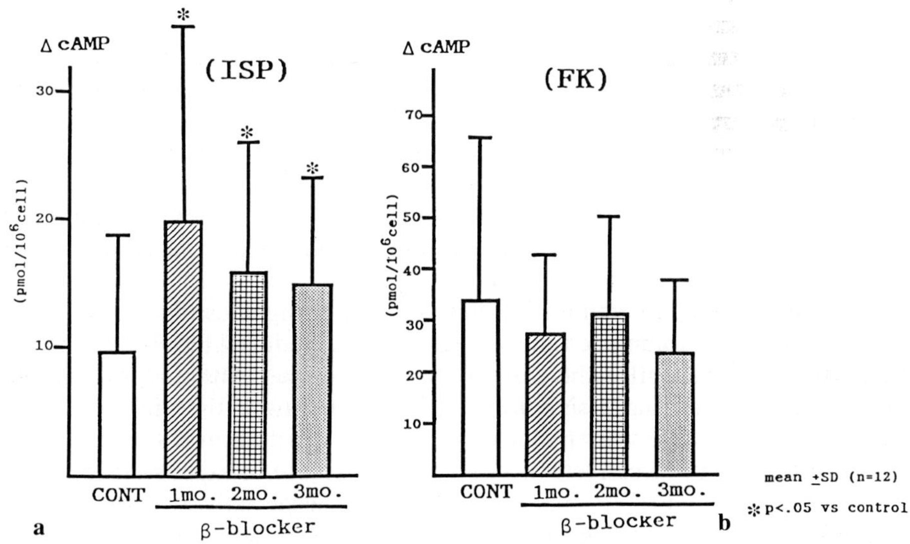

Fig. 6. Serial changes in cyclic AMP production (Δ*cAMP*) of the lymphocyte after loading **a** with 100 μ*M* isoproterenol (*ISP*) and **b** with 100 μ*M* forskolin (*FK*). Note the remarkable increase in cAMP production with ISP, especially at one month after metoprolol administration, without any change in the response to FK loading

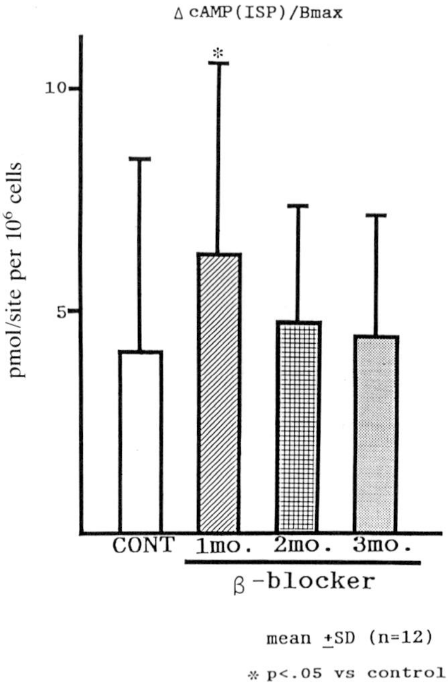

Fig. 7. Serial change in lymphocyte cyclic AMP production after loading with 100 μ *M* isoproterenol, per β-receptor of the lymphocyte ($\Delta cAMP(ISP)/B_{max}$), showing a significant increase only at one month after metoprolol administration. It should be stressed that the efficacy of β-receptor coupling to adenylate cyclase increases soon after treatment with metoprolol, probably leading to β-blocker tolerance

Withdrawal Effect of β-Blocker in DCM

Some investigators have reported an adverse effect of β-blocker withdrawal in patients with DCM [7,8]. We carried out symptom-limited supine biopsy ergometry of three stages (25 W for 4 min, 50 W for 4 min, and 75 W for 4 min or more to the end point), monitoring hemodynamics via a Swan-Ganz catheter before and seven days after withdrawal of metoprolol (60 mg/day) in eight DCM patients who were treated successfully for more than 12 months. HR, BP, PCWP, CO, and plasma norepinephrine (NE) were measured during exercise.

Although NYHA functional class did not change significantly (1.4 ± 0.6 to 1.8 ± 0.5), exercise tolerance time was significantly reduced (15.4 ± 1.3 to 13.6 ± 1.0 min, $P < 0.05$) after the cessation of metoprolol. Although HR at each grade of exercise increased significantly after withdrawal, the increase rate of HR with exercise grade was similar in pre- and post-withdrawal states. CO and stroke work (SW) progressively increased with increase in exercise load in both situations; however, PCWP appeared to increase, especially at early stages in the pre-withdrawal state and at late stages with exercise grading in the post-withdrawal state.

Figure 9 shows the transition of the relationship between PCWP and SW during exercise. Before withdrawal, SW progressively increased without any large rise in PCWP with increasing grade of exercise, although there was an

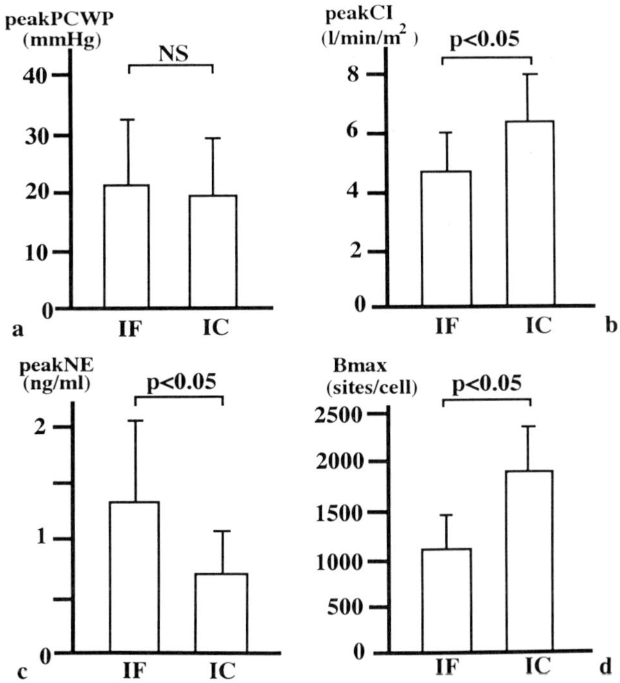

Fig. 8a–d. Differences between the interfascicular dominant type of fibrosis (*IF*) and the intercellular dominant type of fibrosis (*IC*) in hemodynamic parameters during symptom-limited, multistaged, supine ergometry, **a** *Peak PCWP*, the maximal value of pulmonary capillary wedge pressure during exercise; **b** *Peak CI*, the maximal cardiac index during exercise; **c** *Peak NE*, the maximal value of plasma norepinephrine concentration; and **d** β-receptor density (B_{max}) before metoprolol administration. B_{max} was reduced (down-regulation of the β-receptor) in the IF group, probably due to more NE exposure, which is compatible with a smaller increase in CI without a greater change in PCWP in the IF group than in the IC group

initial increase in PCWP. In contrast, after withdrawal, an increase in SW needed a significant increase in PCWP. This result implied that the heart could reach a higher level of the inotropic state during exercise with β-blockade than without it, despite the plasma NE levels during exercise increasing similarly with and without β-blockade. However, at the initial stage of exercise, the heart after withdrawal was more sensitive to increased catecholamine drive by exercise than before withdrawal, probably due to the disappearance of β-receptor competition. The heart with β-blockade reacted more sensitively to the intrinsic sympathetic stimulation than the heart without β-blockade. We believe that these changes in the hemodynamic responses during exercise after withdrawal indicate an adverse effect of withdrawal (a greater increase in PCWP was needed for an increase in SW during exercise).

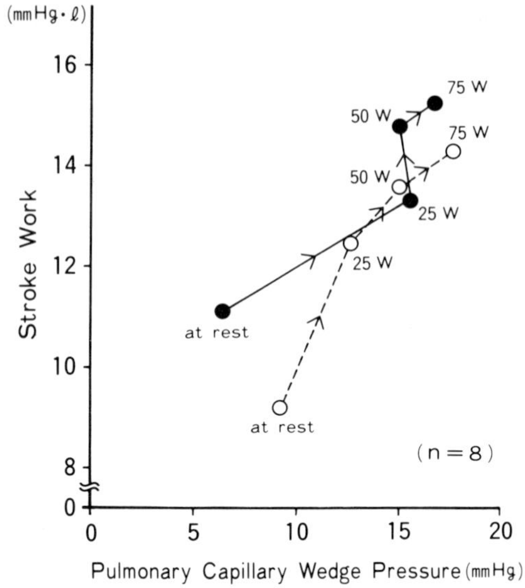

Fig. 9. Serial changes in cardiac inotropic state on the cardiac function curves at rest and during multistage (25 W, 50 W, 75 W; 4 min for each stage) supine bicycle ergometry. Pulmonary artery wedge pressure (*PCWP*)–stroke work (*SW*) relationships are shown with (pre-withdrawal status) and without (post-withdrawal status) β-blockade. *Closed circles* and *open circles* show the mean values of parameters in each stage with and without β-blockade, respectively. The transitions are shown by a *solid line* (pre-withdrawal status) and a *dashed line* (post-withdrawal status). The relative change in stroke work to change in pulmonary artery wedge pressure differs: the increase rate of SW for an increase in PCWP with an increase of exercise grade in pre-withdrawal states becomes higher than that in post-withdrawal status, although it was initially lower

Swedberg et al. [7] demonstrated adverse effects of β-blockade withdrawal, and based on these results, proposed the effectiveness of β-blockade in patients with congestive cardiomyopathy, as in our study. They observed deterioration of clinical conditions in 6 of 15 patients over a wide range of the withdrawal period (7–119 days). We provided a withdrawal period of one week, since one week was long enough to wash out metoprolol (39.0 ± 7.3 to 0.8 ± 0.8 ng/ml) from the circulating blood and enough for the disappearance of the rebound phenomenon [36].

In order to elucidate the mechanism, we also measured the density of β-receptor before and one week after withdrawal [37]. According to the assay, B_{max} was reduced after withdrawal (2505 ± 145 to 2208 ± 187 sites/cell, $P < 0.01$). The reduction of approximately 10% in the density of β-receptors of lymphocytes, predominantly β2-receptors, leads us to speculate that the β1-receptors of the myocardium would be less dense after withdrawal, although there is a limitation on our ability to predict β1-receptor density of the myocardium from β 2-receptor density of peripheral lymphocytes. Nevertheless, this finding implies that down-regulation of the β-receptor after withdrawal may play a role in adversely affecting cardiac function curves during exercise, although the renin–angiotensin system [38] and a subcellular mechanism [39] are also probably involved.

In the early stages of exercise (lower range of plasma NE), cardiac function curves before withdrawal showed lower response to NE than that after withdrawal. This suggests competition between NE and the β-blocker for β-receptor. At a higher range of plasma NE, the cardiac function curve before withdrawal was on the contrary higher (more responsive to catecholamine) than after withdrawal, suggesting an increased β-receptor density (Fig. 10). Such a biphasic cardiac function curve during exercise might be explained by the model of Bristow et al. [40]. According to this model, the percent maximum response of β-agonist plotted against β-agonist concentration generates an S-shaped curve, of which the maximal saturated value is related to the density of β-receptor. The S-shaped curve shifts to the right under β-blockade because of competition for the β-receptor. If it could be considered that the horizontal and vertical lines in their model were analogous to plasma NE level increasing during exercise and the inotropic response on the PCWP–SW relationship during exercise, respectively (Fig. 11), it could be reasonable that the heart with β-blockade shows a lower response to NE in low-grade exercise (lower NE level) and, conversely, a higher response to NE in higher grade exercise (higher NE level) than that without β-blockade.

For How Long Should These Drugs Be Continued?

It remains unknown whether β-blockade is still necessary in patients with DCM whose hearts have already recovered to normal, although it is gradually becoming recognized that long-term β-blockade could provide a favorable effect. Therefore, to clarify how long long-term β-blocker therapy should be continued in DCM, metoprolol administration was twice stopped for a week at the early (within 18 months) phase and the late (after 24 months) phase of treatment in eight patients with DCM. Before and after both withdrawal studies, hemodynamics at rest and during ergometer exercise were again measured via a Swan-Ganz catheter. In the earlier stage, the PCWP–cardiac work (CW) relationship shifted to the upper right, whereas it shifted to the upper left in the late stage, resembling the normal heart (Fig. 12). What is the normalized pattern? Is the drug still necessary even in such a situation? Although some of the patients receiving metoprolol therapy chose to cease being administered, they all eventually deteriorated. Thus, in our hospital the drug is continued at smaller doses for the prevention of sudden death.

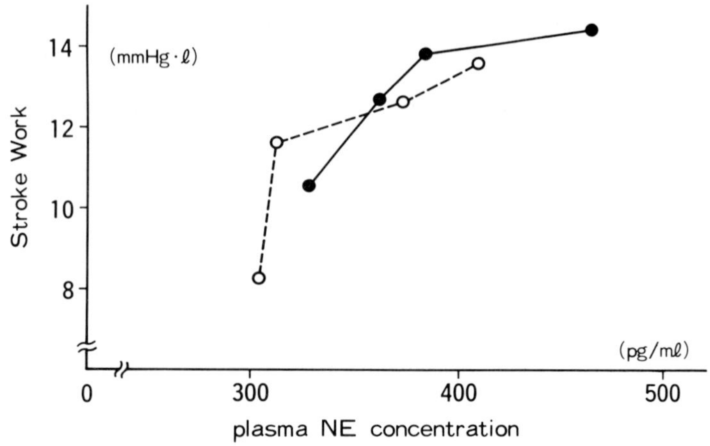

Fig. 10. Plots of stroke work to plasma norepinephrine (*NE*) concentration in pre-withdrawal (*closed circles* and *solid lines*) and post-withdrawal (*open circles* and *dashed lines*) status during multistaged bicycle ergometry. Whereas the response of stroke work to sympathetic drive in the early stage of exercise was higher in pre- than post-withdrawal status, that in the middle and late stages of exercise was lower in pre- than post-withdrawal status

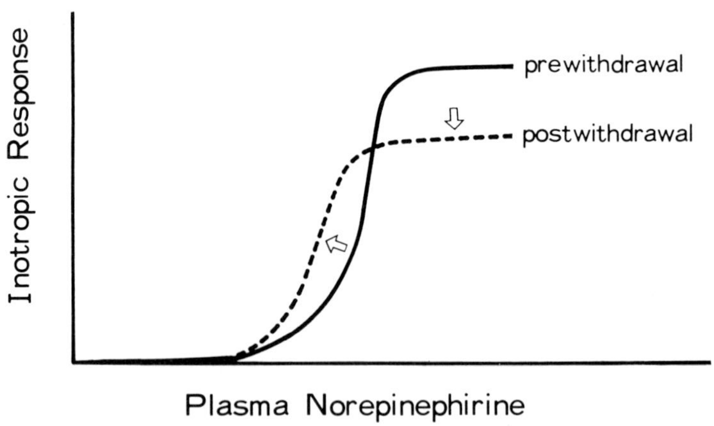

Results : ① catecholamine during exercise pre ≒ post
② inotropic response in lower grade of exercise pre < post
③ inotropic response in higher grade of exercise pre > post
④ β-adrenergic receptor density pre > post

Fig. 12. Changes in pulmonary capillary wedge pressure–cardiac work relationships at rest before (*closed symbols*) and after (*open symbols*) withdrawal of metoprolol. A difference is apparent between the early (*circles*) phase (<18 months after) and the late (*squares*) phase (>24 months after start of metoprolol treatment) when the cardiac function has presumably already improved sufficiently

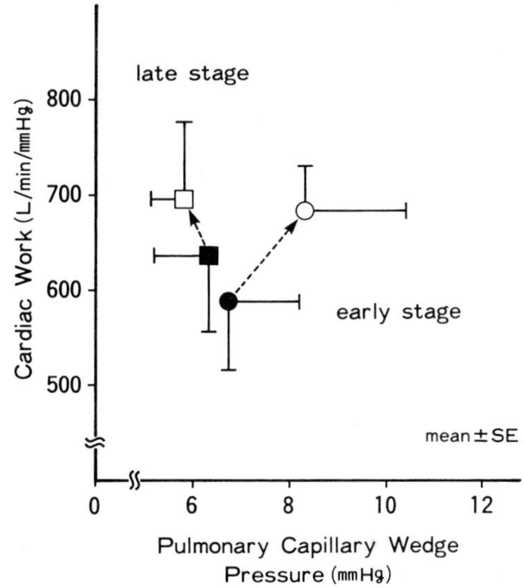

Conclusion

It is concluded that β-blocker therapy is of clinical use for improving exercise capacity not only by protecting the heart from catecholamine, but also by elevating the maximal potency of responce to catecholamine injury. Care must be taken in β-blocker therapy to select the potential candidates from a histological finding by endomyocardial biopsy, or otherwise by estimation of fibrosis using signal-averaged electrocardiography [41], and also to overcome the side effects of β-blocker on the failing heart. Therefore, it is necessary to increase the dose very gradually, so as to be in time for alterations in receptor pathway.

On the other hand, remarkable progress has been made in recent research on the modulation of adrenergic receptors and G protein transduction protein

Fig. 11. Conceptual relationships between plasma norepinephrine (*NE*) level (*x*-axis) and the inotropic response (*y*-axis) derived from the results in Figs. 9 and 10, respectively. The *solid line* shows the catecholamine-response curve in the pre-withdrawal (with β-blockade) state. The *dashed line* shows the catecholamine-response curve in the post-withdrawal (without β-blockade) state. Since the heart has a higher density of β-adrenergic receptor in the pre-withdrawal state than in the post-withdrawal state, the response to catecholamine is depicted as higher than that in the post-withdrawal state. On the other hand, since there is competition by β-blocker for β-adrenergic receptor in the pre-withdrawal state, the curve is expected to shift to the *right*. Note that the catecholamine response in the pre-withdrawal state is greater in the higher range of plasma NE than that in the post-withdrawal state in the failing heart [42,43], including the molecular basis of receptor desensitization [44]. These studies suggest that β 1-selective down-regulation followed by alterations of β1/β2 distribution [45], β2-selective uncoupling [46], enhanced receptor kinase [47], and increased Gi protein [48,49] may be mainly involved in the catecholamine insensitivity of the failing heart. Furthermore, of note is the report of Bristow et al. [50] that potentially important differences exist in the regulatory behavior of components of the β-adrenergic receptor–G protein–adenylate cyclase complex, between idiopathic and ischemic cardiomyopathy.

If further investigation makes the subcellular system of the receptor, including gene expression information [51–53] and other mechanisms of catecholamine injury [54], clear in the clinic and in basic medicine, the mechanism of the beneficial effect of β-blockade in DCM will be elucidated and more patients will benefit from this therapy.

References

1. Reichenbach DD, Benditt EP (1970) Catecholamines and cardiomyopathy: The pathogenesis and potential importance of myofibrillar degeneration. Hum Pathol 1:125–150
2. Bristow MR (1984) The adrenergic nervous system in heart failure. N Engl J Med 311:850–851
3. Cohn JN, Levine TB, Olivari MT, Garberg V, Lura D, Francis GS, Simon AB, Rector T (1984) Plasma norepinephrine as a guide to prognosis in patients with chronic congestive heart failure. N Engl J Med 311:819–823
4. Waagstein F, Hjalmarson A, Varnauskas E, Wallentin I (1975) Effect of chronic beta-adrenergic receptor blockade in congestive cardiomyopathy. Br Heart J 37:1022–1036
5. Swedberg K, Hjalmarson A, Waagstein F, Wallentin I (1979) Prolongation of survival in congestive cardiomyopathy by beta-receptor blockade. Lancet 1:1374–1376
6. Swedberg K, Hjalmarson A, Waagstein F, Wallentin I (1980) Beneficial effects of long-term beta-blockade in congestive cardiomyopathy. Br Heart J 44:117–133
7. Swedberg K, Hjalmarson A, Waagstein F, Wallentin I (1980) Adverse effects of beta-blockade withdrawal in patients with congestive cardiomyopathy. Br Heart J 44:134–142
8. Waagstein F, Caidahl K, Wallentin I, Bergh CH, Hjalmarson A (1989) Long-term β-blockade in dilated cardiomyopathy. Effects of short- and long-term metoprolol treatment followed by withdrawal and readministration of metoprolol. Circulation 80:551–563
9. Andersson B, Blomstrom-Lundqvist C, Hedner T, Waagstein F (1991) Exercise hemodynamics and myocardial metabolism during long-term beta-adrenergic blockade in severe heart failure. J Am Coll Cardiol 18:1059–1066
10. Ikram H, Fitzpatrick D (1981) Double-blind trial of chronic oral beta blockade in congestive cardiomyopathy. Lancet 2:490–492

11. Currie PJ, Kelly MJ, McKenzie A, Harper RW, Lim YL, Federman J, Anderson ST, Pitt A (1984) Oral beta-adrenergic blockade with metoprolol in chronic severe dilated cardiomyopathy. J Am Coll Cardiol 3:203–209
12. Anderson JL, Lutz JR, Gilbert EM, Sorensen SG, Yanowitz FG, Menlove RL, Bartholomew M (1985) A randomized trial of low-dose beta-blockade therapy for idiopathic dilated cardiomyopathy. Am J Cardiol 55:471–475
13. Engelmeier RS, O'Connell JB, Walsh R, Rad N, Scanlon PJ, Gunnar RM (1985) Improvement in symptoms and exercise tolerance by metoprolol in patients with dilated cardiomyopathy. A double-blind, randomized, placebo-controlled trial. Circulation 72:536–546
14. The Xamoterol In Severe Heart Failure Study Group (1990) Xamoterol in severe heart failure. Lancet 336:1–6
15. Heilbrunn SM, Shah P, Bristow MR, Valantine HA, Ginsburg R, Fowler MB (1989) Increased β-receptor density and improved hemodynamic response to catecholamine stimulation during long-term metoprolol therapy in heart failure from dilated cardiomyopathy. Circulation 79:483–490
16. Eichhorn EJ, Bedotto JB, Malloy CR, Hatfield BA, Deitchman D, Brown M, Willard JE, Grayburn PA (1990) Effect of β-adrenergic blockade on myocardial function and energetics in congestive heart failure. Improvements in hemodynamic, contractile, and diastolic performance with bucindolol. Circulation 82:473–483
17. Fukunami M, Hashimura K, Ohmori M, Ikeda T, Umemoto K, Kumagai K, Sakai A, Yamada T, Kondoh N, Minamino T, Nagareda T, Kotoh K, Hoki N (1991) Effectiveness of long-term beta-blocker therapy for dilated cardiomyopathy—Echocardiographical follow-up. Cardiovasc Drugs Ther 5:463–470
18. Yamada T, Fukunami M, Ohmori M, Iwakura K, Kumagai K, Kondoh N, Minamino T, Tsujimura E, Nagareda T, Kotoh K, Hoki N (1993) Which subgroup of patients with dilated cardiomyopathy would benefit from long-term beta-blocker therapy? A histologic viewpoint. J Am Coll Cardiol 21:628–633
19. Fuster V, Gersh BJ, Giuliani ER, Tajik AJ, Brandenburg RO, Frye RL (1981) The natural history of idiopathic dilated cardiomyopathy. Am J Cardiol 47:525–531
20. Anderson KR, Sutton MGS, Lie JT (1979) Histopathological types of cardiac fibrosis in myocardial disease. J Pathol 128:79–85
21. Weibel ER, Gonzagne SK, Walter F (1966) Practical stereological methods for morphometric cytology. J Cell Biol 30:23–37
22. Baandrup U, Florio RA, Rehahn M, Richardson PJ, Olsen EGJ (1981) Critical analysis of endomyocardial biopsies from patients suspected of having cardiomyopathy II: Comparison of histology and clinical/haemodynamic information. Br Heart J 45:487–493
23. Figulla HR, Rahlf G, Nieger M, Luig H, Kreuzer H (1985) Spontaneous hemodynamic improvement or stabilization and associated biopsy findings in patients with congestive cardiomyopathy. Circulation 71:1095–1104
24. Schwarz F, Mall G, Zebe H, et al. (1983) Quantitative morphologic fingings of the myocardium in idiopathic dilated cardiomyopathy. Am J Cardiol 51:501–506
25. Unverferth DV, Fetters JK, Unverferth BJ, et al. (1983) Human myocardial histologic characteristics in congestive heart failure Circulation 68:1194–1200
26. Leung WH, Lau CP, Wong CK, Cheng CH, Tai YT, Lim SP (1990) Improvement in exercise performance and hemodynamics by labetalol in patients with idiopathic dilated cardiomyopathy. Am Heart J 119:884–890

27. Peterson H, Erhardt L (1991) Beta receptor antagonists in the treatment of heart failure. Cardiovasc Drugs Ther 5:589–604
28. Olsen SL, Gilbert EM, Renlund DG, Mealey PC, Tayler DO, Volkman AK, Bristow MR (1993) Carvedilol improves symptoms and left ventricular function in patients with congestive heart failure due to ischemic or idiopathic dilated cardiomyopathy. J Am Coll Cardiol 21:114A
29. Anderson JL, O'Connell JB, Yanowitzs F, Mealey P, Bristow MR (1991) Long-term (2 year) beneficial effects of beta-adrenergic blockade with bucindolol in patients with congestive heart failure due to ischemic or idiopathic dilated cradiomyopathy. J Am Coll Cardiol 17:1373–1381
30. Pollock SG, Lystash J, Tedesco C, Craddock G, Smucker ML (1990) Usefulness of bucindolol in congestive heart failure. Am J Cardiol 66:603–607
31. Anderson JL (1988) Treatment of cardiac myopathies with beta blockers. What do we know, where do we go from here? Postgrad Med 29:104–112
32. Fowler MB, Bristow MR (1985) Rationale for beta-adrenergic blocking drugs in cardiomyopathy. Am J Cardiol 55:120D–124D
33. Fisher ML, Plotnick GD, Peters RW, Carliner NH (1986) Beta-blockers in congestive cardiomyopathy. Conceptual advance or contraindication? Am J Med 80[Suppl 2B]:59–66
34. Bristow MR (1993) Pathophysiologic and pharmacologic rationales for clinical management of chronic heart failure with beta-blocking agents. Am J Cardiol 71:12C–22C
35. Brodde OE, Kretsch R, Ikezono K, Zerkowski HR, Reidemeister JC (1986) Human β-adrenoceptors: Relation of myocardial and lymphocyte β-adrenoceptor density. Science 231:1584–1585
36. Rangno RE, Langlois S, Lutterodt A (1982) Metoprolol withdrawal phenomena: Mechanism and prevention. Clin Pharmacol Ther 31:8–15
37. Fukunami M, Hoki N, Yamada M, Ohmori M, Yamada H, Umemoto K, Sakai A, Ohnishi K (1987) Possible mechanims for the beneficial effect of chronic beta-blockers administration in patients with dilated cardiomyopathy. Circulation 76[Suppl IV]:IV-358
38. Kagiya T, Hori M, Fukunami M, Hoki N, Iwakura K, Kurihara T, Watanabe Y, Kamada T (1987) Role of beta-adrenergic receptors in beta-blocker therapy for chronic heart failure in patients with dilated cardiomyopathy. Circulation 76[Suppl IV]:IV-308
39. Hashimura K, Fukunami M, Ohmori M, Ikeda T, Umemoto K, Kumagai K, Sakai A, Yamada T, Hoki N (1989) Effect of β-blocker withdrawal on β-receptor-adenylate cyclase coupling in patients with dilated cardiomyopathy. Circulation 80[Suppl II]:II-116
40. Bristow MR, Kantrowitz NE, Ginsburg R, Fowler MB (1985) β-adrenergic function in heart muscle disease and heart failure. J Mol Cell Cardiol 17[Suppl 2]:41–52
41. Yamada T, Fukunami M, Ohmori M, Iwakura K, Kumagai K, Kondoh N, Tsujimura K, Abe Y, Nagareda T, Kotoh K, Hoki N (1993) New approach to the estimation of the extent of myocardial fibrosis in patients with dilated cardiomyopathy: Use of signal-averaged electrocardiography. Am Heart J 126:626–631
42. Colucci WS (1993) In situ assessment of α- and β-adrenergic responses in failing human myocardium. Circulation 87[Suppl VII]:VII63–VII67
43. Feldman AM (1993) Modulation of adrenergic receptors and G-transduction proteins in failing human ventricular myocardium. Circulation 87[Suppl IV]:IV-27–IV-34

44. Sibley DR, Lefkowitz RJ (1985) Molecular mechanisms of receptor desensitization using the β-adrenergic receptor-coupled adenylate cyclase system as a model. Nature 317:124–129
45. Bristow MR, Ginsburg R, Fowler M, Minobe W, Rasmussen R, Zera P, Menlove R, Shah P, Stinson E (1986) β1 and β2 adrenergic receptor subpopulations in normal and failing human ventricular myocardium: coupling of both receptor subtypes to muscle contraction and selective β1 receptor down-regulation in heart failure. Circ Res 59:297–309
46. Brodde OE, Schuler S, Kretsch R, Brinkmann M, Borst HG, Hetzer R, Reidemeister JC, Warnecke H, Zerkowski HR (1986) Regional distribution of β-adrenoceptors in the human heart: coexistence of functional β1- and β2-adrenoceptors in both atria and ventricles in severe congestive cardiomyopathy. J Cardiovasc Pharmacol 8:1235–1242
47. Ungerer M, Bohm M, Elce JS, Erdmann E, Lohse MJ (1993) Altered expression of β-adrenergic receptor kinase and β1-adrenergic receptors in the failing human heart. Circulation 87:454–463
48. Neumann J, Schmitz W, Scholz H, von Meyerinck L, Doring V, Kalmar P (1988) Increase in myocardial Gi-proteins in heart failure. Lancet 2:936–937
49. Bohm M, Gierschik P, Jacobs KH, Pieske B, Schnabel P, Ungerer M, Erdmann E (1990) Increase of Gi alpha in human hearts with dilated but not ischemic cardiomyopathy. Circulation 82:1249–1265
50. Bristow MR, Anderson FL, Port JD, Skerl L, Hershberger RE, Larrabee P, O'Connell JB, Renlund DG, Volkman K, Murray J, Feldman AM (1991) Differences in β-adrenergic neuroeffector mechanisms in ischemic versus idiopathic dilated cardiomyopathy. Circulation 84:1024–1039
51. Feldman AM, Ray PE, Silan CM, Mercer JA, Mercer JA, Minobe W, Bristow MR (1991) Selective gene expression in failing human heart: Quantification of steady-state levels of messenger RNA in endomyocardial biopsies using the polymerase chain reaction. Circulation 83:1866–1872
52. Bristow MR, Durham C, Klein J, Rasmussen R, Port JD, Gestiland RR, Barry WH, Feldman AM (1991) Down-regulation of β-adrenergic receptors and receptor mRNA in heart cells chronically exposed to norepinephrine. Clin Res 39:256A
53. Spiegel AM, Weinstein LS, Shenker A (1993) Abnormalities in G protein-coupled signal transduction pathways in human disease. J Clin Invest 92:1119–1125
54. Mann DL, Kent RL, Parsons B, Cooper G IV (1992) Adrenergic effects on the biology of the adult mammalian cardiocyte. Circulation 85:790–804

3.7 Long-Term Effects of Enalapril in Patients with Left Ventricular Dysfunction

The Importance of Assessing Regional Myocardial Function

ISRAEL MIRSKY[1], TERUHIKO AOYAGI[1], TADASHI IHARA[1], CHRISTIAN VAN EYLL[2], MICHEL F. ROUSSEAU[2], and HUBERT POULEUR[2]

Summary. Large-scale drug trials have focused primarily on mortality and morbidity and less on the functional state of the myocardium. A model was developed to assess myocardial contractile state in patients with left ventricular (LV) dysfunction, to address the question of the effects of enalapril, an angiotensin converting enzyme (ACE) inhibitor, and to determine the best predictors of outcome. Pressure–angiographic data were obtained from 16 patients with overt heart failure and 47 without overt heart failure. Repeat studies were conducted in 41 patients after one year's treatment with enalapril or a placebo. Left ventricular silhouettes were divided into 18 segments to evaluate regional ejection fraction (EF), wall stress, and myocardial contractile state which was assessed by EF–preload–afterload relationships. End-diastolic (EDV) and end-systolic volumes (ESV) were significantly greater ($P < 0.001$), and EF lower ($P < 0.009$) in patients with overt heart failure. Enalapril reduced EDV ($P < 0.03$) and ESV ($P < 0.006$), in contrast to the placebo, with which there was an increase in EDV ($P < 0.03$). Diastolic pressure–volume relationships shifted to the left with enalapril, and to the right with the placebo. The best single predictors of post-treatment EF were myocardial contractile state for the enalapril-treated group and ESV for the placebo-treated group. Added benefits of enalapril included the prevention of further dilatation in patients with less-depressed myocardial contractility, and delay in the onset of heart failure. The studies suggest that asymptomatic patients with LV dysfunction should also be considered for ACE inhibitor therapy.

Key words: Myocardial infarction—Contractile state—Left ventricular dysfunction—Enalapril

---

[1] Department of Medicine, Brigham and Women's Hospital and Harvard Medical School, 75 Francis Street, Boston, MA 02115, USA

[2] University of Louvain School of Medicine, av Hippocrate 55, Box 5560, B-1200, Brussels, Belgium

Introduction

Heart failure remains one of the foremost public health problems in the United States and our knowledge of the mechanisms involved in the progression to congestive heart failure is still limited. This is not only due to a lack of appropriate experimental models of chronic congestive heart failure, but also to the lack of attention paid to the development of novel methods for assessing both regional ventricular and myocardial function in the clinical setting.

In recent years, numerous multi-center clinical trials have been conducted to test new drugs; however, many of these trials have focused primarily on the aspects of mortality and morbidity and generally have been based on measurements obtained by noninvasive methods. Such measurements have limitations for the assessment of myocardial function. These trials often revealed that many patients on a placebo responded just as well or even better than those on the drug being tested. The major objectives of the present study were therefore to develop a model for assessing regional and global function in patients with low ejection fraction, and apply the model to data obtained from a subset of patients enrolled in the two "studies of left ventricular dysfunction" (SOLVD) involving the angiotensin converting enzyme (ACE) inhibitor enalapril [1,2]. More specifically, these studies were directed to address several clinical questions including:

1. What are the differences (if any) in the basal hemodynamic and regional myocardial function parameters of patients with overt heart failure (Treatment arm) and without heart failure (Prevention arm)?
2. What are the relative effects of enalapril and a placebo on these functional parameters following a one-year treatment?
3. How important is size and location of the myocardial damage in patients with reduced ejection fraction?
4. Is the contractile state of the myocardium the major determinant of functional outcome in these patients following one year's treatment?

Materials and Methods

Patient Population

Sixty-three patients were studied in the basal state (16 in the Treatment arm with class II–III NYHA heart failure: and 47 in the Prevention arm). The etiology of the left ventricular dysfunction was ischemic heart disease in 55 patients and idiopathic dilated cardiomyopathy in 8 patients. Second studies were also conducted in 41/63 patients after 12.4 months (range 10–17 months).

Catheterization Data and Angiographic Analyses

Left heart catheterization was performed in the fasting state and without premedication as previously described [3]. An 8F pigtal Millar catheter (Millar

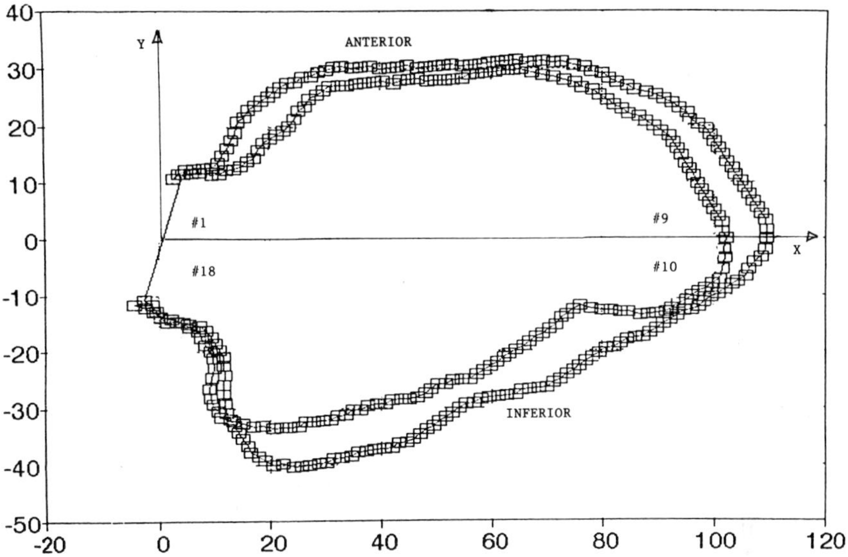

Fig. 1. End-diastolic and end-systolic silhouettes from a patient with an anterior myocardial infarction. The midpoint of the aortic valve plane is the origin of an *x-y* coordinate system with the *x*-axis coinciding with the long axis. Each silhouette is divided into 9 anterior (# 1–9) and 9 inferior segments (#10–18) numbered consecutively from the base

Instruments, Houston, Tex., USA) was introduced through the femoral artery to measure, with high fidelity, left ventricular pressure and to inject contrast material. Angiographic images in the right anterior oblique projection were acquired with Philips Polydiagnost C and DVI systems (Philips Instruments, Best, The Netherlands) at 50 frames/s simultaneously with recordings of the left ventricular pressure and ECG signal on magnetic tape (Honeywell 101, Honeywell Information Systems, Waltham, Mass., USA).

Left ventricular silhouettes were digitized and *x, y* coordinates obtained throughout the cardiac cycle at 50 frames/s. Each silhouette was superimposed so that the long axis and origin (midpoint of the aortic valve plane) coincided with that of the end-diastolic silhouette (Fig. 1). Each silhouette was divided into nine anterior and nine inferior segments. Regional (segmental) cavity areas (Ac) and cavity volumes were evaluated by Simpson's rule.

Evaluation of Left Ventricular Regional Wall Area, Stresses, Volumes, and Myocardial Damage

Since limited thickness data were available, it was necessary to make several simplifying assumptions, namely:

1. At end-diastole, anterior wall thickness in the direction *perpendicular* to the long axis, was assumed to be constant from the base to the point where angiographic thickness was measured, and then to taper towards the apex.
2. For estimation of end-diastolic thickness in the inferior region, it was assumed that global average stresses were equal in the inferior and anterior regions.
3. During systole, segmental geometries were described by truncated cones or by paraboloids in the apical region and the condition of incompressibility invoked.

Regional wall stresses (σ) were estimated by $\sigma \simeq P(Ac/Aw)$, where regional cavity areas (Ac) and wall areas (Aw) were obtained by Simpson's rule. Myocardial damage (% MD_{da}) or "infarct size" was defined as % MD_{da} % (dyskinetic + akinetic wall volume/left ventricular wall volume).

Assessment and Ranking of Regional Myocardial Contractility

Current methods for assessing myocardial contractility are limited since they ignore the effects of preload on the ejection fraction (EF). By omitting dyskinetic and akinetic segments, one can obtain for each patient, a composite regional ejection fraction (EF_r) in the form $EF_r = a + b\,\sigma_{edr} - c\,\sigma_{esr}$ (a,b,c > 0) where σ_{edr}, σ_{esr} are, respectively, the regional end-diastolic and end-systolic stresses (end systole being defined at the time of $(P/V)_{max}$ [3]). By employing a General Linear Models Analysis (SAS, SAS Institute, Carey, NC, USA), these relationships can be compared over common ranges of stress and hence a ranking of contractile state (Rank MC) assigned to each ventricle.

Analysis of Diastolic Pressure–volume (P–V) Relationships

Since sample sizes were small in the various subgroups of patients having two studies, the analysis was conducted for the anterior infarct group (AMI) only. Diastolic pressure–volume (P–V) curves were obtained in the form $P = A\,e^{kV}$ where A,k are regression coefficients [4]. These relationships were used to evaluate volumes at common pressure levels over the range 10–35 mmHg, and by averaging these volumes at given pressure levels, a P–V relationship was obtained for each group before and after one year's treatment.

Predictions of Post Ejection Fraction (EF_{post}) in Patients with AMI Following a One-year Treatment

A detailed Spearman-rank correlation analysis was conducted to determine (a) the associations (if any) between EF_{post} and each of eight functional parameters [end-systolic volume (ESV), end-diastolic volume (EDV), EF, % MD_{da}, end-diastolic pressure (EDP), σ_{ed}, σ_{es}, Rank MC], and (b) the independence of the basal functional parameters. An expression for EF_{post} was then sought in terms of readily attainable parameters.

Results

Baseline Data for Treatment and Prevention Arms

Left ventricular end-diastolic (EDV) and end-systolic (ESV) volumes were significantly greater ($P < 0.001$) in the Treatment arm (EDV: 391 ± 115 *vs* 297 ± 72 mls; ESV: 318 ± 99 *vs* 228 ± 70 mls). This resulted in significantly lower ($P < 0.01$) end-systolic ejection fractions (EF_{es}) in this group (18.1% ± 8.5% *vs* 24.2% ± 7.6%). Left ventricular global average end-diastolic (σ_{ed}) and end-systolic (σ_{es}) stresses were similar in both groups (σ_{ed}: 135 ± 69 *vs* 115 ± 54 g/cm^2; σ_{es}: 483 ± 140 *vs* 458 ± 155 g/cm^2. Myocardial damage also tended to be greater ($P = 0.07$) in the Treatment arm (% MD_{da}: 32 ± 20 *vs* 23 ± 14).

Hemodynamic Responses to Enalapril and Placebo in the Combined Treatment and Prevention Arms

Following a one-year treatment, enalapril significantly reduced both end-diastolic ($P < 0.03$) and end-systolic ($P < 0.006$) volumes in contrast to the placebo which resulted in a significant increase ($P < 0.03$) in EDV and no change in ESV (Table 1). Although no significant differences in these volumes were observed between the two treated groups, there were significant differences in the changes in volume, ΔEDV ($P < 0.002$) and ΔESV ($P < 0.003$). While enalapril improved the ejection fraction ($P < 0.02$), no change was observed with the placebo, and no significant differences were observed between groups after the one-year treatment.

Ejection Fraction Versus Myocardial Damage Relationships for the Treatment and Prevention Arms

Significant inverse relationships between the ejection fraction (EF_{es}) and myocardial damage (% MD_{da}) were obtained for each group, in the forms: $EF_{es} = 29.0 - 0.34$ (% MD_{da}) (Treatment: $n = 16$, $r = -0.814$, $P < 0.001$); and $EF_{es} = 31.4 - 0.32$ (% MD_{da}) (Prevention: $n = 47$, $r = -0.597$, $P < 0.001$). These relationships could be combined, as displayed in Fig. 2.

Multivariate Relationships for Predicting the Ejection Fraction Following a One-year Treatment with Enalapril (E) or Placebo (PL)

$$\text{E: } \ln(EF_{post}) = 4.22 - 0.0030\ ESV_{pre} - 0.00797\ EDP_{pre} \qquad (n = 12,\ r^2 = 0.802)$$

$$\text{PL: } \ln(EF_{post}) = 1.62 - 0.00317\ EDV_{pre} + 0.0825\ EF_{pre} \qquad (n = 8,\ r^2 = 0.979)$$

where the subscript "pre" refers to the basal state.

Table 1. Effects of enalapril *vs* placebo on global function parameters for the combined treatment and prevention arms.

		Baseline	1 year of treatment	Baseline versus 1 year *P*-Value[1]	Enalapril versus placebo *P*-Value[2]
HR (beats/min)	E	84 ± 15	76 ± 16	<0.011	NS
	PL	80 ± 10	78 ± 9	NS	
LVEDP (mmHg)	E	25 ± 10	25 ± 8	NS	NS
	PL	27 ± 11	29 ± 10	NS	
LVPSP (mmHg)	E	136 ± 26	136 ± 21	NS	NS
	PL	138 ± 19	137 ± 20	NS	
EDV (ml)	E	312 ± 85	293 ± 85	<0.03	<0.002
	PL	299 ± 95	321 ± 92	<0.03	
ESV (ml)	E	238 ± 78	213 ± 75	<0.006	<0.003
	PL	229 ± 77	246 ± 93	NS	
SV (ml)	E	74 ± 26	80 ± 26	NS	NS
	PL	70 ± 31	74 ± 26	NS	
EF_{es} (%)	E	24.3 ± 7.8	28.0 ± 8.2	<0.02	NS
	PL	23.5 ± 8.3	24.9 ± 9.7	NS	
σ_{ed} (g/cm^2)	E	103 ± 45	104 ± 42	NS	NS
	PL	118 ± 57	146 ± 103	NS	
σ_{es} (g/cm^2)	E	434 ± 158	421 ± 153	NS	NS
	PL	467 ± 130	528 ± 353	NS	

[1] Paired *t*-test; [2] Statistical significance for difference in treatment (unpaired *t*-test). Values are expressed as mean ± SD E, enalapril (n = 25); PL, placebo (n = 15); HR, heart rate; LVEDP, left ventricular end-diastolic pressure; LVPSP, left ventricular peak systolic pressure; EF_{es}, ejection fraction at end-systole (time of $(P/V)_{max}$); EDV, left ventricular end-diastolic volume; σ_{ed}, left ventricular end-diastolic stress; ESV, left ventricular end-systolic volume; σ_{es}, left ventricular end-systolic stress; SV, stroke volume.

Discussion

The questions posed earlier may now be addressed in more detail. The significantly larger end-diastolic and end-systolic volumes resulting in lower ejection fraction in the Treatment arm, are in agreement with results obtained from the larger double-blind randomized trials [1,2,5] and the recent radionuclide studies [6]. The fact that myocardial damage was greater in the group of patients with congestive heart failure contributed to the lower EF observed in this group (Fig. 2). This inverse relationship between EF and "infarct size" has been observed in both clinical [7] and animal [8] studies and provides a partial validation of the present model. Also of note is the fact that many patients in the Prevention arm (asymptomatic without overt heart failure) were operating at depressed functional levels similar to those in patients with congestive heart failure. Thus, a clinical assessment of heart failure is not always in one-to-one correspondence with a functional assessment.

While enalapril had the effect of reducing both EDV and ESV in contrast to the placebo, the increase in ejection fraction was not significant when com-

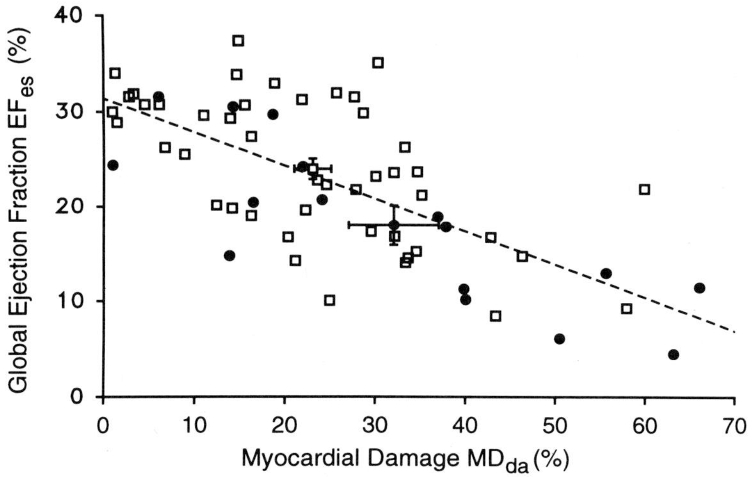

Fig. 2. Ejection fraction–myocardial damage relationship for combined Treatment (*circles*) and Prevention (*squares*) arms. Mean ± SEM values are displayed for each group and indicate that the ejection fraction is significantly lower in the Treatment arm; however, there are many patients without overt heart failure (*squares*) with lower ejection fractions. EF_{es}, global ejection fraction at end-systole; MD_{da}, % myocardial damage based on akinetic and dyskinetic regions

pared to the placebo-treated group. In a recent report [2] it was concluded that patients in the Prevention arm did not benefit as much from enalapril but that the onset of heart failure was delayed. Furthermore, the attenuation of increases in volumes observed in animal and clinical studies [9,10] involving captopril, and its effect in reducing mortality [11], suggest that there is a class effect with regard to ACE inhibitors and that asymptomatic patients with left ventricular (LV) dysfunction might also benefit from ACE inhibitor therapy.

Figure 3 demonstrates that in patients with anterior infarction and on enalapril, the diastolic P–V relationships shift to the left, whereas those on the placebo show shifts to the right. However, because of marked heterogeneity between and within groups observed in large-scale trials, pooling of data may lead to the masking of such shifts for individual cases. When the P–V relationships were examined on an individual basis, it was apparent that the enalapril-treated group responded in a heterogeneous manner and that these responses depended on the range of the operating diastolic volumes. More specifically, in patients with EDV $<$ 300 ml, the P–V relations shifted to the left or were unaltered, whereas for EDV $>$ 300 ml, these shifts occurred to the right. It is noteworthy that EF generally improved (or the relatively high basal EF values were maintained) in the patients treated with enalapril and having EDV $<$ 300 ml, while 50% of the patients on the placebo maintained their high basal values. In almost all cases, these responses were closely associated with their basal contractile state.

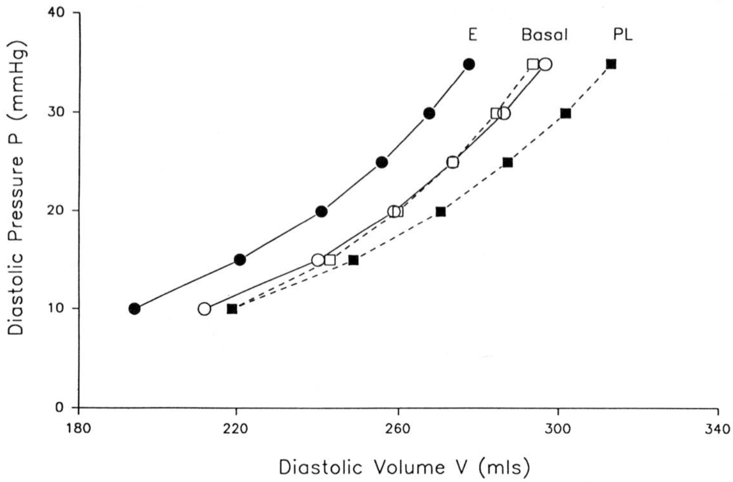

Fig. 3. Diastolic pressure–volume relationships (P–V) for patients with anterior myocardial infarction (AMI) before and one year following treatment with enalapril (*E*) or a placebo (*PL*). With enalapril, the P–V curves shift to the left, in contrast to placebo treatment which tends to shift curves to the right. In both groups, significant variability occurs in the shift of the P–V curve, and this shift depends on the range of end-diastolic volume

A possible mechanism explaining the improvement in pump function generally in the enalapril group is as follows. The vasodilatory effects of the drugs administered early after infarction in addition to enalapril, may have partially restored coronary flow to portions of the infarcted region. This could have led to a reduction in the degree of asynchrony of contraction and hence a load redistribution resulting in a more efficient use of the viable myocardium. In the case of anterior infarction, the reduction in wall stress would occur predominantly in the anterior region, and this would result in a less uniform stress distribution. On the other hand, the placebo-treated group would experience an increase in systolic stress, a greater degree of asynchrony, and a more uniform stress distribution, indicating that the ventricles assume a more spherical configuration.

Current methods for assessing myocardial contractility in the clinical setting have focused on ejection fraction–afterload relationships ($EF_{es}-\sigma_{es}$) which are based on single point calculations of EF_{es} and σ_{es} for each patient. Since these methods ignore the preload effect, they are limited, at best, to assessing changes in the contractile state on a group basis but not on an individual basis. Figure 4 displays a weak but significant relationship between EF_{es} and afterload for patients in the combined Treatment and Prevention arms. On the other hand, the ejection fraction displays a much stronger relationship with preload (Fig. 4) and this emphasizes the importance of reducing end-diastolic volumes in patients with LV dysfunction.

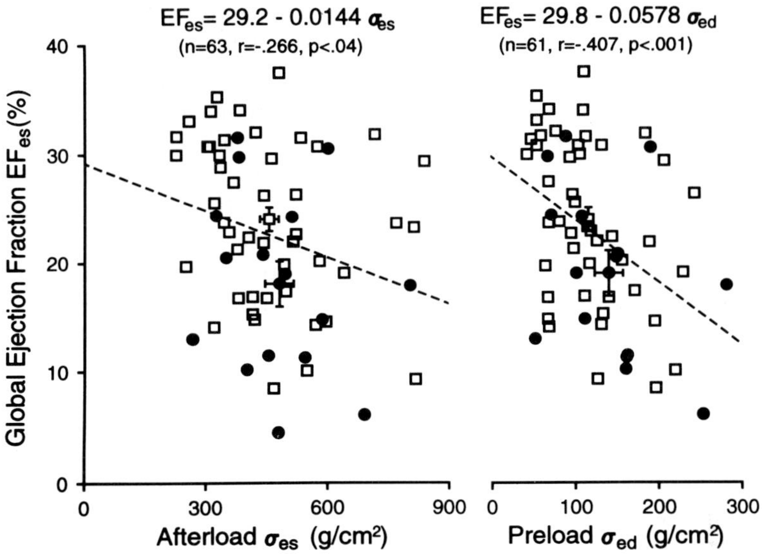

Fig. 4. Ejection fraction–afterload ($EF_{es}-\sigma_{es}$; *left panel*) and ejection fraction–preload ($EF_{es}-\sigma_{ed}$; *right panel*) relationships for patients in combined Treatment (*circles*) and Prevention (*squares*) arms. There was a weak but significant inverse relationship with afterload; however, the relationship was much stronger with preload. Mean ± SEM values are presented for both Treatment and Prevention arms and indicate, on a group basis, that global myocardial contractility is more depressed in the Treatment arm

On a group basis, it would appear that global contractility is more depressed in the Treatment arm since ejection fraction is significantly different at common preload and afterload. Furthermore, with enalapril the EF is increased from the baseline state in the presence of preload and afterload levels similar to those in the baseline state. Although this may suggest an enhancement of intrinsic global contractility, an alternative explanation is that it is due to a load rearrangement.

It is generally recognized that anterior myocardial infarction (AMI) results in a greater depression of LV function than in patients with inferior infarcts (IMI). This is a consequence of increased "infarct size" [7] and relatively higher systolic stresses being present in AMI patients. However, in these studies [7], the mean values of the ejection fraction in the AMI and IMI groups were 35% and 60%, respectively, and their ranges did not overlap. A reanalysis of their data revealed that the EF *vs* infarct size relationships were either nonsignificant for AMI or borderline significant for IMI. In the present studies, there appeared to be no functional difference between the AMI and IMI groups based on EF *vs* myocardial damage relationships (AMI: $EF_{es} = 23.3 \pm 8.9$, $\% \ MD_{da} = 24 \pm 19$, $n = 33$; IMI: $EF_{es} = 25.8 \pm 6.9$, $\% \ MD_{da} = 28 \pm 13$, $n = 15$).